SOUNDING SENSORY PROFILES IN THE ANCIENT NEAR EAST

ANCIENT NEAR EAST MONOGRAPHS

General Editors
Jeffrey Stackert
Juan Manuel Tebes

Editorial Board
Reinhard Achenbach
Jeffrey L. Cooley
C. L. Crouch
Roxana Flammini
Christopher B. Hays
Emanuel Pfoh
Andrea Seri
Bruce Wells

Number 25

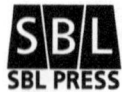

SOUNDING SENSORY PROFILES IN THE ANCIENT NEAR EAST

Edited by
Annette Schellenberg and Thomas Krüger

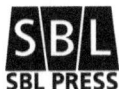

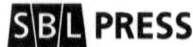 PRESS

Atlanta

Copyright © 2019 by SBL Press

All rights reserved. No part of this work may be reproduced or transmitted in any form or by any means, electronic or mechanical, including photocopying and recording, or by means of any information storage or retrieval system, except as may be expressly permitted by the 1976 Copyright Act or in writing from the publisher. Requests for permission should be addressed in writing to the Rights and Permissions Office, SBL Press, 825 Houston Mill Road, Atlanta, GA 30329 USA.

Library of Congress Control Number: 2019940320

Printed on acid-free paper.

Contents

Preface   vii

Abbreviations   ix

Methodology

Sounding Sensory Profiles
David Howes and Constance Classen   3

Resounding Sensory Profiles: Sensory Studies Methodologies
David Howes   43

Ancient Israel

Empiricism or Rationalism in the Hebrew Bible?
Some Thoughts about Ancient Foxes and Hedgehogs
Jan Dietrich   57

Moving and Thinking: Kinesthesis and Wisdom in the Book of Proverbs
Greg Schmidt Goering   69

On the Sense of Balance in the Hebrew Bible
Thomas Krüger   87

Tasting Metaphor in Ancient Israel
Pierre Van Hecke   99

Feces: The Primary Disgust Elicitor in the Hebrew Bible
and in the Ancient Near East
Thomas Staubli   119

Senses Lost in Paradise? On the Interrelatedness of Sensory
and Ethical Perceptions in Genesis 2–3 and Beyond
Dorothea Erbele-Küster   145

Home but Not Healed: How the Sensory Profiles of Prophetic
Utopian Visions Influence Presentations of Disability
Kirsty L. Jones   161

The Role of Senses in Lamentations 4
Marianne Grohmann   181

Senses, Sensuality, and Sensory Imagination:
On the Role of the Senses in the Song of Songs
Annette Schellenberg   199

ANCIENT MESOPOTAMIA

"Rude Remarks Not Fit to Smell": Negative Value Judgements
Relating to Sensory Perceptions in Ancient Mesopotamia
Nicla De Zorzi   217

Laying Foundations for Eternity: Timing Temple Construction in Assyria
Kiersten Neumann   253

The Doors of Perception: Senses and Their Variations in Akkadian Texts
Anne-Caroline Rendu Loisel   279

Sensing Nature in the Neo-Assyrian World
Allison Thomason   293

ANCIENT EGYPT

Sound Studies and Visual Studies Applied to Ancient Egyptian Sources
Dorothée Elwart and Sibylle Emerit   315

Fish, Fowl, and Stench in Ancient Egypt
Dora Goldsmith   335

Smelling Fat and Hearing Flame: Sensory Experience of Artificial
Light in Ancient Egypt
Meghan E. Strong   361

Contributors   381

Index of Ancient Sources   383

Index of Modern Authors   396

Preface

The senses have attracted much attention in cultural studies in recent times. Which senses are important in different cultures? What is the relationship between sensory experience and reasoning? Which senses are considered reliable sources of knowledge? Which senses are linked to emotions like love or disgust? With which senses are gods or angels perceived? Which experiences of the senses have a part to play in festivals and religious celebrations? How do theory and practice of the senses relate to each other?

In the last few years, questions about the senses have also started to attract the interest of scholars in the fields of Hebrew Bible and ancient Near Eastern studies, which is the focus of this volume. For example, since 2009 there has been a program unit on Senses, Cultures, and the Biblical World at the Annual Meeting of the Society of Biblical Literature; in 2012 Yael Avrahami published a monograph on *The Senses of Scripture: Sensory Perception in the Hebrew Bible* (New York: T&T Clark); 2015 marked the beginning of the interdisciplinary *synaesthesia* project at the University of Toulouse; since 2016 there have been sessions on Senses and Sensibility in the Near East at the Annual Meeting of the American Schools of Oriental Research; and in 2017 Nicole L. Tilford authored the book *Sensing World, Sensing Wisdom: The Cognitive Foundation of Biblical Metaphors* (Atlanta: SBL Press).

So far, the respective discussions are still very fresh, and most of them take place outside Europe. This prompted us to organize an international and interdisciplinary conference on the topic, inviting many of the pioneers behind the development mentioned above. The conference took place at the University of Vienna on March 23–25, 2017. Its title, and thus the title of this volume, was inspired by an article by David Howes and Constance Classen, "Conclusion: Sounding Sensory Profiles" (pages 257–88 in *The Varieties of Sensory Experience: A Sourcebook in the Anthropology of the Senses*, ed. David Howes [Toronto: University of Toronto Press, 1991]), which is reprinted in this volume.

The present volume brings together most of the contributions to this meeting, supplemented by a few other articles on the subject. It offers insights into the meaning of the senses in ancient Israel, Mesopotamia, and Egypt and shows various questions and methods with which this topic can be approached. We hope that this will provide a stimulus and a basis for further exploration of the senses in the ancient Near East.

We would like to thank the Universities of Vienna and Zurich for funding the conference and the publication of this volume. Our thanks go to everyone who contributed a paper to the conference and to this volume, to Alan Lenzi, Jeffrey Stackert, and the editorial board of the Ancient Near East Monographs for the inclusion of this volume in this series, and to Nicole Tilford and the SBL Press staff for their excellent editorial work. Special thanks are due to Jeanine Lefèvre, Nina Beerli, Christian Sichera, and Sarah Herzog for their help in the preparation of the manuscript.

Annette Schellenberg and Thomas Krüger

Abbreviations

AB	Anchor Bible
AbB	Kraus, Fritz R., ed. *Altbabylonische Briefe in Umschrift und Übersetzung.* Leiden: Brill, 1964–.
ABL	Harper, Robert F., ed. *Assyrian and Babylonian Letters Belonging to the Kouyunjik Collections of the British Museum.* 14 vols. Chicago: University of Chicago Press, 1892–1914.
AeL	*Ägypten und Levante*
AfK	*Archiv für Keilschriftforschung*
AfOB	Archiv für Orientforschung: Beiheft
AHR	*American Historical Review*
AHw	Von Soden, Wolfram. *Akkadisches Handwörterbuch.* 3 vols. Wiesbaden, 1965–1981.
AIL	Ancient Israel and Its Literature
AJA	*American Journal of Archaeology*
AJP	*American Journal of Philology*
AnBi	Analecta Biblica
AOAT	Alter Orient und Altes Testament
AOS	American Oriental Series
AR	*Archiv für Religiongeschichte*
ARM	Archives royales de Mari
AS	Assyriological Studies
ASAW	Abhandlungen der Sächsischen Akademie der Wissenschaften zu Leipzig
ASOR	American Schools of Oriental Research
ATD	Das Alte Testament Deutsch
BASOR	*Bulletin of the American Schools of Oriental Research*
BDB	Brown, Francis, S. R. Driver, and Charles A. Briggs. *A Hebrew and English Lexicon of the Old Testament.* Oxford: Clarendon, 1907.
BETL	Bibliotheca Ephemeridum Theologicarum Lovaniensium
Bib	*Biblica*
BibInt	*Biblical Interpretation*
BibOr	Biblica et Orientalia

BHQ	*Biblia Hebraica Quinta*
B.J.	Josephus, *Bellum judaicum*
BKAT	Biblischer Kommentar, Altes Testament
BM	British Museum
BTS	Biblical Tools and Studies
BZAW	Beihefte zur Zeitschrift für die alttestamentliche Wissenschaft
BZRGG	Beihefte der Zeitschrift für Religions- und Geistesgeschichte
CAD	Gelb, Ignace J., et al., eds. *The Assyrian Dictionary of the Oriental Institute of the University of Chicago*. Chicago: The Oriental Institute of the University of Chicago, 1956–2006.
CBQ	*Catholic Biblical Quarterly*
CBS	Tablets in the collections of the University Museum of the University of Pennsylvania, Philadelphia
CCP	Cuneiform Commentaries Project
CDCH	Clines, David J. A, ed. *A Concise Dictionary of Classical Hebrew*. Sheffield: Sheffield Phoenix, 2009.
CHANE	Culture and History of the Ancient Near East
CM	Cuneiform Monographs
CT	Cuneiform Texts from Babylonian Tablets in the British Museum
D	*piel*
Dp	*pual*
DCH	Clines, David J. A., ed. *Dictionary of Classical Hebrew*. 9 vols. Sheffield: Sheffield Phoenix, 1993–2016.
DDD	Van der Toorn, Karel, Bob Becking, and Pieter W. van der Horst, eds. *Dictionary of Deities and Demons in the Bible*. Leiden: Brill, 1995. 2nd rev. ed. Grand Rapids: Eerdmans, 1999.
DMOA	Documenta et Monumenta Orientis Antiqui
EA	Egyptian Antiquities (British Museum)
Erm	Ermitage Museum
ESV	English Standard Version
ETCSL	Electronic Text Corpus of Sumerian Literature
FAT	Forschungen zum Alten Testament
FRLANT	Forschungen zur Religion und Literatur des Alten und Neuen Testaments
G	*qal*
H	*hiphil*
Hp	*hophal*
HtD	*hithpael*

HAL	Koehler, Ludwig, Walter Baumgartner, and Johann J. Stamm. *Hebräisches und aramäisches Lexikon zum Alten Testament.* 3rd ed. Leiden: Brill 1995, 2004.
HANE/M	History of the Ancient Near East/Monographs
HAT	Handbuch zum Alten Testament
HBAI	*Hebrew Bible and Ancient Israel*
HBM	Hebrew Bible Monographs
HBS	Herders Biblische Studien
HCOT	Historical Commentary on the Old Testament
HdO	Handbuch der Orientalistik
HThKAT	Herders Theologischer Kommentar zum Alten Testament
HUCA	*Hebrew Union College Annual*
IOS	Israel Oriental Studies
JAEI	*Journal of Ancient Egyptian Interconnections*
JALSupp	Supplements to the Journal of Arabic Literature
JANER	*Journal of Ancient Near Eastern Religions*
JANES	*Journal of the Ancient Near Eastern Society*
JAOS	*Journal of the American Oriental Society*
Jastrow	Jastrow, Marcus. *A Dictionary of the Targumim, the Talmud Babli and Yerushalmi and the Midrashic Literature.* Leipzig: Drugulin, 1926.
JBL	*Journal of Biblical Literature*
JCS	*Journal of Cuneiform Studies*
JHI	*Journal of the History of Ideas*
JHS	*Journal of Hellenic Studies*
JJS	*Journal of Jewish Studies*
JNES	*Journal of Near Eastern Studies*
JPS	*Tanakh: The Holy Scriptures: The 1917 Edition according to the Masoretic Text*
JSOT	*Journal for the Study of the Old Testament*
JSOTSup	Journal for the Study of the Old Testament Supplement Series
JSSEA	*Journal of the Society for the Study of Egyptian Antiquities*
JSS	*Journal of Semitic Studies*
Joüon Muraoka	Joüon, Paul, and Takamitsu Muraoka. *A Grammar of Biblical Hebrew.* SubBi 27. Rome: Pontifical Biblical Institute, 2006.
K	cuneiform tablets in the Kouyunjik Collection of the British Museum
KAR	Ebeling, Erich, ed. *Keilschrifttexte aus Assur religiösen Inhalts.* Leipzig: Hinrichs, 1919–1923.
KBo	*Keilschrifttexte aus Boghazköi.* Leipzig: Hinrichs, 1916–1923; Berlin: Gebr. Mann, 1954–.
KRI	Kitchen, Kenneth Anderson. *Ramesside Inscriptions.* 9 vols. Oxford: Blackwell, 1975–2018.

LAOS	Leipziger altorientalische Studien
Lane	Lane, Edward William, ed. *An Arabic-English Lexicon*. 8 vols. London: Williams & Norgate, 1863–1893.
LHBOTS	The Library of Hebrew Bible/Old Testament Studies
LKA	Ebeling, Erich. *Literarische Keilschrifttexte aus Assur*. Berlin: Akademie-Verlag, 1953.
LSJ	Liddell, Henry George, Robert Scott, and Henry Stuart Jones. *A Greek-English Lexicon*. 9th ed. With revised supplement. Oxford: Clarendon, 1996.
MAD	Materials for the Assyrian Dictionary
MAJA	Münchner Arbeitskreises Junge Aegyptologie
MÄS	Münchner ägyptologische Studien
MC	Mesopotamian Civilizations
MDOG	Mitteilungen der Deutschen Orient-Gesellschaft
MIFAO	Mémoire publiés par les membres de l'institut Français d'Archéologie Orientale
MSL	*Materialien zum sumerischen Lexikon/Materials for the Sumerian Lexicon*. 17 vols. Rome: Pontifical Biblical Institue, 1937–2004.
N	*niphal*
NABU	*Nouvelles assyriologiques brèves et utilitaires*
NAC	New American Commentary
NBL	Görg, Manfred, and Bernhard Lang, eds. *Neues Bibel-Lexikon*. 3 vols. Zurich: Benziger, 1988–2001.
NCB	New Century Bible
NEB.T	Neue Echter Bibel. Themen
NICOT	New International Commentary on the Old Testament
NIV	New International Version
NJPS	*Tanakh: The Holy Scriptures: The New JPS Translation according to the Traditional Hebrew Text*
NRSV	New Revised Standard Version
NSKAT	Neuer Stuttgarter Kommentar, Altes Testament
o.	obverse
OBC	Orientalia Biblica et Christiana
OBO	Orbis Biblicus et Orientalis
OBT	Overtures to Biblical Theology
OIP	Oriental Institute Publications
OLA	Orientalia Lovaniensia Analecta
OLP	Orientalia Lovaniensia Periodica
Or	*Orientalia (NS)*
OTL	Old Testament Library
OtSt	*Oudtestamentische Studiën*

PAe	Probleme der Ägyptologie
PBS	University of Pennsylvania, Publications of the Babylonian Section
PNAS	*Proceedings of the National Academy of Sciences of the United States of America*
Poet.	Aristotle, *Poetics*
r.	reverse
RBS	Resources for Biblical Study
RA	*Revue d'assyriologie et d'archéologie orientale*
RAI	Rencontre assyriologique internationale
RAPH	Recherches d'archéologie, de philologie et d'histoire
Rhet.	Aristotle, *Rhetoric*
RIM	The Royal Inscriptions of Mesopotamia Project. Toronto
RIMA 1	Grayson, A. Kirk. *Assyrian Rulers of the Third and Second Millennia BC (To 1115 BC)*. RIMA 1. Toronto: University of Toronto Press, 1987.
RIMA 2	Grayson, A. Kirk *Assyrian Rulers of the Early First Millennium BC Part 1 (1114–859 BC)*. RIMA 2. Toronto; Buffalo: University of Toronto Press, 1991.
RIMA 3	Grayson, A. Kirk. *Assyrian Rulers of the Early First Millennium BC Part II (858–745 BC)*. RIMA 3. Toronto; Buffalo: University of Toronto Press, 1996.
RIMB 2	Frame, Grant. *Rulers of Babylonia: From the Second Dynasty of Isin to the End of Assyrian Domination (1157–612 BC)*, RIMB 2. Toronto: University of Toronto Press, 1995.
RINAP 3.1	Grayson, A. K., and J. Novotny. *The Royal Inscriptions of Sennacherib, King of Assyria (704–681 BC), Part 1*. RINAP 3.1. Winona Lake, IN: Eisenbrauns, 2012.
RINAP 3.2	Grayson, A. K., and J. Novotny. *The Royal Inscriptions of Sennacherib, King of Assyria (704–681 BC), Part 2*. RINAP 3.2. Winona Lake, IN: Eisenbrauns, 2014.
RINAP 4	Leichty, E. *The Royal Inscriptions of Esarhaddon, King of Assyria (680–669 BC)*. RINAP 4. Winona Lake, IN: Eisenbrauns, 2011.
RlA	Ebeling, Erich, et al., eds. *Reallexikon der Assyriologie*. Berlin: de Gruyter, 1928–.
SAA	State Archives of Assyria
SAAB	*State Archives of Assyria Bulletin*
SAACT	State Archives of Assyria Cuneiform Texts
SAAS	State Archives of Assyria Studies
SAK	*Studien zur altägyptischen Kultur*
SAK.B	Studien zur altägyptischen Kultur. Beihefte
SAOC	Studies in Ancient Oriental Civilizations

SBTU	Spätbabylonische Texte aus Uruk
SEAL	Sources of Early Akkadian Literature
SHR	Studies in the History of Religions (supplements to *Numen*)
StBibLit	Studies in Biblical Literature (Lang)
StMes	Studia Mesopotamica
StPohl	Studia Pohl
STT	Oliver Robert Gurney, Jacob J. Finkelstein, and P. Hulin, *The Sultantepe Tablets*, 1–2 (= OccPubl. BIAA 3 and 7, 1957/1964).
SubBi	Subsidia Biblica
TAD	Textbook of Aramaic Documents from Ancient Egypt. 1986 (= TAD A); 1989 (= TAD B); 1993 (= TAD C)
TAPS	Transactions of the American Philosophical Society
TDOT	Johannes Botterweck, G., and Helmer Ringgren, eds. *Theological Dictionary of the Old Testament.* Translated by John T. Willis et al. 8 vols. Grand Rapids: Eerdmans, 1974–2006.
ThWAT	Johannes Botterweck, G., and Helmer Ringgren, eds. *Theologisches Wörterbuch zum Alten Testament.* Stuttgart: Kohlhammer, 1970–.
TLA	Thesaurus Linguae Aegyptiae
TUAT	Kaiser, Otto, ed. *Texte aus der Umwelt des Alten Testaments.* Gütersloh: Mohn, 1984–.
UAVA	Untersuchungen zur Assyriologie und vorderasiatischen Archäologie
UF	*Ugarit-Forschungen*
WAW	Writings from the Ancient World
Wb	Erman, Adolf, and Hermann Grapow. *Wörterbuch der ägyptischen Sprache.* 5 vols. Leipzig: Hinrichs; Berlin: Akademie, 1926–1931. Repr., 1963.
WBC	Word Biblical Commentary
WiBiLex	Das Wissenschaftliche Bibellexikon im Internet
WMANT	Wissenschaftliche Monographien zum Alten und Neuen Testament
WO	*Die Welt des Orients*
VT	*Vetus Testamentum*
VTSup	Supplements to Vetus Testamentum
VWGTh	Veröffentlichungen der Wissenschaftlichen Gesellschaft für Theologie
YOS	Yale Oriental Series, Texts
ZA	*Zeitschrift für Assyriologie*
ZAW	*Zeitschrift für alttestamentliche Wissenschaft*
ZBK	Zürcher Bibelkommentare
ZTK	*Zeitschrift für Theologie und Kirche*

METHODOLOGY

SOUNDING SENSORY PROFILES

David Howes and Constance Classen

The purpose of this chapter is to present a paradigm for sensing and making sense of other cultures. We want to emphasize the practical and open-ended nature of the discussion that follows. It sums up some of the main points of the chapters in *The Varieties of Sensory Experience: A Sourcebook in the Anthropology of the Senses* but is equally concerned to open up new directions and questions for research.

The chapter begins with a discussion of some general considerations which ought to be borne in mind when studying the sensorium. The next two parts are concerned with field research and library research respectively. They offer practical advice on, among other things, how best to clear one's senses for purposes of sensory analysis, and how to read between the lines of an ethnography for information on a culture's "way of sensing" or "sensory profile." The fourth part is called "A Paradigm for Sensing." It is divided into ten sections. The sections are entitled: (1) language, (2) artefacts and aesthetics, (3) body decoration, (4) childrearing practices, (5) alternative sensory modes, (6) media of communication, (7) natural and built environment, (8) rituals, (9) mythology, and (10) cosmology. These headings refer to those cultural domains which, in our experience, have proved the most informative with regard to eliciting a given culture's "sensory profile."

SOME GENERAL CONSIDERATIONS

Other cultures do not necessarily divide the sensorium as we do. The Hausa recognize two senses;[1] "the Javanese have five senses (seeing, hearing, *talking*, smelling and feeling), which do not coincide exactly with our five."[2] In short, there

---

Reprinted (with some minor corrections and adaptations) from David Howes, ed., *The Varieties of Sensory Experience: A Sourcebook in the Anthropology of the Senses* (Toronto: University of Toronto Press, 1991), 257–88.

[1] Ian Ritchie, "Fusion of the Facilities: A Study of the Language of the Senses in Hausaland," in Howes, *Varieties of Sensory Experience*, 192–202.

[2] Alan Dundes, "Seeing Is Believing," in *Interpreting Folklore* (Bloomington: Indiana University Press, 1980), 92.

may be any number of "senses," including what we would classify as extrasensory perception—the "sixth sense."[3] According to the Peruvian curer interviewed by Douglas Sharon in *Wizard of the Four Rinds*, for example, a sixth clairvoyant sense opens up when all five other senses have been stimulated through the use of hallucinogens and other ritual elements.[4] Eduardo, the curer, describes this sixth sense as "a 'vision' much more remote ... in the sense that one can look at things that go far beyond the ordinary or that have happened in the past or can happen in the future."[5]

The senses interact with each other first, before they give us access to the world; hence, the first step, the indispensable starting point, is to discover what sorts of relations between the senses a culture considers proper. One commonly finds that when a particular sense is emphasized by a culture, some other sense emerges as its opposite, and becomes the target of repression. It is also quite common to find one sense substituting for another, more dangerous, sense. For example, Desana men, who manifest a high degree of anxiety regarding sexual contact, would appear to use sight as a substitute for touch when they relive birth and other sexually related experiences through the visual imagery of hallucinations.[6] In Islamic society, the repression of sight which results from the prohibition on the visual representation of God or creation, and the fear of being accused of casting the "evil eye," would seem to be designed to emphasize hearing (and obeying or "submitting" to) the *word* of God.

Senses which are important for practical purposes may not be important culturally or symbolically. For instance, while sight is greatly valued by the Inuit for hunting and other activities, it does not have the symbolic importance of hearing and sound, which are associated with creation. Language, in fact, is likened by the Inuit to the knife of the carver which creates form out of formlessness. Sight can thus be said to be of practical value for the Inuit because it perceives form, but

---

[3] The idea that human beings are equipped with five senses might seem obvious and beyond dispute, but it is in fact no less symbolic than other numerations. According to the latest scientific estimates there are seventeen senses, see Robert Rivlin and Karen Gravelle, *Deciphering the Senses: The Expanding World of Human Perception* (New York: Simon & Schuster, 1984).

[4] Douglas Sharon, *Wizard of the Four Winds: A Shaman's Story* (New York: Free Press, 1978), 117.

[5] Sharon, *Wizard of the Four Winds*, 115.

[6] Gerardo Reichel-Dolmatoff, "The Cultural Context of an Aboriginal Hallucinogen: Banisteriopsiscaapi," in *Flesh of the Gods: The Ritual Use of Hallucinogens*, ed. Peter T. Furst (New York: Praeger, 1972), 84–113; Reichel-Dolmatoff, *Basketry as Metaphor: Arts and Crafts of the Desana Indians of the Northwest Amazon*, Occasional Papers of the Museum of Cultural History (Los Angeles: University of California, 1985), 4.

sound has cultural priority because it *creates* form.⁷ An analogous profile is presented by the Suya of Brazil who privilege speech and hearing:⁸

> In discussion of Suya ideas about vision, the ability to see must be distinguished from the symbolic meaning of the eyes. Good everyday sight, in the sense of accurate reception of visual stimuli, is apparently unrelated to the other modes [i.e., speaking and hearing] because it is not symbolically elaborated. The Suya prize a good hunter who can accurately shoot fish and game. It is not his sight that is stressed but the accuracy of his shooting. Hunting medicines are applied to the forearm to make a man a good shot, not to his eyes.⁹

Sensory orders are not static: they develop and change over time, just as cultures do. Some of the sensory expressions of a society, manifested in its language, rituals, and myths, may be relics or survivals from an earlier sensory order. This is particularly evident in societies "with history" (i.e., where records of earlier ways of life are extant). For example, Mackenzie Brown gives a fascinating account of how visuality came to dominate aurality in the history of the Hindu tradition, based on a reading of India's sacred texts.¹⁰ As another example, the Latin-based word "sagacious," which now means only "wise," originally, at a more olfactory-conscious period, meant "keen-scented" as well. In societies "without history" (i.e., those for which earlier records do not exist), this kind of sensory layering is more difficult to discern, but not impossible. In *Do Kamo: Person and Myth in the Melanesian World*,¹¹ Maurice Leenhardt was able to trace the origin of certain olfactory and visual representations of the body to different stages of Melanesian civilization by relating the representations in question to evolving concepts of space.¹² In such cases, the contemporary relevance of a given sensory expression can only be determined by relating it to the *total sensory dynamic* of the culture.

---

⁷ Edmund Carpenter, *Eskimo Realities* (New York: Holt, Rinehart & Winston, 1973), 33, 43.

⁸ See the discussion in David Howes, "Sensorial Anthropology," in Howes, *Varieties of Sensory Experience*, 167–91.

⁹ Anthony Seeger, "The Meaning of Body Ornaments," *Ethnology* 14.3 (1975): 215.

¹⁰ Cheever Mackenzie Brown, "Purana as Scripture: From Sound to Image of the Holy Word in the Hindu Tradition," *History of Religions* 26.1 (1986): 69–86. For a tasteful critique of the Mackenzie Brown article see Sylvain Pinard, "L'Economie des sens en Inde: Exploration des thèses de Walter Ong," *Anthropologica* 32.1 (1990): 75–99.

¹¹ Maurice Leenhardt, *Do Kamo: Person and Myth in the Melanesian World*, trans. B. Miller Gulati (Chicago: University of Chicago Press, 1979).

¹² See further David Howes, "On the Odour of the Soul: Spatial Representation and Olfactory Classification in Eastern Indonesia and Western Melanesia," *Bijdragen tot de Taal-, Land- en Volkenkunde* 144 (1988): 84–113.

There may be different sensory orders for different groups within a society, for example, women and men, children and adults, leaders and workers, people in different professions, as will be discussed below in the section on alternative sensory modes.

Doing Field Research

If one's research involves participant observation, then the question to be addressed is this: *Which senses are emphasized and which senses are repressed, by what means and to which ends?* This complex question can be broken down into a variety of subsidiary questions, which range from the particular to the general. Particular questions would include: Is there a lot of touching or very little? Is there much concern over body odours? What is the range of tastes in foods and where do the preferences tend to centre? At a more general level: Does the repression of a particular sense or sensory expression correspond to the repression of a particular group within society? Or, how does the sensory order relate to the social and symbolic order?

Every culture strikes its own balance among the senses. While some cultures tend toward an equality of the senses, most cultures manifest some bias or other, either privileging a particular sense or some cluster of senses. In order successfully to fathom the sensory biases of another culture, it is essential for the researcher to overcome, to the extent possible, his or her own sensory biases. The first and most crucial step in this process is to discover one's personal sensory biases.[13] The second step involves training oneself to be sensitive to a multiplicity

---

[13] How can one become aware of what one's own sensory biases are? The simplest exercise for this purpose is the one initially popularized by Galton. The exercise involves recalling the scene at breakfast, describing it, and then analysing the extent to which you depend on each of your senses in memory. For example, is it the words for each of the objects on the table that come to you, or their visual images, or the motions you performed in grasping them, etc. The labels for these three pre-dispositions are "verbalizer," "visualizer," and "kinesthete"; see William James, *Psychology: The Briefer Course* (New York: Harper, 1961), 169–77. More comprehensive discussions of how to discover your own sensing pattern and how to control as well as use it for purposes of cultural analysis can be found in Rhoda Métraux, "Resonance in Imagery," in *The Study of Culture at a Distance*, ed. Margaret Mead and Rhoda Métraux (Chicago: University of Chicago Press, 1953), 343–62; Edward T. Hall, *Beyond Culture* (New York: Anchor Books, 1977), 169–87; and Manda Cesara, *No Hiding Place: Reflections of a Woman Anthropologist* (New York: Academic Press, 1982), 48, 109–11. Other techniques for enhancing sensory awareness include the "spiritual exercises" first proposed by Loyola (see Anthony Synnott, "Puzzling over the Senses: From Plato to Marx," in Howes, *Varieties of Sensory Experience*, 61–76), and developed to an excessive degree by James Joyce (*The Portable James Joyce*, introduced by H. Levin [New York: Viking Press, 1946], 109–12). It is also helpful to consider

of sensory expressions. This kind of awareness can be cultivated by taking some object in one's environment and disengaging one's attention from the object itself so as to focus on how each of its sensory properties would impinge on one's consciousness were they not filtered in any way.[14] The third step involves developing the capacity to be "of two sensoria" about things,[15] which means being able to operate with complete awareness in two perceptual systems or sensory orders simultaneously (the sensory order of one's own culture and that of the culture studied), and constantly comparing notes.

The procedure sketched above may be illustrated by taking the example of blood. Blood has a variety of sensory properties: it is warm, viscous, red, salty, and odorous. The salience of these properties, however, depends on the sensory order within which they are perceived. Thus, North Americans tend to think of blood in terms of its visual appearance, its redness. In South India, practitioners of Siddha medicine give priority to the tactile dimension of blood, the pulse it produces within the body.[16] This holds true in Guatemala as well, although there the pulse is said to be the "voice" of blood, suggesting an audio-tactile perceptual framework.[17] Among the Ainu of Japan, it is the odour of blood that is most salient, as the smell of blood is thought to repel spirits.[18] In the myth of the Wauwalak sisters as told in northern Australia, there is reference to both the smell of blood and to "blood containing sound,"[19] which implies an audio-olfactory bias.

---

the work of the musicologist R. Murray Schafer (*The Tuning of the World* [New York: Knopf, 1977]) on "soundscapes" and the geographer J. Douglas Porteous (*Landscapes of the Mind: Worlds of Sense and Metaphor* [Toronto: University of Toronto Press, 1990]) on "smellscapes" and "bodyscapes" by way of sensitizing oneself to the limits of "the tourist perspective" (Kenneth Little, "On Safari: The Visual Politics of a Tourist Representation," in Howes, *Varieties of Sensory Experience*, 148–63), and coming to perceive how sounds, smells, and textures really *matter* in the environment of a given culture.

[14] See Maurice Merleau-Ponty, *Phenomenology of Perception* (London: Routledge and Kegan Paul, 1962); Andrew Rawlinson, "Yoga Psychology," in *Indigenous Psychologies: The Anthropology of the Self*, ed. Paul Heelas and Andrew Lock (London: Academic Press, 1981), 247–63.

[15] David Howes, "Beyond Textualism and Hermeneutics in Cultural and Religious Studies," *Journal of Religion and Culture* 4.2 (1990): 1–8.

[16] E. Valentine Daniel, "The Pulse as an Icon in Siddha Medicine," in Howes, *Varieties of Sensory Experience*, 100–110.

[17] Barbara Tedlock, *Time and the Highland Maya* (Albuquerque: University of New Mexico Press, 1982), 53, 134.

[18] Emiko Ohnuki-Tierney, *Illness and Healing among the Sakhalin Ainu* (Cambridge: Cambridge University Press, 1981), 97.

[19] Ronald M. Berndt, *Kunapipi* (New York: International Universities Press, 1951), 44.

As this brief survey illustrates, a single substance or object may figure very differently in different sensory imaginaries. But by using one's imagination judiciously, which is to say multi-modally, it is possible to bracket or suspend one's "natural" way of perceiving the world and allow these other ways of sensing, with their own biases, to inform one's consciousness. That is the essence of "being of two sensoria" about things. Developing such a capacity can be a source of many delights, as well as insights into how other cultures construct the world.

Doing Library Research

If one's research is to be based on textual sources, the best method is to select an ethnography, or other piece of literature (e.g., an African novel, a life history), or even a film, and proceed as follows:

(1) Extract all the references to the senses or sensory phenomena from the source in question.

(2) Divide the references into intra-modal sets, and analyse the data pertaining to each modality individually after the manner of the essays by Steven Feld,[20] Valentine Daniel,[21] and Joel Kuipers[22] in part 2 of *The Varieties of Sensory Experience*.

(3) Analyse the relations between the modalities with regard to how each sense contributes to the meaning of experience in the culture, using the questions in "A Paradigm for Sensing" (see the following section) as a guide.

(4) Conclude with a statement of the hierarchy or order of the senses for the culture. Andermann's reading of Evon Vogt's *Tortillas for the Gods*[23] is exemplary in all of these respects. Note especially how the sketch of the Zinacanteco sensory order with which she concludes her piece allows for comparison with other sources on the Zinacanteco, as well as other cultures.

If one is relying on a text, there is always the problem of how the ethnographer's own sensory biases may have influenced the selection and presentation of the material. Such biases are, at times, evident in the particular focus of the ethnography; for example, it may be a monograph on linguistics, or music, or the visual arts. At other times, one can see that the ethnographer has emphasized certain of the culture's sensory expressions and excluded others according to the sensory model of his or her own culture. In such cases one will only be able to analyse the role of those senses which were brought out by the ethnographer. Such

---

[20] Steven Feld, "Sound as a Symbolic System: The Kaluli Drum," in Howes, *Varieties of Sensory Experience*, 79–99.

[21] Daniel, "Pulse as an Icon in Siddha Medicine."

[22] Joel C. Kuipers, "Matters of Taste in Wajéwa," in Howes, *Varieties of Sensory Experience*, 111–27.

[23] Lisa Andermann, "'The Great Seeing': The Senses in Zinacanteco Ritual Life," in Howes, *Varieties of Sensory Experience*, 231–38.

a problem can sometimes be resolved by examining other ethnographies on the same culture, as Pinard does in his critical reading of Diana Eck's book *Darsan*.[24]

A Paradigm for Sensing

In this part, each section will begin with a series of questions which introduce the sorts of considerations one would want to bear in mind in turning to examine a given cultural domain, such as language, body decoration, or the built environment, for information on a culture's sensory profile. The questions are followed by commentaries which elaborate on some of the ways in which the facts revealed in the course of a sensory analysis of a culture might be interpreted.

1. Language

- What words exist for the different senses?
- Which sensory perceptions have the greatest vocabulary allotted them (sounds, colours, odours)?
- How are the senses used in metaphors and expressions?

The way the senses are used in the language of a culture can reveal a good deal about that culture's sensory model. In the following discussion, we shall focus on the similarities and differences between Quechua, the language spoken in the central Andes, and English.[25]

The level of onomatopoeia in a language may indicate the relative importance of aurality. In some cases the onomatopoeia is obvious, for example, *achini* in Quechua, "to sneeze," while in other cases it is more difficult to determine: Is the word *otoronco*, Quechua for jaguar, meant to imitate the jaguar's roar? In any event, it appears customary in most languages for words which represent sounds to imitate those sounds, as in "crack" or "thud." When an object or action which is multisensory, however, such as an animal, is represented by a word which mimics the sound it makes, this would seem to point to an auditory bias in that culture. Similarly, if things are usually named according to their visual appearance this indicates a visual bias, and so on. In Western languages words for objects are usually not based on any of their sensory qualities, or if they originally were, they

---

[24] Sylvain Pinard, "A Taste of India: On the Role of Gustation in the Hindu Sensorium," in Howes, *Varieties of Sensory Experience*, 221–30.

[25] The Quechua material is derived from Diego González Holquín, *Vocabulario de la lengua general de todo el Perú llamada lengua quichua* (Lima: Universidad Nacional Mayor de San Marcos, 1952; originally published in 1608); for further background see Constance Classen, *Inca Cosmology and the Human Body* (Salt Lake City: University of Utah Press, 1993).

no longer evoke these qualities for us. Perhaps this indicates a "de-sensualizing" and "abstracting" of the environment in order to render it more accessible to detached manipulation.

Some words imitate the sound supposedly produced by a certain sensation, for example, "ugh" and "ugly." In many cases this may be cross-cultural. For instance, the word "aha" is used to express a sudden experience of enlightenment in Quechua and in Western languages. Other words try to convey certain kinetic sensations, such as "slip." Visual qualities can also be indicated; for example, the word "glossy" is probably meant to convey the impression of a shiny surface. In *The Unity of the Senses*,[26] Lawrence Marks refers to studies which show that people associate certain vowel sounds with "brightness" and others with "dullness." It is difficult to find examples of this happening with tastes or smells. Does "sweet" have a sweet sound? Most examples of this kind of synaesthesia in English apparently occur with words referring to tactile sensations: "prickly," "smooth," "mush." This suggests that tactile and aural sensations have a certain closeness for English-speakers. Finally, certain sounds may be used to express value judgments. In English, for instance, many words starting with "sl" have the sense of a metaphorical slippage, as in "slut" and "sly."

The importance of a sensory organ can be revealed in part by the number of words used to describe it. In Quechua there are separate terms for outer ear, inner ear, upper ear, and lower ear; outer and inner mouth and upper and inner lip, etc. The spaces between the sensory organs—that is, the space between the nose and the mouth and the space between the eyes—also have their own terms. This may simply express a preoccupation with spatial divisions; however, it likely affects the understanding of the senses as well. The concern for in-between spaces in Quechua, for example, suggests a parallel concern for how the senses relate to each other, rather than an emphasis on sensory organs as independent entities.

Terms which are used for the different senses provide the most basic source of knowledge on how the senses are understood through language. In Quechua there is a special word to indicate one who uses his senses sharply, and verbs to express the subtle use of all of the senses—*ccazcachini rrtallini*, "to taste subtly"; *ccazcachini uyarini*, "to near subtly"; etc. Undoubtedly, keen sensory ability is of importance in this culture. There are also words to express the loss of each of the senses through old age.

The number of terms for each of the senses is an indicator of the relative importance of that sense, or else of the different ways in which it is understood to operate. In Quechua there are verbs meaning "to smell any smell," "to smell a good smell," "to smell a bad smell," "to give a bad smell to others," "to smell naturally bad," "to leave a good smell," "to come across the remains of a smell,"

---

[26] Lawrence Marks, *The Unity of Senses: Interrelations among the Modalities* (New York: Academic Press, 1982).

"to let oneself be smelled," etc. This implies that smell is highly important for Quechua speakers. However, the virtual absence of reference to smell in Andean myths indicates that, while smell may be important on a practical or popular level, it is less so at the level of symbols.

Metaphors for the senses provide further information on how they are perceived and valued. In Quechua these metaphors generally follow those in Western languages; for example, "to smell" can mean "to discover." Of particular importance in this regard is to determine which sense is most associated with knowledge and understanding.

The structure of the verbs used for the different senses can also be informative. Does each sense have a separate single word? Are compound words used for some of the senses? Finally, it can be useful to look at related words. In Quechua, for instance, the verb "to see," *ricuni*, is very close to the verb "to go," *riccuni*. This perhaps expresses the distance involved in sight, or that seeing is a kind of vicarious going. As always, sensory metaphors must be understood within the cultural context. An association between "hearing" and "obeying," for example, might indicate a positive valuation of hearing in a culture in which obedience is highly valued, but a negative valuation in one in which individual initiative is stressed.

2. Artefacts and Aesthetics

- What do a culture's aesthetic ideals suggest about the value it attaches to the different senses?
- How are the senses represented and evoked in or by a culture's artefacts?
- How may other senses be involved in the coding, or essential to the decoding, of representations that appear primarily visual or auditory?
- What does putting a non-Western artefact "on display" in a museum do to its sense(s)? How should such artefacts be presented?

In the West, aesthetic ideals are primarily visual: beauty is first and foremost beauty of appearance.[27] In other cultures the concept of beauty may involve various senses. For the Shipibo-Conibo of Eastern Peru, for instance, an aesthetic experience, denoted by the term *quiquin* which means both "aesthetic" and "appropriate," involves pleasant auditory, olfactory, or visual sensations.[28]

---

[27] Anthony Synnott, "Truth and Goodness, Mirrors and Masks: A Sociology of Beauty and the Face, Part I," *British Journal of Sociology* 39.4 (1989): 607–36; Synnott, "Truth and Goodness, Mirrors and Masks: A Sociology of Beauty and the Face, Part II," *British Journal of Sociology* 40.1 (1990): 55–76.

[28] Angelika Gebhart-Sayer, "The Geometric Designs of the Shipibo-Conibo in Ritual Context," *Journal of Latin American Lore* 11.2 (1985): 143–75.

Although all cultures would seem to have some concept *of* beauty, most non-Western cultures have no term for "art," nor do they privilege the attitude of detached contemplation once thought so essential to the "aesthetic experience" by Western art critics. "Art" is used rather than viewed, and the conception of beauty which goes along with this is dynamic rather than static.[29] Navajo sand paintings are a case in point. Photographs of these paintings taken by tourists or art collectors capture the whole of the design from above. The Navajo, however, never see the paintings from that perspective. They situate themselves *within* the painting. When a sand painting is used in a healing ritual, the person to be healed, or "recreated" as the Navajo say, actually sits in the painting. Sand is taken from the bodies of the holy people represented in the drawing and pressed on the body of the ill person.[30] Thus, while outside observers see the sand paintings as visual objects, for the Navajo their tactile dimension is, in fact, more important.

The idea of sensing a painting "from within it, being surrounded by it,"[31] as the Navajo do, is foreign to conventional Western aesthetic sensibilities. Contemplation is encouraged (at the expense of participation) by rules like: "Do not touch the exhibit!" The disengagement of all the senses, save for sight, is also encouraged by the technique of linear perspective drawing, as discussed by Howes in the Introduction to *The Varieties of Sensory Experience*.[32] This technique is foreign to most non-Western cultures. Among the Tsimshian of the Northwest Coast, for example, one finds a style, known as "split-representation," that is the complete antithesis of linear perspective vision. Consider the representation of "bear" taken from a Tsimshian housefront in figure 1 (below).

If we ask "What is the point of view expressed in this representation?" we are forced to admit that it does not have one, but many, as many as there are sides to Bear. The animal has, in fact, been cut from back to front and flattened so that we see both sides of Bear at once, as well as the back, which is indicated by the jagged outlines meant to represent its hair.[33] Since we know that one cannot see an object from all sides at once, we conclude that the artist "lacked perspective." But what we ought to be asking ourselves, following Carpenter,[34] is how the artist's hand might

---

[29] Gary Witherspoon, *Language and Art in the Navajo Universe* (Ann Arbor: University of Michigan Press, 1977).

[30] Sam D. Gill, *Native American Religious Action: A Performative Approach* (Columbia: University of South Carolina Press, 1987), 37–40.

[31] Gill, *Native American Religious Action*, 39.

[32] David Howes, "Introduction: 'To Summon All the Senses,'" in Howes, *Varieties of Sensory Experience*, 3–21.

[33] Franz Boas, *Primitive Art* (New York: Dover, 1955), 225.

[34] Edmund Carpenter, *Oh, What a Blow That Phantom Gave Me!* (Toronto: Bantam Books, 1972).

have been guided by the multidirectional "perspective" of the ear rather than the unidirectional "perspective" of the eye, given that his culture is an oral-aural one.

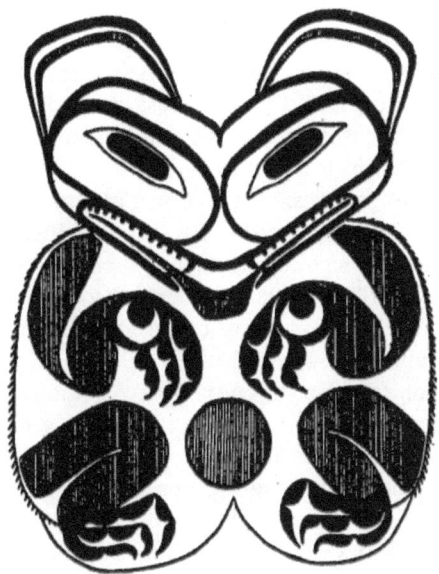

Figure 1. Tsimshian representation of Bear, after Franz Boas, *Primitive Art* (New York: Dover, 1955), 225.

In effect, the Tsimshian "wraparound" representation of Bear corresponds to the experience of sound, which also envelops and surrounds one.[35] The "ear-minded" Tsimshian would thus seem to transpose visual imagery into auditory imagery in their visual art. To understand that art involves what Edmund Carpenter has described as "hearing with the eye."[36]

A more explicit example of an auditory-based visual representation is found in the intricate geometric designs of the Shipibo-Conibo. These designs, which are kept by the Shipibo-Conibo in glyphic books and used extensively in the decoration of artefacts and clothes, are said to embody songs. During the healing ritual the shaman, in a hallucinogenic trance, perceives these designs floating downwards. When the designs reach the shaman's lips he sings them into songs. On coming into contact with the patient, the songs once again turn into designs

---

[35] Don Ihde, *Listening and Voice: A Phenomenology of Sound* (Athens: Ohio University Press, 1976).

[36] Carpenter, *Oh, What a Blow*, 30.

which penetrate the patient's body and heal the illness. These design-songs also have an olfactory dimension, as their power is said to reside in their "fragrance."[37]

Geometric designs are also used extensively by the Desana of Colombia, who, like the Shipibo-Conibo, associate them with a series of sensory manifestations. The symbolic significance of Desana baskets and mats, for instance, lies not only in the design of their weave, but also in their specific odour and texture.[38] It is telling of the extent to which we in the West live under the thrall of the visual that, although the multisensory nature of Desana baskets is evident, while that of the Shipibo-Conibo designs is not, most Westerners would be as unlikely to pick up on the extra-visual significance of the former as they would that of the latter.

Just as artefacts and designs can have sensory significance beyond the visual, so can music have sensory significance beyond the auditory. One example of this is the design-songs described above. Another is that of Desana instrumental music, discussed by Classen.[39] Desana music interrelates all of the senses. The music of the Kogi of Colombia has a specifically tactile aspect, because, for the Kogi, sacred songs are "threads" which tie one to benevolent forces.[40] Artefacts and aesthetic manifestations, therefore, may well evoke sensory associations or resonances far beyond those immediately apparent to the outside observer.

Masks provide other kinds of information about a culture's sensory order. As Edmund Carpenter[41] notes with regard to the use of masks in West Africa: "West African dancers and singers close their eyes partially or wholly. The masks they wear are similarly carved. Masks with open, staring eyes are rare and usually covered by hanging hemp or fur. Sight is deliberately muted." By way of contrast to the downplaying of vision evidenced by West African masks, a positive emphasis on vision is manifested by the paper figures used ritually by the Otomi of Mexico. The Otomi only give eyes to those figures representing good beings, such as humans, thus according a high moral value to eyesight.[42] Yet another contrast is presented by the masks which the Kalapalo of Brazil make to represent powerful spirits. Kalapalo spirit masks emphasize all of the senses: eyes are fashioned from mother-of-pearl, ears protrude, noses are long, and the tongue and breath are represented by a pair of red cotton strings hanging from the mouth. This is because

---

[37] Gebhart-Sayer, "Geometric Designs."

[38] Reichel-Dolmatoff, *Basketry as Metaphor*.

[39] Constance Classen, "Creation by Sound/Creation by Light: A Sensory Analysis of Two South American Cosmologies," in Howes, *Varieties of Sensory Experience*, 239–55.

[40] Gerardo Reichel-Dolmatoff, "Funerary Customs and Religious Symbolism among the Kogi," in *Native South Americans*, ed. Patricia J. Lyon (Boston: Little, Brown, 1974), 298.

[41] Carpenter, *Oh, What a Blow*, 22.

[42] James Dow, *The Shaman's Touch: Otomi Indian Symbolic Healing* (Salt Lake City: University of Utah Press, 1986), 103.

powerful spirits are said to be "hyperanimate" and thus possess extraordinary sensory powers. The particular auditory bias of the Kalapalo is evidenced, however, in the fact that the most important distinguishing characteristic of powerful spirits is their ability to create music.[43]

Given all that has just been said, it should be apparent that when artefacts are put on display in museums they are stripped of much of their sense. Can their sense be preserved rather than reified in museum exhibits? If so, how? Would it help to affix a note explaining the other sensory dimensions of the artefact? Or, should curators stop at nothing less than re-creating the total sensory environment in which the artefact was originally used? What might be the drawbacks of providing simulations of the latter sort?[44] The problem raised here can be focused by setting oneself the task of designing an exhibit for a Kaluli drum, bearing in mind everything noted by Steven Feld.[45]

The preceding discussion is somewhat one-sided, insofar as it has concentrated on how non-Western artefacts are perceived by Western observers. In the interest of balance, one should also examine how Western artefacts are perceived according to the sensory models of other cultures. In *A Musical View of the Universe*, for instance, Ellen Basso relates that her glasses were understood by a member of the "ear-minded" Kalapalo, not in terms of their visual function, but in terms of the sound they made on being put on: "nngnruk."[46]

3. Body Decoration

- What can the ways in which a culture decorates and deforms (reforms) the human body tell us about that culture's sensory order?
- Are any of the sense organs physically emphasized through the use of earrings, nose-rings, scarification, paint, etc.?
- Which senses figure foremost in cultural ideals of personal beauty?

The topic of body decoration is closely related to the previous section on artefacts and aesthetics. A culture's ideals of personal beauty are influenced by its aesthetic ideals, and the ways in which bodies are decorated are often similar to the ways in which artefacts are decorated. The designs which the Shipibo-Conibo use to

---

[43] Ellen Becker Basso, *A Musical View of the Universe: Kalapalo Myth and Ritual Performance* (Philadelphia: University of Philadelphia Press, 1985), 70, 245–47.

[44] See Jean Baudrillard, *Simulations*, trans. P. Foss, P. Patton, and P. Beitchman (New York: Semiotext[e], 1983); Michael M. Ames, *Museums, the Public and Anthropology* (New Delhi: Concept Publishing; Vancouver: University of British Columbia Press, 1985), 10.

[45] Feld, "Sound as a Symbolic System."

[46] Basso, *Musical View*, 64.

decorate artefacts and clothes, for instance, are also painted on the faces of members of the tribe for healing and festive purposes.[47]

Body decorations (ornaments, scars) can seem purely "cosmetic," but they frequently convey information about group identity and social status as well. At a deeper level, they may serve to "embody" a particular sensory order, as Seeger found among the Suya of Brazil.[48] As will be recalled from the discussion in Howes, "Sensorial Anthropology," among the Suva ear-discs serve to emphasize the cultural importance of hearing and moral behaviour while lip-discs are associated with speaking, singing, and aggression.

An interesting variation on the Suya example is presented by the Dogon of Mali. Among the Dogon, a girl's "education in speaking" begins at age three with the piercing of a hole and the insertion of a metal ring in her lower lip. This is followed by the piercing of her ears at age six. If she continues to make grammatical errors or utter uncouth remarks by age twelve, then rings are inserted in the septum and wings of her nose.[49] For those who come from cultures which do not postulate any connection between the organ of smell and that of speech, this practice will be found difficult to comprehend. For the Dogon, however, "Despite its invisible nature, [speech] has material properties that are more than just sound … [it] has an 'odour'"; "sound and odour having vibration as their common origin are so near to one another that the Dogon speak of 'hearing a smell.'"[50] Thus, according to Dogon conceptions, words may be classified by smell. Good words smell "sweet," and bad words smell "rotten," which explains the practice of operating on the nose so as to encourage the reception and utterance of "good-smelling words" and the repression or deflection of bad ones. We may conclude that the Dogon (unlike the Suya) regard smell, speech, and hearing as equally "social faculties." At least ideally: "the mouth too ready to speak is likened to the rectum."[51] In other words, bad or impetuous speech is synonymous with flatulence.[52]

Sometimes it may take some probing to discover the deeper sense of what are ostensibly "beauty marks." To take an example from Western culture, the artificial beauty spots which were so popular in Enlightenment France, and which we think

---

[47] Gebhart-Sayer, "Geometric Designs."

[48] Seeger, "Meaning of Body Ornaments."

[49] Geneviève Calame-Griaule, *Words and the Dogon World*, trans. D. La Pin (Philadelphia: Institute for the Study of Human Issues, 1986), 308–10.

[50] Calame-Griaule, *Words and the Dogon World*, 39 and 48, n. 69.

[51] Calame-Griaule, *Words and the Dogon World*, 320.

[52] Like the Suya, however, the Dogon would seem to regard sight as an "antisocial" or pre-social faculty. For example, it is by means of graphic symbols (paw marks) that Fox communicates with human beings in the context of Dogon divination. The dreams inspired in people by Fox are also silent. The reason for this is that Fox's tongue was severed by the Creator Amma, as punishment for resisting the latter's cosmic plan and bringing death into the world (Calame-Griaule, *Words and the Dogon World*, 102–3, 146).

of as purely visual, were in fact always dipped in perfume giving them an olfactory dimension.[53] In modern Africa, the Tiv of Nigeria have a special marking called "catfish" which is incised on a young woman's belly. When confronted with the suggestion that the designs were not purely decorative, but rather symbolic of the girls' biological roles as wives and mothers (i.e., their fertility), the Tiv more or less agreed: "They said that the scars are tender for some years after they are made and these artificial erogenous zones make women sexier and hence more fertile."[54] Note how the Tiv give a tactile meaning to the visual marks. What we would also note is that the heightened cutaneous awareness such markings make possible is consistent with other facts about Tiv society. Kinaesthetic awareness also appears to have been developed to a remarkably high degree in this culture: "Those of us brought up in the northern European tradition are underdeveloped rhythmically. We have a single beat that we dance to, whereas the Tiv ... have four drums, *one for each part of the body.* Each drummer beats out a different rhythm; talented dancers move to all four."[55] Is the Tiv case unique, or are scarification and related forms of body decoration normally found in those cultures which place a premium on "bodily intelligence"?

4. Child-Rearing Practices

- Which of the senses do caretakers stress or repress the most in raising children? Touch, taste, hearing?
- Do the socialization practices emphasize self-control or self-indulgence, individuality or conformity?
- Are these emphases reversed or altered at any stage of a child's development?
- Is the primary means of education visual, oral, kinaesthetic? How are children taught to conform to their culture's sensory order?

The first moments and months of a child's existence are of paramount importance with respect to shaping the sensory orientation that individual will manifest for the rest of his or her life. In North American society, it is customary for the newborn to be separated from its mother, swaddled, and put to sleep in a crib. In other cultures, infants are virtually always in contact with the skin of some caretaker or other. The communication styles of adults have been shown to reflect these early

---

[53] Roy Genders, *A History of Scent* (London: Hamish Hamilton, 1972), 129.
[54] Robert Brain, *The Decorated Body* (New York: Harper & Row, 1979), 78.
[55] Hall, *Beyond Culture*, 77–78.

childhood experiences.[56] For example, North American society is an extreme example of a "non-contact culture," in that there is considerably less sensory involvement, eye contact, and touching, and relatively greater interpersonal distance, during social interaction, than in, for example, most African societies, where child-rearing practices tend to be more tactile.

Socialization practices have also been found to influence "perceptual style."[57] For example, the Inuit perform better on Witkin's Embedded Figures Test, and thus manifest greater "field independence," than the Temne of Sierra Leone. Temne child-rearing practices tend to be strict and emphasize conformity; those of the Inuit are more lenient and foster individuality. The greater ability on the part of Inuit subjects to disembed figures from surrounding fields (i.e., to experience items as separate from context) may thus be related to the greater likelihood for a sense of separate identity to emerge in Inuit society than in Temne society.[58]

Of course, the Embedded Figures Test only pertains to differentiation in the visual field. As far as the Temne are concerned, it may simply be that vision is not a field of "productive specialization" (in Ong and Wober's sense) for them, because they attach more importance to discrimination in the auditory or proprioceptive field. This possibility must always be borne in mind. It is best gauged by examining the full range of educational practices in place in the society, as well as the amount of time allotted to each of them. Thus, in some cultures children are taught how to dance from an early age, in others to recite sacred texts from memory.[59] Or again, in some cultures children (and adults) are told what to do, in others they are shown what to do. Thomas Gregor writes of the Mehinaku of the Brazilian Amazon: "The villagers are given to the use of visual aids in teaching. Whenever I failed to follow, an explanation of a ritual or custom, I was urged to wait until I could see it; then I would understand. The Mehinaku teach physical skills ... by having the pupil look on as the work is performed. There are ... occasional verbal explanations but these are a relatively small part of the teaching

---

[56] Ashley Montagu, *Touching: The Human Significance of the Skin*, 2nd ed. (New York: Harper & Row, 1978).

[57] J. Mallory Wober, "The Sensotype Hypothesis," in Howes, *Varieties of Sensory Experience*, 31–42.

[58] John W. Berry, "Temne and Eskimo Perceptual Skills," *International Journal of Psychology* 1.3 (1966): 207–29.

[59] In North American society, such skills are relatively underdeveloped, because of the paramount value attached to learning to read and write, which entails shutting up and sitting still. On the cognitive implications of the amount of stress different cultures attach to the development of different faculties, such as to read, to recite, or to dance, see Howard Gardner, *Frames of Mind: The Theory of Multiple Intelligences* (New York: Basic Books, 1983).

process."⁶⁰ Different techniques may be used according to the nature of the material which is being communicated. Among the Yanomama of the Brazilian Amazon, for example, shamanistic knowledge can only be communicated in the darkness; thus a shaman speaks only at night.⁶¹

Children do not always manifest the same sensory order as adults. For example, it has often been observed that North American children have a greater interest in odours and tastes than do North American adults.⁶² Among the Inuit, the self-control manifested by adults contrasts with the self-indulgence of infants. Inuit children are characterized by their "touchability." They are "cuddled, cooed at, talked to and played with endlessly."⁶³ When they cry they are instantly comforted, either through touch or through food. Indeed, nearly all delicacies are saved to be given to children for this purpose. Touch and taste, therefore, are given free rein in infancy.

As an Inuit child passes infancy, she or he is expected to learn to suppress the senses of taste and touch. Jean Briggs notes several examples of this among the Utku. When a new child is born, its older sibling is discouraged from breastfeeding by the mother as follows: "Your little sister has nursed and gotten the breast and the inside of the parka all shitty and stinky; it smells [and tastes, one word has both meanings] horrible."⁶⁴ Similarly, being poked in various parts of the body is a favourite game with infants. Older children, however, are warned: "Watch out, your uncle's going to poke you if you don't cover up and get dressed!"⁶⁵ Thus, older children are taught to regard as unpleasant sensations which they formerly regarded as highly pleasurable. Touch, in particular, is greatly restricted after the period of infancy. Briggs writes: "Utku husbands and their wives, children older than five or six and their parents, never embrace or kiss ... and rarely touch one another in any way, except insofar as they lie under the same quilts at night."⁶⁶

Among the Utku, the senses which are developed in adults are sight, so necessary for hunting and other practical endeavours, and above all hearing, by which oral traditions are passed on.⁶⁷ People in Inuit society are therefore trained to grow out of the "infantile" senses of touch and taste into the "practical" sense of sight and the "social" sense of hearing. Many cultures mark such an entrance

---

⁶⁰ Thomas Gregor, *Mehinaku* (Chicago: University of Chicago Press, 1977), 40.
⁶¹ Ettore Biocca, *Yanoama* (New York: Dutton, 1970), 72.
⁶² Porteous, *Landscapes of the Mind*, 145-73.
⁶³ Jean L. Briggs, *Never in Anger: Portrait of an Eskimo Family* (Cambridge: Harvard University Press, 1970), 71.
⁶⁴ Briggs, *Never in Anger*, 158.
⁶⁵ Briggs, *Never in Anger*, 149.
⁶⁶ Briggs, *Never in Anger*, 117.
⁶⁷ Carpenter, *Eskimo Realities*, 26, 33.

into the adult sensory and social order by a specific rite, as in the case of the Barasana male puberty rite described in the section on cosmology (see below).

5. Alternative Sensory Modes

- What exceptions to the dominant sensory model exist within a society?
- Are different ways of sensing attributed to or manifested by women or men?
- How are persons with sensory handicaps treated?

In the previous section we saw that children sometimes manifest a markedly different sensory order than adults. Women also frequently manifest a sensory order which differs from the dominant one. Women and men are commonly held to perceive the world in different ways, with the male way usually being normative and the female way a complementary adjunct at best, and an aberration at worst. Different sensory characteristics are often attributed to men and women as well. Among the Hua of Papua New Guinea, for instance, the inside of the male body is considered to be white, hard, and odourless, that of the female body to be dark, juicy, and fetid.[68] In the Amazon, men are commonly thought to be cold and women to be hot,[69] while the reverse holds true for the indigenous cultures of Mexico.[70] All of these characteristics, of course, are associated with fundamental cultural values.

Those rites which initiate a girl or boy into the adult world often serve as initiations into a particular, gender-determined sensory order. The Yanoama, for instance, believe that a woman should not speak with a louder voice than a man's, that is, that she should not assert herself.[71] During the female puberty rite, consequently, a girl will be shut in a cage and not allowed to speak for three weeks. After this time, she may begin to speak, but only very softly. At the moment of reemergence, her lips and ears are pierced,[72] which undoubtedly serves to mark the socialization of her speech and hearing according to the "correct" female sensory order.

Aside from, but related to, these sensory differences arbitrarily imposed upon the sexes by culture, are the differences in sensory orders which women and men

---

[68] Anna Stokes Meigs, *Food, Sex and Pollution: A New Guinea Religion* (New Brunswick: Rutgers University Press, 1984), 127.

[69] E.g., Stephen Hugh-Jones, *The Palm and the Pleiades: Initiation and Cosmology in Northwest Amazonia* (Cambridge: Cambridge University Press, 1979), 111.

[70] E.g., Alfredo López Austin, *The Human Body and Ideology: Concepts of the Ancient Nahuas*, vol. 1 (Salt Lake City: University of Utah Press, 1988), 53.

[71] Biocca, *Yanoama*, 136.

[72] Biocca, *Yanoama*, 82.

may actually (as opposed to theoretically) manifest. Among the Desana, for instance, the male sensory order is characterized by an emphasis on transcendent sight acquired through narcotic visions. Women, who are not allowed to take narcotics, appear to have a sensory order which emphasizes senses other than sight—in particular, touch.[73]

Such sensory distinctions are invariably related to the social distinctions made by a culture between different groups, as well as to the different practices of such groups. Some of the groups within society which may manifest alternative sensory modes include: religious specialists, outcasts, and, in larger societies, the ruling and working classes and ethnic groups. Among the ancient Nahuas of Mexico, for example, nobles had "the right to eat human flesh, to drink pulque and cacao, to smell fragrant flowers, and to be given the gift of aromatic burning incense."[74]

The reactions displayed by a culture to the real or imagined sensory differences of persons from other cultures can also prove revealing of local sensory preferences. The Sharanahua of Peru, for example, see westernized Peruvians as "speakers of another language, eaters of disgusting animals like cows, potential cannibals with enormous sexual appetites."[75] Anthony Seeger reports that the Suya regarded his practice of taking notes as evidence that his ears were "swollen," for the Suya believe that knowledge is acquired and retained by the ear, not the eye.[76]

The treatment a culture accords to persons with sensory handicaps, notably the blind and the deaf, is especially revealing. While one must keep in mind that blindness is a handicap even in the most auditory of societies (because of the practical value of sight), it may be much less of a handicap in some cultures than in others. In certain cultures blind persons may be thought to compensate for their sightlessness by being clairvoyant, or by having supernatural powers of hearing.[77] Indeed, the different modes of perceiving of persons with sensory handicaps can in themselves form the basis of a fascinating study.[78]

Finally, alternative sensory modes often come into play when people are rebelling against some aspect of their existence. Among the Inuit, for example, who regard excessive emotions of all kinds as dangerous, anger is usually expressed

---

[73] Classen, "Creation by Sound."

[74] López Austin, *Human Body and Ideology*, 393.

[75] Janet Siskind, *To Hunt in the Morning* (New York: Oxford University Press, 1973), 49.

[76] Anthony Seeger, *Why Suya Sing: A Musical Anthropology of an Amazonian People* (Cambridge: Cambridge University Press, 1987), 11.

[77] William Paulson, *Enlightenment, Romanticism and the Blind in France* (Princeton: Princeton University Press, 1987), 5–6.

[78] See Oliver W. Sacks *The Man Who Mistook His Wife for a Hat and Other Clinical Tales* (New York: Harper & Row, 1985); Sacks, *Seeing Voices: A Journey into the World of the Deaf* (Berkeley: University of California Press, 1989).

by withdrawal and rejection of all sensory stimuli. Jean Briggs gives an example of this among the Utku Inuit of the Northwest Territories: "In such moods [of anger] Raigili might stand for an hour or more facing the wall, her arms withdrawn from her sleeves the latter pose a characteristic Utku expression of hunger, cold, fatigue, and grief. If her mother tried to tempt her with a piece of jammy bannock [cake] she dropped it or ignored it. If her father tried to move her she was limp in his hands."[79] Another example of this rejection of external stimuli is the case of an adolescent girl in the same community who, intensely unhappy, pretended to be deaf for a summer.[80] Such withdrawal can also take the form of sleep. Sleeping long hours is a characteristic sign among the Inuit of an emotional disturbance.[81] Varieties of sensory experience thus exist not only among cultures, but also within cultures.

6. Media of Communication

- What media does a society use for communication? Is the dominant medium the spoken word, the written word, the printed word, or the electronic bit? What other kinds of sensory codes are employed?
- How do members of the culture react when exposed to new communications media?
- If the culture manifests a preference for some media of communication over others, which senses are engaged the most and how?

It is important to analyse the *full* range of media used for communication in the culture—music, dance, food, perfumes, designs, writing, television, etc.—and not simply those which have to do with the transmission of "the Word."[82] The so-called "orality/literacy divide" has been shown to be misleading. As the essays in *The Varieties of Sensory Experience* attest, oral cultures can be quite diverse in their sensory and symbolic systems, as can literate cultures. Furthermore, not all cultures which possess writing are literate to the same degree or in the same

---

[79] Briggs, *Never in Anger*, 137.

[80] Briggs, *Never in Anger*, 137.

[81] Briggs, *Never in Anger*, 281.

[82] Indeed, why the fascination in Communications Studies departments with "the technologizing of the word" (Walter J. Ong, *Orality and Literacy* [New York: Methuen, 1982])? Might this verbocentrism have something to do with the religious orientation of those who laid the groundwork for this discipline (i.e., McLuhan and Ong)?

ways.[83] Among the Hanunoo of the Philippines, for instance, writing is used almost exclusively for romantic purposes.[84] In general, one may expect a culture which is predominantly oral to manifest an auditory bias and one which is predominantly literate to manifest a visual bias. However, this is at best a preliminary typology which must be supplemented by the study of the full range of media used in a society and how they interact with one another.[85]

Reactions upon first exposure to Western communications media can serve as a litmus test of a culture's sensory order. Thus, a Tully River Aborigine, seeing whites communicate with each other by means of a letter (i.e., written marks on paper), put a letter to his ear to "see if he could understand anything by that method."[86] As one would expect, in the local language, "to understand" is expressed by the same verb as "to hear." Such reactions can also shed light on our own sensory order. For example, the naivety of the Western belief in the "truth of photography" is nicely brought out in the story of the Tanzanian chief who, when shown various photos, "recognized some of the pictures of animals ... but invariably looked at the back of the paper to see what was there, and remarked that he did not consider them finished since they did not give the likeness of the other side of the animal."[87] This clash of expectations is instructive: the chief expected the picture to show what he *knew* about the animal in question (namely, that it has more than one side), whereas Westerners are satisfied with being shown only what one can *see*.

---

[83] Sylvia Scribner and Michael Cole, *The Psychology of Literacy* (Cambridge: Harvard University Press, 1981).

[84] Charles Frake, "Did Literacy Cause the Great Cognitive Divide?," *American Ethnologist* 10 (1983): 368–71.

[85] While anthropologists normally search for "consonance" across media (Mary Douglas, *Natural Symbols* [New York: Pantheon, 1982], 68), dissonances can be equally revealing. Paul Stoller and Cheryl Olkes ("La Sauce épaisse: Remarques sur les relations sociales songhaïs," *Anthropologie et Sociétés* 14.2 [1990]: 57–76) have shown how messages in one medium, say the verbal message "This is a formal (read: 'thick') social occasion," may be contradicted by those in another; for example, a woman serving a "thin" (meatless, hence informal) sauce on the occasion in question (see further Arjun Appadurai, "Gastro-politics in Hindu South Asia," *American Ethnologist* 8 [1981]: 494–511). Similarly, documentary producers have been known to get a point across by, for example, playing "Rule Britannia" while images of London slums, as opposed to Buckingham Palace, pass by on the screen (John Morgan and Peter Welton, *See What I Mean: An Introduction to Visual Communication* [New York: Edward Arnold, 1986]).

[86] Alexander Chamberlain, "Primitive Hearing and Hearing-Words," *American Journal of Psychology* 16 (1905): 126.

[87] J. Mallory Wober, *Psychology in Africa* (London: International African Institute, 1975), 80.

Such inventions as the telephone and television might seem to have extended the scope of human communication to an unprecedented degree, but it is important to recognize how they also limit human communication by occluding certain channels of sensory awareness—most notably smell and taste and touch. Cultures which do without these particular means of communication exploit other media—that is, they extend their senses in other ratios, which may be equally complex. Odour communication is very important to the Desana, for instance, who admire and elaborate on the use of odours by animals.[88] The Murngin of northern Australia have evolved an intriguing "audio-olfactory" technique for communicating with whales. As one informant told Warner: "we can take sweat from under our arms and put our hands in the water, and we can put that water in our mouths and sing out the power names of that whale. It is just the same as if we were asking him for something."[89] In a related form of communication found among a neighbouring people, the members of one moiety rub the sweat from their armpits on the eyes of the other moiety to enable the latter to "see with sacredness."[90] This form of communication could be considered either a form of haptic visuality or, in the alternative, olfacto-visual.

As these examples suggest, there exist many possible ways of combining the senses for purposes of communication, and the audio-visual is but one among them.[91] The extent to which this particular combination (the audio-visual) has been developed in the West reflects the depth of our commitment to a particular "regime of sensory values,"[92] one which, significantly, privileges the distance senses. The Murngin and their neighbours have experimented with other ratios, the audio-olfactory and the olfacto-visual, and they evidently enjoy a very different mode of relating self to self, and self to world, in consequence.

7. Natural and Built Environment

- Does the natural environment call for the exercise of some senses more than others, and if so in what ways?

---

[88] Gerardo Reichel-Dolmatoff, "Tapir Avoidance in the Colombian Northwest Amazon," in *Animal Myths and Metaphors*, ed. Gary Urton (Salt Lake City: University of Utah Press, 1985), 104–43.

[89] William Lloyd Warner, *A Black Civilization: A Study of an Australian Tribe* (New York: Harper & Row, 1958), 354–57.

[90] Berndt, *Kunapipi*, 44.

[91] Of course, Western culture also employs non-audio-visual media of communication, such as food codes, but these are rarely explicit and are completely overshadowed by the dominant media.

[92] Alain Corbin, *The Foul and the Fragrant: Odor and the French Social Imagination*, trans. M. Kochan, R. Porter, and C. Prendergast (Cambridge: Harvard University Press, 1986).

- How does the layout of the community influence sensory perception? Is the home sealed off from the outside world, or is there an interchange of sensory perceptions?
- Does the home consist of only one room, or are there separate rooms for different activities? Does the family sleep together or separately?

Perception, like cognition, must be studied in its "natural setting."[93] Perceptual experiments carried out in psychology laboratories yield clear results. Try carrying out the same experiment in the midst of a Moroccan bazaar, the Arctic tundra, the Sepik River region of Papua New Guinea and, suffice it to say, the results will not be the same. The point here is that the natural environment does influence perception. It may call for the use of some senses more than others, or in any event in different ways from our own, as Gilbert Lewis found in the course of his fieldwork among the Gnau of Papua New Guinea:

> Although it is usually easy to walk through the forest, there are no perspectives, no open views.... The light is dimmed and greenish. Occasionally one passes through a path of unmoving air faintly scented by some plant like honey-suckle; one passes transient smells, of humus, of moist rotting wood or bruised fruits. The Gnau people are alert to smell ... in some cases they use scent to decide the identification of trees or shrubs, scraping or cutting the bark.... The canopy and confusion of trees alters sounds and calls, limiting and muffling them, but as though enclosed in a leafy hall; the sharp screech or squawks from a nearby bird sound echoes in one's ears. I found the localization of forest sounds difficult, ... although the native people were accurate in pointing to the direction and finding them. They excel in identifying bird calls.[94]

Lewis's account of how the environment affects the senses agrees in an interesting way with the privileging of the auditory and olfactory modalities in the context of ritual communication, and as metaphors for cognition, in other New Guinea societies.[95] However, as Classen points out,[96] cultures may seek to compensate for the

---

[93] John W. Berry, Sidney H. Irvine, and Earl B. Hunt, eds., *Indigenous Cognition: Functioning in Cultural Context* (Dordrecht: Nijhoff, 1988).

[94] Gilbert Lewis, *Knowledge of Illness in a Sepik Society: A Study of the Gnau, New Guinea* (London: Athlone Press; Atlantic Highlands, NJ: Humanities Press, 1975), 46.

[95] See Howes, "Sensorial Anthropology." One also wants to be attentive to how the different environmental niches spanned by a culture (for example, sea and land) give rise to different sorts of sense perceptions (such as wet/dry, or feeling buoyant and moving speedily/feeling heavy and slow), and how these are valued and elaborated upon in the culture's symbolic system, as Nancy D. Munn so well demonstrates in *The Fame of Gawa: A Symbolic Study of Value Transformation in a Massim (Papua New Guinea) Society* (New York: Cambridge University Press, 1986); see also Ohnuki-Tierney, *Illness and Healing*.

[96] Classen, "Creation by Sound."

restrictions imposed upon the senses by the environment. A society in which the availability of odours and flavours is limited by nature, for example, may value these all the more because of their scarcity. Witness the high value accorded to Eastern spices in the Europe of the Middle Ages.[97] Therefore, contrary to Berry,[98] we would hold that there is no one-to-one correspondence between the characteristics of a culture's physical environment (e.g., arctic tundra vs. tropical forest) and its cognitive style (e.g., field-independent vs. field-dependent).

The built environment also influences perception. In a classic study, Segal et al.[99] demonstrated that the fact of living in a "carpentered world" as opposed to a "circular world" (like that of the Zulu of South Africa, with their oval huts and compounds) makes a person more susceptible to the Sander Parallelogram illusion (see figure 2).

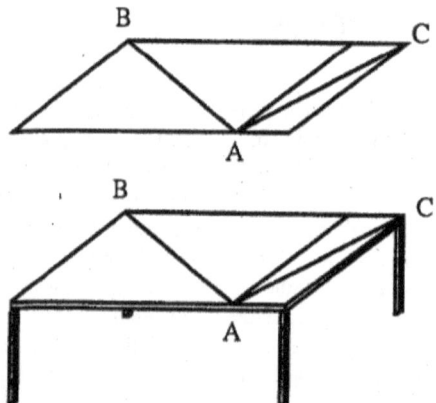

Figure 2. The Sander parallelogram, after Jan B. Deregowski, *Illusions, Patterns and Pictures: A Cross-Cultural Perspective* (New York: Academic Press, 1980), 14.

In experiments involving the Sander parallelogram, the respondent is asked: "Which of the two lines, AB or AC, is shorter?" Respondents raised in a carpentered environment usually say "AC" even though AC is, in fact, 15 per cent *longer* than AB. Respondents raised in a circular environment, like that of the Zulu, do not usually make this error. The reason for this misperception may

---

[97] Colin Clair, *Of Herbs and Spices* (London: Abelard Schuman, 1961), 15.

[98] Berry, "Temne and Eskimo Perceptual Skills"; Berry, *Human Ecology and Cognitive Style: Comparative Studies in Cultural and Psychological Adaptation* (Beverly Hills: Sage, 1976).

[99] Marshall H. Segal, Donald T. Campbell, and Melville J. Herskovits, *The Influence of Culture on Visual Perception* (Chicago: Bobbs-Merrill, 1966).

have to do with the Western subject automatically interpreting the two-dimensional representation as if it were three-dimensional (i.e., as if it were drawn on the surface of a rectangular table).

The built environment can also be analysed as a projection of a given culture's sensory profile. We think of Michel Foucault's insightful analysis of how Bentham's design for a prison, the Panopticon, has been generalized to encompass other spaces (the hospital, the school), such that we moderns live in a "society of surveillance."[100] By contrast, for the Suya, "the sonic transparency of their community makes of their village a concert hall."[101] For the Inuit, "visually and acoustically the igloo is 'open,' a labyrinth alive with the movements of crowded people."[102]

The construction of the built environment in the image of a culture's sensory profile is apparent in the nineteenth-century English and French bourgeois fetish for balconies: "From the balcony, one could gaze, but not be touched."[103] It is also apparent in the proliferation of rooms within the bourgeois dwelling. This multiplication had the effect of privatizing what were once more social functions (the preparation and consumption of food, the elimination of bodily wastes, sleeping) by confining each to a separate room.[104] The fragmented (as opposed to synaesthetic) understanding of the sensorium with which we moderns operate is at least partly attributable to this great nineteenth-century repartition of space and bodily functions. Imagine the intermingling of sensations that would result from simply removing some of the inner walls we have built up.

8. Rituals

- In ritual settings, is any sense usually more engaged than others, for example, sight by costumes and dance, hearing by speeches and music?
- Are any senses suppressed in order to privilege other senses?
- Is there a sequence to how the senses are engaged or alternately extinguished in a ritual?
- Is the ritual specialist distinguished by the use of any one sense or particular combination of senses?

---

[100] Michel Foucault, *Discipline and Punish: Birth of the Prison*, trans. A. Sheridan (New York: Vintage Books, 1979).

[101] Seeger, *Why Suya Sing*, xiv.

[102] Carpenter, *Eskimo Realities*, 25.

[103] Peter Stallybrass and Allon White, *The Politics and Poetics of Transgression* (Ithaca: Cornell University Press, 1986), 132.

[104] Corbin, *Foul and the Fragrant*; David Howes, "Scent and Sensibility," *Culture, Medicine and Psychiatry* 13 (1989): 121–29.

It has frequently been noted that ritual communication takes place through physical demonstration: "it concretely enacts assertions rather than simply referring to them in discourse."[105] Many anthropologists have also drawn attention to the "multi-channel character" of ritual communication.[106] As Fredrik Barth observes of ritual performance among the Baktaman of Papua New Guinea: "Different aspects of a ritual performance reach the participant by way of each of his different senses; and the diversity of meaningful features and idioms is very great."[107]

Ideally, the ethnographer wants to attend to each and every message in each and every channel: for example, among the Baktaman, the smell of burning marsupial, the redness of the dancers, the different drum rhythms each invoking a different spirit, all contribute to the total meaning of the event. Regrettably, it is rarely possible for the ethnographer to attend to all these sensations at once. However, cultures also tend to be selective regarding the media they emphasize. The Suya, for instance, perform their major rituals at night, thereby excluding the significant participation of vision and giving prominence to their ceremonial singing.[108] The Bosotho of southern Africa resort to "played aurality" (as a matter of conscious preference to other sensory modes) to resolve situations of crisis.[109] The Moroccan ritual of silent wishes described by Griffin,[110] where even speech is proscribed and everything centres around the burning of the seven kinds of incense, is a further example of a ritual which augments some meanings at the expense of others by restricting the number of sensory channels in use.

In addition to rituals which stimulate all the channels of sensory awareness at once,[111] and those which restrict them to a few, there are rituals that accentuate

---

[105] Bruce M. Knauft, *Good Company and Violence: Sorcery and Social Action in a Lowland New Guinea Society* (Berkeley: University of California Press, 1985), 247.

[106] Edmund Leach, *Culture and Communication* (Cambridge: Cambridge University Press, 1976); Ruth Stone, *Let the Inside Be Sweet: The Interpretation of Music Event among the Kpelle of Liberia* (Bloomington: Indiana University Press, 1986).

[107] Fredrik Barth, *Ritual Knowledge among the Baktaman of New Guinea* (New Haven: Yale University Press, 1975), 223.

[108] Anthony Seeger, *Nature and Society in Central Brazil: The Suya Indians of Mato Grosso* (Cambridge: Harvard University Press, 1981), 87.

[109] Charles Adams, "Aurality and Consciousness: Basotho Production of Significance," in *Essays in Humanistic Anthropology*, ed. Bruce T. Grindal and Dennis M. Warren (New York: University Press of America, 1986) 303–26.

[110] Kit Griffin, "The Ritual of Silent Wishes: Notes on the Moroccan Sensorium," in Howes, *Varieties of Sensory Experience*, 210–20.

[111] Perhaps the most splendid example of stimulating all the senses to the same extent at the same time is provided by the traditional Indian courts: "The fulfillment of every sense was considered an art in the Indian courts.... Scents were blended to suit moods and seasons and were believed to complement the colour of clothing—thus, musk was worn

and suppress different modalities according to a certain sequence. We think of the Japanese midday tea ceremony (*shogo chaji*), a minutely prescribed rite, which takes from three to five hours to complete. In the tea ceremony, the "progressive induction into ritual time is reflected in an increasing emphasis on non-verbal modes of communication."[112] Thus, conversation is permitted upon first entering the tea garden, but in the tea hut itself it is the burning incense, scrolls, and flower arrangements that set the tone. The moment of greatest symbolic intensity—imbibing the tea—is surrounded by silence. The whole purpose of this ritual is to instill a mental attitude of introspective "emptiness";[113] hence the sequencing of the sensations. In Japan to be introspective (which is *the* Zen state) is to close one's ears but keep one's other senses open. We close our eyes.

At the opposite extreme from the Japanese tea ceremony, which celebrates the senses in a determinate order, are those rituals designed to "overcome" or "vanquish" them and thus pave the way for a transcendental experience. Valentine Daniel describes one such rite in *Fluid Signs*.[114] The ritual involved an arduous six-mile pilgrimage in honour of Lord Ayyappan (that was supposed to help the devotee achieve union with the deity). Daniel undertook this pilgrimage with some Tamil friends. There is a definite sequence to the order in which the senses are "merged" or "collapsed" in the course of this ritual. As Daniel recounts, first hearing goes, then smell, then sight, then "the sense organ *the mouth*" (taste and possibly speech), and finally, all these organs having "merged" into the sense of touch (which itself feels nothing besides pain as of this late point), that sense too "disappears," along with any sense of self.[115] This sequence may be read as an expression of the sensory profile of the Tamil culture of South India, hearing and touch being at opposite ends of the Tamil sensorium, the other senses in between.

---

with winter silks; vetiver was associated with lemon scent, and gossamer went with summer garments" (Naveen Patnaik, *A Second Paradise: Indian Courtly Life, 1590–1947* [London: Sidgwick & Jackson, 1985], 68). The complex combinatorics of emotions, seasons, and sensations played out daily in these courts has no western equivalent. Baudelaire's *Correspondances* pales by comparison (see David Howes, "Le sens sans parole: Vers une anthropologie de l'odorat," *Anthropologie et Sociétés* 10.3 [1986]: 42–43).

[112] Dorinne Kondo, "The Way of Tea: A Symbolic Analysis," *Man* 20 (1983): 297.

[113] Kondo, "The Way of Tea," 301.

[114] E. Valentine Daniel, *Fluid Signs: Being a Person the Tamil Way* (Berkeley: University of California Press, 1984).

[115] Daniel, *Fluid Signs*, 270–76. To illustrate, midway through the third stage of the trek, an informant told Daniel: "I stopped smelling things after Aruda Nati." To which Daniel responded: "Did you not even smell the camphor and incense sticks offered at the various shrines on the way after Aruda?" His informant replied: "You might say I felt it. I didn't smell it" (Daniel, *Fluid Signs*, 272). Incidentally, when the last of the senses, that of pain, "goes" or "dissolves" close to the end of the trek, "love" is said to take its place.

The rituals described above can be said to use techniques of "sensory deprivation," to achieve their effects. As the sensory deprivation literature attests, restricting sensation in one channel enhances sensitivity in other channels as the sensorium seeks to recover "sensoristasis"—that is, to compensate for the deficit.[116] When all the senses are occluded, experimental subjects have been known to hallucinate sensations, or produce percepts from within, so as to fill the void. There is a further body of literature, less well known than the above, which concerns how applying a stimulus to one sensory channel can enhance perception in some other. For example, exposing subjects to the scent of cassia or vanillin facilitates the perception of the colour green while at the same time inhibiting the perception of red or violet.[117]

It would be interesting to analyse accounts of vision quests, shamanic flight, possession dances, and the like in the light of this literature on the application of sensory restriction and cross-modal enhancement techniques to human subjects. Lisa Andermann's analysis of how the senses are combined in Ndembu rituals of divination is a step in this direction.[118] Another account is provided by Gerardo Reichel-Dolmatoff, who describes the ways in which the Tukano restrict and stimulate the senses in order to have bright and pleasant narcotic visions:

> In the first place, the participants should have observed sexual abstinence for several days before the event and should have consumed only a very light diet, devoid of peppers and other condiments. In the second place, physical exercise and profuse perspiration are thought to be necessary for the visionary experience.... Next, the amount and quality of light are said to influence the sensitiveness of the participants who occasionally should stare for a while into the red glow of the torch.... Finally, acoustical stimulations are said to be of importance. The sudden sound of the seed rattles, the shrill notes of a flute, or the long-drawn wails of the clay trumpets are said to release or to modify the luminous images.[119]

Lastly, the sensory specializations of a culture's ritual experts can indicate which senses are considered most important by that culture. Classen[120] explores this topic in relation to the ritual experts of the Andes, who are characterized by their orality, and those of the Desana, who are characterized by their penetrating gaze.

---

[116] John Zubek, ed., *Sensory Deprivation: Fifteen Years of Research* (New York: Appleton-Century-Crofts, 1969).

[117] Frank Allan, "The Influence of the Senses on One Another: Responses of the Organism to Stimulation" (unpublished manuscript; University of Manitoba: Department of Psychology, 1971).

[118] Andermann, "'Great Seeing.'"

[119] Gerardo Reichel-Dolmatoff, *Beyond the Milky Way: Hallucinatory Images of the Tukano Indians* (Los Angeles: UCLA Latin American Center Publications, 1978), 11.

[120] Classen, "Creation by Sound."

By contrast, the healers of the olfactory-conscious Warao of Venezuela must possess an acute sense of smell, as both diseases and the medicinal herbs which cure them are distinguished by their odours.[121] In cases where shamans or sorcerers are believed to stand outside society, their particular sensory characteristics can be considered to contradict the normative sensory model, as among the Suya of Brazil and the Wolof of Senegal.[122]

9. Mythology

- How is the world created? By sound, light, touch?
- What kinds of sensory descriptions are contained in the myths? Is there much visual description, interaction involving touch, dialogue? How are the senses of the first human beings portrayed? If there is a "fall from grace," does this come about through the misuse of any particular sense?
- Does a culture hero have acute eyesight, a keen sense of smell, superior strength, or any particular physical characteristics?
- How are myths passed on? Are they told or acted?

The "sensory codes" of diverse South American Indian myths have been analysed by Lévi-Strauss, and he has shown how the contrasts in one sensory modality can be transposed into those of another, after the manner of a fugue. What this form of analysis unfortunately leaves out is the whole question of the *value* attached to the different modalities in different societies; if factored in, these values might explain why, for example, in one of the myths discussed by Lévi-Strauss, the Opaye myth of "How Men Lost Their Immortality," death came because they smelled its stench, while in a Shipaya myth it came because people failed to detect its odour.[123]

A sensorial (as opposed to structural) anthropological analysis of myth would be attentive not only to how a culture "thinks with" smells and tastes, and textures and sounds or colours, but also "thinks in" or "through" such media.[124] Since Plato,[125] but particularly since the "Enlightenment,"[126] the idiom of Western

---

[121] Werner Wilbert, "The Pneumatic Theory of Female Warao Herbalists," *Social Sciences and Medicine* 25.10 (1987): 1139–46.

[122] Howes, "Sensorial Anthropology."

[123] See Claude Lévi Strauss, *The Raw and the Cooked: Introduction to a Science of Mythology*, trans. J. and D. Weightman vol. 1 (New York: Harper & Row, 1969), 147–63.

[124] See Michael Jackson, *Paths toward a Clearing: Radical Empiricism and Ethnographic Inquiry* (Bloomington: Indiana University Press, 1989), 137–55.

[125] As Synnott shows in "Puzzling over the Senses."

[126] Walter J. Ong, *The Presence of the Word* (New Haven: Yale University Press, 1967), 63, 221.

thought has been ocular.[127] It is hard for us to imagine the world in any other light.[128]

The Hopi do, however. The Hopi think "in sound," as Kathleen Buddle has shown in a recent article called "Sound Vibrations,"[129] which analyses the Hopi Myth of Creation. In the myth, Spider Woman brings the Twins into being by chanting the Song of Creation over them and then commands one of them to "Go about all the world and send out sound so that it may be heard throughout all the land." The Twin goes out, and "all the vibratory centres along the earth's axis from pole to pole resounded his call; the whole earth trembled; the universe quivered in tune. Thus he made the whole world an instrument of sound."[130] It is consistent with Buddle's analysis that there are no "things"—no tables or chairs, to use the standard example of Western philosophers—in the Hopi universe, only vibrations; hence the fact that in the Hopi language one speaks of "tabling," not "a table," and "chairing," not "a chair."[131]

In the Hopi cosmogony the world is created by sound, whereas in the Desana cosmogony the world is created by the light of the sun. The emphasis on light in the latter myth agrees with the great importance the Desana accord to sight. However, in the Desana case, the sense which is most emphasized in creation is not the one most valued in society. Sight is the subject of immense symbolic elaboration in Desana culture, because of its prominent role in creation and perception, but hearing is ultimately of greater importance because of its association with

---

[127] For an intriguing account of French thought in the sixteenth century, when the sensorium appears to have been more balanced and "thoughts existed in a more clouded and less purified atmosphere" than they have since the "Enlightenment," see Lucien Febvre, *The Problem of Unbelief in the Sixteenth Century: The Religion of Rabelais*, trans. B. Gottlieb (Cambridge: Harvard University Press, 1982). According to Febvre (*Problem of Unbelief*, 432) "The sixteenth century did not see first: it heard and smelled, it sniffed the air and caught sounds."

[128] Indeed, we are positively hindered from so doing by the glare of the television screen: "On the television screen, the world, broken down at its source, is reassembled as dots of light, and in this respect the television screen is everyone's personal converter of light back into matter which originally has been decomposed as light." The television screen makes the world "matter as a matter of light," and that is all (Robert D. Romanyshyn, *Technology as Symptom and Dream* [London: Routledge, 1989], 186).

[129] Kathleen Buddle, "Sound Vibrations: An Exploration of the Hopi Sensorium," *Journal of Religion and Culture* 4.2 (1990): 9–19.

[130] Waters quoted by Buddle, "Sound Vibrations," 10.

[131] See further Benjamin Lee Whorf, *Language, Thought and Reality: Selected Writings of Benjamin Lee Whorf*, ed. John B. Carroll (New York: John Wiley; Cambridge: MIT Press, 1956).

comprehension.[132] Thus, the study of cosmogonies can provide a basis for a fuller, more nuanced understanding of the meaning of the senses in society.

Other kinds of myths can be read for information on a culture's sensory priorities in other ways. In many myths from the Massim region of Papua New Guinea, the ancestors of humanity lack mouths or digestive tracts. Food is simply dropped in a hole on top of the head and comes out of the anus still whole. These ancestral beings only become human when their mouths (and genital orifices) are cut or burst open, which normally occurs at the same time they acquire "culture" or rules. Thus, according to Melanesian notions, the sensory order and the social order emerged together, and "orality" is equally central to both. Put simply, "to have a mouth" is to be "civilized the Melanesian way."[133] As Melanesian ethnographer Michael Young observes: "The mouth, from which issues the magic which controls the world and into which goes the food which the world is manipulated to produce, is the principal organ of man's social being, the supremely instrumental orifice and channel for the communication codes of language and food."[134]

A culture's ideal sensory model can sometimes be inferred from the sensory abilities and qualities manifested by its culture heroes. In a Desana myth, for instance, Megadiame, an ant-man, is presented as eating only pure foods, having perfect face paintings, giving off the odour of herbs that induce respect and love, making clear sounds while bathing, and singing and dancing well.[135] In the myths of other cultures, a hero may display one or two outstanding sensory qualities, such as a beautiful appearance, clever speech, or remarkable sexual powers. In the case of a hero who is quick-witted, but has no particular sensory characteristics, one is led to wonder whether this may not be indicative of a certain "desensualization" in the culture concerned. It is not only the direct employment of the senses and sensory stimuli in myths which should be attended to, but also their indirect use or exclusion. For example, a lack of visual description, such as we find in the Hausa "Tale of Daudawar Batso,"[136] implies a corresponding lack of interest in (or repression of) the visual.

Finally, it is essential to consider the means by, and context in which, myths are passed on. Are they read in private or told to a group? If the latter, are they

---

[132] As shown by Classen, "Creation by Sound." Of course, oral communication usually forms an important part of education in our society as well. It is not essential, however, as the existence of "correspondence courses" attests.

[133] Miriam Kahn, *Always Hungry, Never Greedy: Food and the Expression of Gender in a Melanesian Society* (Cambridge: Cambridge University Press, 1986), 171–73.

[134] Michael W. Young, *Magicians of Manumanua: Living Myth in Kalauna* (Berkeley: University of California Press, 1938), 172.

[135] Gerardo Reichel-Dolmatoff, *Amazonian Cosmos: The Sexual and Religious Symbolism of the Tukano Indians* (Chicago: University of Chicago Press, 1971), 267.

[136] Ritchie, "Fusion of the Facilities."

usually told in the dark or in the light? Are they told before meals, during meals, after meals? Are they danced? Sung? Represented in Pictures? What other sensors phenomena accompany their communication? Are the myths understood differently by different groups within society?

9. Cosmology

- How are sensory data used to order the world? Are things classified by their colour, shape, smell, texture, sound, taste?
- What symbolic use is made of the imagery of the senses?
- How are the "soul" and "mind" conceptualized? In which part of the body is the soul or mind thought to reside?
- What are the sensory characteristics of good or evil spirits?
- How are the senses elaborated in the afterlife? Is there a different sensory order from that of earthly life? Are sweet fragrances or good foods emphasized? Is there any sensory deprivation, such as darkness, silence, hunger?

It has often been noted that non-Western cultures classify things by sound to a much greater extent than do Western cultures.[137] Even more pronounced, at least in certain parts, is the classification of things by smell or taste. The Batek Negrito of peninsular Malaysia classify virtually everything in their environment by smell, including the sun and the moon. The sun is said to have a bad smell, "like that of rare meat," while the moon has a good smell, "like that of flowers."[138]

This is not so much a case of the "classificatory urge"[139] gone wild as an index of the centrality of smell in the Batek sensorium. This smell-mindedness also distinguishes the Batek as a people from the other people of the Malay Peninsula (in a manner analogous to the way the differential extension of the senses by means of body decoration functions as a means of cultural differentiation in the Mato Grosso region of Brazil).[140] For example, the neighbouring Chewong also pay close attention to odours. However, unlike the Batek, they have only to be careful that no two different foodstuffs be present *in the stomach* at the same time.[141] The Batek must never so much as cook meat from different species at the

---

[137] Ohnuki-Tierney, *Illness and Healing*; Edward L. Schieffelin, *The Sorrow of the Lonely and the Burning of the Dancers* (New York: St. Martins Press, 1976).

[138] Kirk M. Endicott, *Batek Negrito Religion* (Oxford: Clarendon, 1979), 39.

[139] Claude Lévi-Strauss, *The Savage Mind* (Chicago: University of Chicago Press, 1966).

[140] See Seeger, "Meaning of Body Ornaments."

[141] Signe Howell, *Society and Cosmos: Chewong of Peninsular Malaysia* (Oxford: Oxford University Press, 1984), 231.

same time for fear that the mixing of smells would offend the nostrils of the Thunder deity and bring calamity.[142] Thus, the order of both peoples' universes depends on keeping the categories of creation separate; but whereas in the Batek case the distinctions are expressed primarily in terms of ethereal odours, in the Chewong case the categories are more substantive, having to do with stuffs. The greater substantivism of the Chewong cosmology is perhaps consistent with the heightened visualism of Chewong epistemology, as discussed by Howes.[143]

In the previous section on myths, the importance of examining how a culture thinks "in" or "through" the senses was underlined. To grasp the indigenous epistemology it also helps to study how the culture conceptualizes and localizes the "soul" or "mind" within the body. Not all cultures are agreed in this regard. The ancient Greeks associated the soul with the breath, the Mehinaku of Brazil place the soul in the eye,[144] the Zinacanteco of Mexico, in the blood.[145] In, the West, we think of the mind as residing in the head; the Uduk of the Sudan locate it in the stomach.[146] According to the Aguaruna of the Amazon: "The people who say that we think with our heads are wrong because we think with our hearts. The heart is connected to the veins, which carry the thoughts in the blood through the entire body. The brain is only connected to the spinal column, isn't it? So if we thought with our brains; we would only be able to move the thought as far as our anus?"[147] What different sensory priorities and modes of thinking are produced by these different localizations of being and thought within the body?

A culture's representations of spirits can be a good source of information on its sensory model. In cultures with a pronounced olfactory sensitivity, good spirits are often associated with good odours and evil spirits with bad odours.[148] Care must be taken in analysing such material, however, for a one-to-one correspondence between the sensory profile of spiritual beings, and the sensory order of human beings cannot be assumed. The fact that the chief deity of the Tarahumara of Mexico is blind, for instance, might lead one to think that the Tarahumara do not value sight. On the contrary, sight is of the utmost importance to the Tarahumara, since it enables them to provide the deity with game (which his blindness

---

[142] Endicott, *Batek Negrito Religion*, 74.

[143] Howes, "Sensorial Anthropology."

[144] Thomas Gregor, *Anxious Pleasures: The Sexual Lives of an Amazonian People* (Chicago: University of Chicago Press, 1985), 152.

[145] Carol Karasik, ed., *The People of the Bat: Mayan Tales and Dreams from Zinacantan*, trans. W. Laughlin (Washington: Smithsonian Institution Press, 1988), 5.

[146] Wendy James, *The Listening Ebony: Moral Knowledge, Religion and Power among the Uduk of Sudan* (Oxford: Clarendon, 1988), 69.

[147] Michael Brown, *Tsewa's Gift: Magic and Meaning in an Amazonian Society* (Washington: Smithsonian Institution Press, 1985), 19.

[148] See Griffin, "Ritual of Silent Wishes."

makes him unable to hunt for himself) and thus maintain a harmonious relationship between the supernatural and natural worlds.[149]

The same caveat holds for the analysis of the rote of the senses in the afterlife. Sometimes the imagined sensory gratifications and/or deprivations of the afterlife replicate the ideal sensory model, at others they invert it, while in still other cases the afterlife is simply a projection of what a culture imagines the sensory existence of a corpse or disembodied spirit to be. The Barasana of the Amazon, for instance, consider the world of the dead to be characterized by coldness, hardness, a strong odour, the separation of the sexes, and the consumption of "spiritual" foods, such as coca, beer, and tobacco. To some degree this represents an ideal male sensory order, as men are supposed to be cold and hard. The complete realization of this sensory order, however, occurs only in the context of the male initiation rite. During this rite, initiates must have no contact with fire or women, only tobacco, coca, and beer are consumed, and strong-smelling beeswax is burnt. During ordinary life, the ideal sensory order in fact consists of a combination of hot and cold, regular foods and spiritual foods, and so on.[150]

It is of particular interest to examine representations of the afterlife in relation to the liturgy, or ritual life, of a given community. Sometimes it is possible to detect a sort of balance of opposites between the quality of worship and the vision of the afterlife. We think of the contrast between Islam, on the one hand, and Hinduism, on the other—Islam with its austere worship and sensual heaven, Hinduism with its sensual worship and ultimate transcendence or escape from sensation. Other religions appear to fall in-between these two extremes, such as some of the varieties of Christianity, where earthly liturgy and heavenly bliss mirror each other. Understanding the role of the senses in the afterlife postulated by a culture, therefore, requires first understanding the role of the afterlife in that culture.

BIBLIOGRAPHY

Adams, Charles. "Aurality and Consciousness: Basotho Production of Significance." Pages 303–26 in *Essays in Humanistic Anthropology*. Edited by Bruce T. Grindal and Dennis M. Warren. New York: University Press of America, 1986.

Allan, Frank. "The Influence of the Senses on One Another: Responses of the Organism to Stimulation." Unpublished manuscript. University of Manitoba: Department of Psychology, 1971.

---

[149] John G. Kennedy, *Tarahumara of the Sierra Madre: Beer, Ecology and Social Organization* (Arlington Heights, IL: AHM Press, 1978), 130.

[150] Christine Hugh-Jones, *From the Milk River: Spatial and Temporal Processes in Northwest Amazonia* (Cambridge: Cambridge University Press, 1979); Hugh-Jones, *Palm and the Pleiades*.

Ames, Michael M. *Museums, the Public and Anthropology*. New Delhi: Concept Publishing; Vancouver: University of British Columbia Press, 1985.
Andermann, Lisa. "'The Great Seeing': The Senses in Zinacanteco Ritual Life." Pages 231–38 in *The Varieties of Sensory Experience: A Sourcebook in the Anthropology of the Senses*. Edited by David Howes. Toronto: University of Toronto Press, 1991.
Appadurai, Arjun. "Gastro-politics in Hindu South Asia." *American Ethnologist* 8 (1981): 494–511.
Barth, Fredrik. *Ritual Knowledge among the Baktaman of New Guinea*. New Haven: Yale University Press, 1975.
Basso, Ellen Becker. *A Musical View of the Universe: Kalapalo Myth and Ritual Performance*. Philadelphia: University of Philadelphia Press, 1985.
Baudrillard, Jean. *Simulations*. Translated P. Foss, P. Patton, and P. Beitchman. New York: Semiotext(e), 1983.
Berndt, Ronald M. *Kunapipi*. New York: International Universities Press, 1951.
Berry, John W. *Human Ecology and Cognitive Style: Comparative Studies in Cultural and Psychological Adaptation*. Beverly Hills: Sage, 1976.
———. "Temne and Eskimo Perceptual Skills." *International Journal of Psychology* 1.3 (1966): 207–29.
Berry, John W., Sidney H. Irvine, and Earl B. Hunt, eds. *Indigenous Cognition: Functioning in Cultural Context*. Dordrecht: Nijhoff, 1988.
Biocca, Ettore. *Yanoama*. New York: Dutton, 1970.
Boas, Franz. *Primitive Art*. New York: Dover, 1955.
Brain, Robert. *The Decorated Body*. New York: Harper & Row, 1979.
Briggs, Jean L. *Never in Anger: Portrait of an Eskimo Family*. Cambridge: Harvard University Press, 1970.
Brown, Michael. *Tsewa's Gift: Magic and Meaning in an Amazonian Society*. Washington: Smithsonian Institution Press, 1985.
Buddle, Kathleen. "Sound Vibrations: An Exploration of the Hopi Sensorium." *Journal of Religion and Culture* 4.2 (1990): 9–19.
Calame-Griaule, Geneviève. *Words and the Dogon World*. Translated by D. La Pin. Philadelphia: Institute for the Study of Human Issues, 1986.
Carpenter, Edmund. *Eskimo Realities*. New York: Holt, Rinehart & Winston, 1973.
———. *Oh, What a Blow That Phantom Gave Me!* Toronto: Bantam Books, 1972.
Cesara, Manda. *No Hiding Place: Reflections of a Woman Anthropologist*. New York: Academic Press, 1982.
Chamberlain, Alexander. "Primitive Hearing and Hearing-Words." *American Journal of Psychology* 16 (1905): 119–30.
Clair, Colin. *Of Herbs and Spices*. London: Abelard Schuman, 1961.
Classen, Constance. "Creation by Sound/Creation by Light: A Sensory Analysis of Two South American Cosmologies." Pages 239–55 in *The Varieties of Sensory Experience: A Sourcebook in the Anthropology of the Senses*. Edited by David Howes. Toronto: University of Toronto Press, 1991.
———. *Inca Cosmology and the Human Body*. Salt Lake City: University of Utah Press, 1993.

Corbin, Alain. *The Foul and the Fragrant: Odor and the French Social Imagination.* Translated by M. Kochan, R. Porter, and C. Prendergast. Cambridge: Harvard University Press, 1986.
Daniel, E. Valentine. *Fluid Signs: Being a Person the Tamil Way.* Berkeley: University of California Press, 1984.
———. "The Pulse as an Icon in Siddha Medicine." Pages 100–110 in *The Varieties of Sensory Experience: A Sourcebook in the Anthropology of the Senses.* Edited by David Howes. Toronto: University of Toronto Press, 1991.
Deregowski, Jan B. *Illusions, Patterns and Pictures: A Cross-Cultural Perspective.* New York: Academic Press, 1980.
Douglas, Mary. *Natural Symbols.* New York: Pantheon, 1982.
Dow, James. *The Shaman's Touch: Otomi Indian Symbolic Healing.* Salt Lake City: University of Utah Press, 1986.
Dundes, Alan. "Seeing Is Believing." Pages 86–92 in *Interpreting Folklore.* Bloomington: Indiana University Press, 1980.
Endicott, Kirk M. *Batek Negrito Religion.* Oxford: Clarendon, 1979.
Febvre, Lucien. *The Problem of Unbelief in the Sixteenth Century: The Religion of Rabelais.* Translated by B. Gottlieb. Cambridge: Harvard University Press, 1982.
Feld, Steven. "Sound as a Symbolic System: The Kaluli Drum." Pages 79–99 in *The Varieties of Sensory Experience: A Sourcebook in the Anthropology of the Senses.* Edited by David Howes. Toronto: University of Toronto Press, 1991.
Foucault, Michel. *Discipline and Punish: Birth of the Prison.* Translated by A. Sheridan. New York: Vintage Books, 1979.
Frake, Charles. "Did Literacy Cause the Great Cognitive Divide?" *American Ethnologist* 10 (1983): 368–71.
Gardner, Howard. *Frames of Mind: The Theory of Multiple Intelligences.* New York: Basic Books, 1983.
Gebhart-Sayer, Angelika. "The Geometric Designs of the Shipibo-Conibo in Ritual Context." *Journal of Latin American Lore* 11.2 (1985): 143–75.
Genders, Roy. *A History of Scent.* London: Hamish Hamilton, 1972.
Gill, Sam D. *Native American Religious Action: A Performative Approach.* Columbia: University of South Carolina Press, 1987.
González Holquín, Diego. *Vocabulario de la lengua general de todo el Perú llamada lengua quichua.* Lima: Universidad Nacional Mayor de San Marcos, 1952.
Gregor, Thomas. *Anxious Pleasures: The Sexual Lives of an Amazonian People.* Chicago: University of Chicago Press, 1985.
———. *Mehinaku.* Chicago: University of Chicago Press, 1977.
Griffin, Kit. "The Ritual of Silent Wishes: Notes on the Moroccan Sensorium." Pages 210–20 in *The Varieties of Sensory Experience: A Sourcebook in the Anthropology of the Senses.* Edited by David Howes. Toronto: University of Toronto Press, 1991.
Hall, Edward T. *Beyond Culture.* New York: Anchor Books, 1977.
Howell, Signe. *Society and Cosmos: Chewong of Peninsular Malaysia.* Oxford: Oxford University Press, 1984.
Howes, David. "Beyond Textualism and Hermeneutics in Cultural and Religious Studies." *Journal of Religion and Culture* 4.2 (1990): 1–8.

———. "Introduction: 'To Summon All the Senses.'" Pages 3–21 in *The Varieties of Sensory Experience: A Sourcebook in the Anthropology of the Senses*. Edited by David Howes. Toronto: University of Toronto Press, 1991.

———. "Le sens sans parole: Vers une anthropologie de l'odorat." *Anthropologie et Sociétés* 10.3 (1986): 29–46.

———. "On the Odour of the Soul: Spatial Representation and Olfactory Classification in Eastern Indonesia and Western Melanesia." *Bijdragen tot de Taal-, Land- en Volkenkunde* 144 (1988): 84–113.

———. "Scent and Sensibility." *Culture, Medicine and Psychiatry* 13 (1989): 121–29.

———. "Sensorial Anthropology." Pages 167–91 in *The Varieties of Sensory Experience: A Sourcebook in the Anthropology of the Senses*. Edited by David Howes. Toronto: University of Toronto Press, 1991.

Howes, David, and Constance Classen. "Sounding Sensory Profiles." Pages 257–88 in *The Varieties of Sensory Experience: A Sourcebook in the Anthropology of the Senses*. Edited by David Howes. Toronto: University of Toronto Press, 1991.

Hugh-Jones, Christine. *From the Milk River: Spatial and Temporal Processes in Northwest Amazonia*. Cambridge: Cambridge University Press, 1979.

Hugh-Jones, Stephen. *The Palm and the Pleiades: Initiation and Cosmology in Northwest Amazonia*. Cambridge: Cambridge University Press, 1979.

Ihde, Don. *Listening and Voice: A Phenomenology of Sound*. Athens: Ohio University Press, 1976.

Jackson, Michael. *Paths toward a Clearing: Radical Empiricism and Ethnographic Inquiry*. Bloomington: Indiana University Press, 1989.

James, Wendy. *The Listening Ebony: Moral Knowledge, Religion and Power among the Uduk of Sudan*. Oxford: Clarendon, 1988.

James, William. *Psychology: The Briefer Course*. New York: Harper, 1961.

Joyce, James. *The Portable James Joyce*. Introduced by H. Levin. New York: Viking Press, 1946.

Kahn, Miriam. *Always Hungry, Never Greedy: Food and the Expression of Gender in a Melanesian Society*. Cambridge: Cambridge University Press, 1986.

Karasik, Carol, ed. *The People of the Bat: Mayan Tales and Dreams from Zinacantan*. Translated by W. Laughlin. Washington: Smithsonian Institution Press, 1988.

Kennedy, John G. *Tarahumara of the Sierra Madre: Beer, Ecology and Social Organization*. Arlington Heights, IL: AHM Press, 1978.

Knauft, Bruce M. *Good Company and Violence: Sorcery and Social Action in a Lowland New Guinea Society*. Berkeley: University of California Press, 1985.

Kondo, Dorinne. "The Way of Tea: A Symbolic Analysis." *Man* 20 (1983): 287–306.

Kuipers, Joel C. "Matters of Taste in Wajéwa." Pages 111–27 in *The Varieties of Sensory Experience: A Sourcebook in the Anthropology of the Senses*. Edited by David Howes. Toronto: University of Toronto Press, 1991.

Leach, Edmund. *Culture and Communication*. Cambridge: Cambridge University Press, 1976.

Leenhardt, Maurice. *Do Kamo: Person and Myth in the Melanesian World*. Translated by B. Miller Gulati. Chicago: University of Chicago Press, 1979.

Lévi Strauss, Claude. *The Raw and the Cooked: Introduction to a Science of Mythology*. Translated by J. and D. Weightman. Vol. 1. New York: Harper & Row, 1969.

———. *The Savage Mind*. Chicago: University of Chicago Press, 1966.
Lewis, Gilbert. *Knowledge of Illness in a Sepik Society: A Study of the Gnau, New Guinea*. London: Athlone Press; Atlantic Highlands, NJ: Humanities Press, 1975.
Little, Kenneth. "On Safari: The Visual Politics of a Tourist Representation." Pages 148–63 in *The Varieties of Sensory Experience: A Sourcebook in the Anthropology of the Senses*. Edited by David Howes. Toronto: University of Toronto Press, 1991.
López Austin, Alfredo. *The Human Body and Ideology: Concepts of the Ancient Nahuas*. Vol. 1. Salt Lake City: University of Utah Press, 1988.
Mackenzie Brown, Cheever. "Purana as Scripture: From Sound to Image of the Holy Word in the Hindu Tradition." *History of Religions* 26.1 (1986): 69–86.
Marks, Lawrence. *The Unity of Senses: Interrelations among the Modalities*. New York: Academic Press, 1982.
Meigs, Anna Stokes. *Food, Sex and Pollution: A New Guinea Religion*. New Brunswick: Rutgers University Press, 1984.
Merleau-Ponty, Maurice. *Phenomenology of Perception*. London: Routledge and Kegan Paul, 1962.
Métraux, Rhoda. "Resonance in Imagery." Pages 343–62 in *The Study of Culture at a Distance*. Edited by Margaret Mead and Rhoda Métraux. Chicago: University of Chicago Press, 1953.
Montagu, Ashley. *Touching: The Human Significance of the Skin*. 2nd ed. New York: Harper & Row, 1978.
Morgan, John, and Peter Welton. *See What I Mean: An Introduction to Visual Communication*. New York: Edward Arnold, 1986.
Munn, Nancy D. *The Fame of Gawa: A Symbolic Study of Value Transformation in a Massim (Papua New Guinea) Society*. New York: Cambridge University Press, 1986.
Ohnuki-Tierney, Emiko. *Illness and Healing among the Sakhalin Ainu*. Cambridge: Cambridge University Press, 1981.
Ong, Walter J. *Orality and Literacy*. New York: Methuen, 1982.
———. *The Presence of the Word*. New Haven: Yale University Press, 1967.
Patnaik, Naveen. *A Second Paradise: Indian Courtly Life, 1590–1947*. London: Sidgwick & Jackson, 1985.
Paulson, William. *Enlightenment, Romanticism and the Blind in France*. Princeton: Princeton University Press, 1987.
Pinard, Sylvain. "A Taste of India: On the Role of Gustation in the Hindu Sensorium." Pages 221–30 in *The Varieties of Sensory Experience: A Sourcebook in the Anthropology of the Senses*. Edited by David Howes. Toronto: University of Toronto Press, 1991.
———. "L'Economie des sens en Inde: Exploration des thèses de Walter Ong." *Anthropologica* 32.1 (1990): 75–99.
Porteous, J. Douglas. *Landscapes of the Mind: Worlds of Sense and Metaphor*. Toronto: University of Toronto Press, 1990.
Rawlinson, Andrew. "Yoga Psychology." Pages 247–63 in *Indigenous Psychologies: The Anthropology of the Self*. Edited by Paul Heelas and Andrew Lock. London: Academic Press, 1981.
Reichel-Dolmatoff, Gerardo. *Amazonian Cosmos: The Sexual and Religious Symbolism of the Tukano Indians*. Chicago: University of Chicago Press, 1971.

———. *Basketry as Metaphor: Arts and Crafts of the Desana Indians of the Northwest Amazon*. Occasional Papers of the Museum of Cultural History. Los Angeles: University of California, 1985.

———. *Beyond the Milky Way: Hallucinatory Images of the Tukano Indians*. Los Angeles: UCLA Latin American Center Publications, 1978.

———. "The Cultural Context of an Aboriginal Hallucinogen: Banisteriopsiscaapi," Pages 84–113 in *Flesh of the Gods: The Ritual Use of Hallucinogens*. Edited by Peter T. Furst. New York: Praeger, 1972.

———. "Funerary Customs and Religious Symbolism among the Kogi." Pages 289–301 in *Native South Americans*. Edited by Patricia J. Lyon. Boston: Little, Brown, 1974.

———. "Tapir Avoidance in the Colombian Northwest Amazon." Pages 104–43 in *Animal Myths and Metaphors*. Edited by Gary Urton. Salt Lake City: University of Utah Press, 1985.

Ritchie, Ian. "Fusion of the Facilities: A Study of the Language of the Senses in Hausaland." Pages 192–202 in *The Varieties of Sensory Experience: A Sourcebook in the Anthropology of the Senses*. Edited by David Howes. Toronto: University of Toronto Press, 1991.

Rivlin, Robert, and Karen Gravelle, *Deciphering the Senses: The Expanding World of Human Perception*. New York: Simon & Schuster, 1984.

Romanyshyn, Robert D. *Technology as Symptom and Dream*. London: Routledge, 1989.

Sacks, Oliver W. *The Man Who Mistook His Wife for a Hat and Other Clinical Tales*. New York: Harper & Row, 1985.

———. *Seeing Voices: A Journey into the World of the Deaf*. Berkeley: University of California Press, 1989.

Schafer, R. Murray. *The Tuning of the World*. New York: Knopf, 1977.

Schieffelin, Edward L. *The Sorrow of the Lonely and the Burning of the Dancers*. New York: St. Martins Press, 1976.

Scribner, Sylvia, and Michael Cole. *The Psychology of Literacy*, Cambridge: Harvard University Press, 1981.

Seeger, Anthony. "The Meaning of Body Ornaments." *Ethnology* 14.3 (1975): 211–24.

———. *Nature and Society in Central Brazil: The Suya Indians of Mato Grosso*. Cambridge: Harvard University Press, 1981.

———. *Why Suya Sing: A Musical Anthropology of an Amazonian People*. Cambridge: Cambridge University Press, 1987.

Segal, Marshall H., Donald T. Campbell, and Melville J. Herskovits. *The Influence of Culture on Visual Perception*. Chicago: Bobbs-Merrill, 1966.

Sharon, Douglas. *Wizard of the Four Winds: A Shaman's Story*. New York: Free Press, 1978.

Siskind, Janet. *To Hunt in the Morning*. New York: Oxford University Press, 1973.

Stallybrass, Peter, and Allon White. *The Politics and Poetics of Transgression*. Ithaca: Cornell University Press, 1986.

Stoller, Paul, and Cheryl Olkes. "La Sauce épaisse: Remarques sur les relations sociales songhaïs." *Anthropologie et Sociétés* 14.2 (1990): 57–76.

Stone, Ruth. *Let the Inside Be Sweet: The Interpretation of Music Event among the Kpelle of Liberia*. Bloomington: Indiana University Press, 1986.

Synnott, Anthony. "Puzzling over the Senses: From Plato to Marx." Pages 61–76 in *The Varieties of Sensory Experience: A Sourcebook in the Anthropology of the Senses.* Edited by David Howes. Toronto: University of Toronto Press, 1991.

———. "Truth and Goodness, Mirrors and Masks: A Sociology of Beauty and the Face, Part I." *British Journal of Sociology* 39.4 (1989): 607–36.

———. "Truth and Goodness, Mirrors and Masks: A Sociology of Beauty and the Face, Part II." *British Journal of Sociology* 40.1 (1990): 55–76.

Tedlock, Barbara. *Time and the Highland Maya.* Albuquerque: University of New Mexico Press, 1982.

Warner, William Lloyd. *A Black Civilization: A Study of an Australian Tribe.* New York: Harper & Row, 1958.

Whorf, Benjamin Lee. *Language, Thought and Reality: Selected Writings of Benjamin Lee Whorf.* Edited by John B. Carroll. New York: John Wiley; Cambridge: MIT Press, 1956.

Wilbert, Werner. "The Pneumatic Theory of Female Warao Herbalists." *Social Sciences and Medicine* 25.10 (1987): 1139–46.

Witherspoon, Gary. *Language and Art in the Navajo Universe.* Ann Arbor: University of Michigan Press, 1977.

Wober, J. Mallory. *Psychology in Africa.* London: International African Institute, 1975.

———. "The Sensotype Hypothesis." Pages 31–42 in *The Varieties of Sensory Experience: A Sourcebook in the Anthropology of the Senses.* Edited by David Howes. Toronto: University of Toronto Press, 1991.

Young, Michael W. *Magicians of Manumanua: Living Myth in Kalauna.* Berkeley: University of California Press, 1938.

Zubek, John, ed. *Sensory Deprivation: Fifteen Years of Research.* New York: Appleton-Century-Crofts, 1969.

RESOUNDING SENSORY PROFILES: SENSORY STUDIES METHODOLOGIES

David Howes

I feel deeply honored that Annette Schellenberg and Thomas Krüger chose to call this book *Sounding Sensory Profiles*, and asked to reprint the chapter by the same name from *The Varieties of Sensory Experience*.[1] That chapter, which I wrote together with Constance Classen, set out a methodology for the practice of the anthropology of the senses or "sensory ethnography" involving fieldwork and for the history of the senses, or sensory history, involving bibliographic or archival research.

"Participant sensation" is the hallmark of sensory ethnography. It differs from "participant observation," the standard anthropological methodology, by virtue of its emphasis on sensing along with one's informants, and relinquishing the status of the observer. The French anthropologist François Laplantine sums up this approach nicely when he writes, in *The Life of the Senses*:

> The experience of fieldwork is an experience of sharing in the sensible [*partage du sensible*]. We observe, we listen, we speak with others, we partake of their cuisine, we try to feel along with them what they experience.[2]

The hallmark of sensory history, on the other hand, is "sensing between the lines"—as opposed to merely "reading between the lines"—of historical sources. There is no finer practitioner of this art than my coauthor, Constance Classen,

---

This essay is a product of an ongoing program of research sponsored by the Social Sciences and Humanities Research Council of Canada and the Fonds de Recherche du Québec—Société et Culture.

[1] David Howes, ed., *The Varieties of Sensory Experience: A Sourcebook in the Anthropology the Senses* (Toronto: University of Toronto Press, 1991).

[2] François Laplantine, *The Life of the Senses: Toward a Modal Anthropology* (London: Bloomsbury, 2015), 2.

whose many books all attest to her highly refined capacity to summon up the sensory worlds of past societies.[3] This is actually history as Johan Huizinga, the founder of cultural history, conceived it: the historian should give us the "historical sensation" of a period, he suggested.[4]

Sensory ethnography or sensory anthropology (the terms are used interchangeably) has evolved dramatically since we first attempted to articulate a framework for its practice. Antonius C. G. M. Robben and Jeffrey A. Slukka dedicate a whole section of *Ethnographic Fieldwork*, which is a bible for many anthropologists, to what they call "sensorial fieldwork,"[5] and the term "sensory ethnography" has come to cover a wide spectrum of research and communication practices. For example, it figures in the name of an ethnographic film lab at Harvard University directed by Lucien Castaing-Taylor, which is committed to expanding the frontiers of media anthropology. It appears in the title of a manual of fieldwork practice by Sarah Pink,[6] which advocates intensive use of audiovisual media but also acknowledges the usefulness of the unaided senses. It applies to Kathryn Geurts's in-depth ethnographic study of the enculturation of the senses among the Anlo-Ewe of Ghana, and it is very much in evidence in the collection, edited by Denielle Elliott and Dara Culhane.[7] The latter book contains chapters on "Sensing," "Recording and Editing" (i.e., using film and audio recordings), "Walking," and "Performing" (i.e., staging one's own and/or other cultures), as well as "Writing."

As reflected in *A Different Kind of Ethnography*, the space and the attention devoted to writing has shrunk substantially since the onset of "the sensory turn" in anthropology in the early 1990s. In the preceding decade, the focus was squarely on issues of "representation" and writing (with only scant attention paid

---

[3] See Constance Classen, *The Color of Angels: Cosmology, Gender and the Aesthetic Imagination* (London: Routledge, 1998); Classen, *The Deepest Sense: A Cultural History of Touch*, Studies in Sensory History (Urbana: University of Illinois Press, 2012); Classen, *The Museum of the Senses: Experiencing Art and Collections*, Sensory Study Series (New York: Bloomsbury Academic, 2017).

[4] See Frank Ankersmit, "Huizinga on Historical Experience," in *History and Sociology*, vol. 2 of *Senses and Sensation: Critical and Primary Sources*, ed. David Howes (London: Bloomsbury, 2018), 23–38.

[5] Antonius C. G. M. Robben and Jeffrey A. Sluka, eds., *Ethnographic Fieldwork: An Anthropological Reader* (Oxford: Blackwell: 2007), 441–510.

[6] Sarah Pink, *Doing Sensory Ethnography* (Los Angeles: SAGE, 2009).

[7] Kathryn Linn Geurts, *Culture and the Senses: Bodily Ways of Knowing in an African Community*, Ethnographic Studies in Subjectivity 3 (Berkeley: University of California Press, 2002); Denielle Elliott and Dara Culhane, eds., *A Different Kind of Ethnography: Imaginative Practices and Creative Methodologies* (Toronto: University of Toronto Press, 2017).

to perception or sensing). *Writing Culture: The Politics and Poetics of Ethnography* occupied the whole of anthropology,[8] and having an "experimental style" of writing was all important. But the standards of ethnography have changed. "Authority" is no longer the central preoccupation it was in the 1980s. Good ethnography is increasingly seen as going beyond representation and beyond poetics to engage with culturally mediated sensory experiences and modes of expression.[9]

In what follows, I would like to sketch some of the intellectual context to the invention of the construct of the "sensory profile" of a culture and then offer a reading—or rather sensing—of Thorleif Boman's classic study, *Hebrew Thought Compared with Greek*.[10] The ancient Hebrew tradition is of interest because here we have a so-called Religion of the Book, yet the characteristics of the Hebrew sensorium defy interpretation in terms of standard Western theories of the impact of the technology of writing on modes of thought and expression.

I

What set me off on the path of the senses was attending a lecture by Marshall McLuhan in the Senior Common Room of Trinity College in 1979. At the time, I was an undergraduate student in anthropology at the University of Toronto. McLuhan was then working on the book that became *Laws of Media*, written together with Eric McLuhan.[11] He famously argued that media should be seen as "extensions of the senses." Each new medium (e.g., writing relative to speech, or print relative to writing) alters the ratio or balance of the senses and impacts not only the sensory order but the social order and rationality of a culture, too. Thus, the adoption of writing and *a fortiori* the printing press brought about the "substitution of an eye for an ear" and promoted linearity, objectivity, and (individual) point of view as dominant modes of thought.

---

[8] James Clifford and George E. Marcus, eds., *Writing Culture: The Politics and Poetics of Ethnography* (Berkeley: University of California Press, 1986).

[9] See Paul Stoller, *Sensuous Scholarship*, Contemporary Ethnography (Philadelphia: University of Pennsylvania Press, 1997); Michael Herzfeld, *Anthropology: Theoretical Practice in Culture and Society* (Oxford: Blackwell, 2000), 240–54; David Howes, *Sensual Relations: Engaging the Senses in Culture and Social Theory* (Ann Arbor: University of Michigan Press, 2003); David Howes and Constance Classen, *Ways of Sensing: Understanding the Senses in Society* (London: Routledge, 2014); and, especially, Rupert Cox, Andrew Irving, and Chris Wright, eds., *Beyond Text? Critical Practices and Sensory Anthropology* (Manchester: Manchester University Press, 2016).

[10] Thorleif Boman, *Hebrew Thought Compared with Greek* (New York: Norton, 1970).

[11] Marshall McLuhan and Eric McLuhan, *Laws of Media: The New Science* (Toronto: University of Toronto Press, 1988).

Another influence was the image of the sensory homunculus inspired by the neurosurgeon Wilder Penfield's research into the representation of the body on the brain. The image of the sensory homunculus provided a means of visualizing McLuhan's notion of the ever-shifting ratio of the senses. The cortical magnification of some body parts and constriction of others was very suggestive (see fig. 1. The Sensory Homunculus). One could readily imagine the proportional representation of the different sense organs changing as one went from the study of one culture, say an oral culture, to another, say a print culture, or an electronic culture.[12]

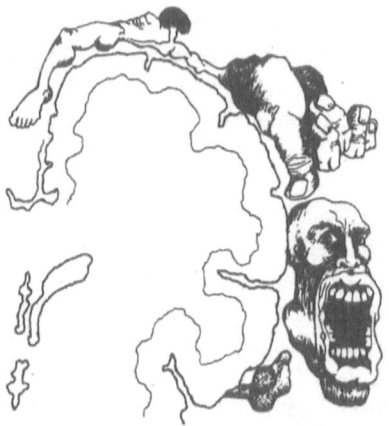

Fig. 1. The Sensory Homunculus (after Wilder Penfield and Theodore Rasmussen, *The Cerebral Cortex of Man: A Study of Localization of Function* [New York: Macmillan, 1950], 119).

Consideration of the work of the cross-cultural psychologist Mallory Wober added a further dimension to the developing notion of the sensory profile—the dimension of practice. Wober elaborated what he called the "sensotype hypothesis" to explain why it was that British subjects performed better on tasks involving visual discrimination than West African subjects (e.g., Witkins's Embedded Figures Test), while West African subjects performed better on tests requiring proprioceptive discrimination than their British counterparts (e.g., the Rod-and-Frame Test). Wober's hypothesis was indebted to McLuhan's theory of the mediated sensorium. It held that sensory acuity or "analytic functioning" varies with the dominant medium of communication, whether speech or writing, orality or

---

[12] By way of analogy, see Carl Zimmer on the sensory maps of moles in "Mouseunculus: How the Brain Draws a Little You," *Phenomena: A Science Salon*, 24 July 2013, https://tinyurl.com/SBL2827a.

literacy. But it also highlighted the sense in which perception is a practice or skill: that is, Wober's hypothesis directed attention to the *exercise* of the senses and not simply their extension via diverse media. Thus, he suggested that the differential performance of West African subjects was due not only to the absence of writing but, more positively, to "an elaboration of the proprioceptively and aurally perceived world. Thus, music is an extension of speech, rhythm an extension of movement, beauty a function of grace of movement as much as of configuration of visage, and dance is a regular and favoured form of elaboration of activity, started at an early age."[13]

Further research revealed that, contrary to McLuhan's great divide theory of mentalities, which turned on the distinction between oral and literate culture, there is as much sensory diversity among societies that may be classified as "oral" as there is between oral cultures and literate cultures. This point was brought home to me in the course of my field research in Papua New Guinea in 1990. This research involved a comparative study of the sensory orders of two (so-called) oral cultures. The culture of the coastal Massim region was decidedly ear-minded and confirmed McLuhan's predictions, but the culture of the Middle Sepik River region was surprisingly eye-minded. Thus, among the Kwoma of the Middle Sepik, it was the visual aspects of society and the cosmos that figured foremost. The visual culture of the Kwoma, which consisted of sculptures and bark paintings of spirits, was highly elaborated compared to the relative dearth of visual representation in the Massim world. Also of significance: among the Kwoma, social status was dependent on visual revelation whereas at Budoya, in the Massim region, the most important status marker was to have a name that was spoken far and wide and resounded like thunder.[14]

Perhaps the greatest difficulty facing the scholar desirous of studying the life of the senses across cultures stems from all the assumptions regarding the "nature" of the senses embedded in conventional Western constructions of the sensorium, such as the distinction between proximity and distance senses, or the idea of sight being active and hearing passive, or the notion of some senses being more "emotional" or "subjective" than others. The first task of the anthropology of the senses is to clear the mind of all such assumptions and redirect attention to finding out how the senses are constructed and lived locally, in the culture one studies. For example, while visuality is normally associated with rationality and objectivity in Western culture, in other cultures visuality is suspect (e.g., the widespread belief in the evil eye), and tactility, which occupies the lowest rung in the conventional

---

[13] Mallory Wober, "The Sensotype Hypothesis," in Howes, *Varieties of Sensory Experience*, 33.

[14] Howes, *Sensual Relations*, 81–85. There are various initiatory grades in Kwoma society, which are marked by the degree to which an initiate is permitted to see the tribal sacra.

Western hierarchy of the senses and is subject to heavy restriction, is instead regarded as the most sociable of the senses, to be cultivated instead of repressed. Furthermore, in many non-Western cultures, touch is held to operate at a distance. It is not the proximity sense it is supposed to be in the West.[15]

The preceding litany of considerations led Classen and I to insist on the necessity of pluralizing the range of cultural domains to be examined in the effort to arrive at a composite understanding of a given society's sensory model. These other domains, besides communications technology, include childrearing practices (the socialization of the senses), linguistics (the language of the senses), ritual life (the celebration of the senses), aesthetic sensibilities (the full gamut of artistic forms and practices, and not merely the visual arts), and the natural and built environment or "sensescape."

II

Anthropologists can depend on the deliverances of their own senses when studying the sensory profile of a culture and may also put questions to their informants—the answers to which will shed additional light on how the senses are constructed and lived locally. Historians, by contrast, have to rely on written sources. This is problematic, for much happens in any society that is not talked about or written down, either because it is suppressed or taken for granted or because language is not considered the proper medium for its expression. Furthermore, when primary sources are translated there is often the problem that the material gets re-written according to the sensory and social biases of the translator's own time and culture. Translations of the Bible presents many examples of elisions of this sort. For example, the passage in Isa 11, which originally stated that the messiah would judge people by smell, is stripped of any olfactory reference in modern translations in order to cater to an odor-denying contemporary public.[16] The historian may nevertheless gain insights into the unvoiced and unwritten or manage to see through a translator's bowdlerizations, by examining other material, such as outsiders' accounts (e.g., travel writings often make note of practices left undescribed in local accounts), or by studying the material culture of a period (e.g., the artifacts contained in museum collections), or by inferring

---

[15] David Howes, "Afterword: The Skinscape; Reflections on the Dermalogical Turn," *Body and Society* 24.1–2 (2018): 225–39.

[16] Ian Ritchie, "The Nose Knows: Bodily Knowing in Isaiah 11:3," *JSOT* 87 (2000): 59–73; Susan Ashbrook Harvey, *Scenting Salvation: Ancient Christianity and the Olfactory Imagination* (Berkeley: University of California Press, 2006).

the nonvisual sensations of a period from a careful, sensorially mined consideration of the objects depicted in contemporary paintings.[17]

Apart from the challenge of translation, the historian of the senses must contend with the equally pernicious problem of working around or perceiving through the ingrained biases of the historical actors who "bequeath" their writings to history. in "Histoire et anthropologie sensorielle," Alain Corbin warned of the dangers of "confusing the reality of the employment of the senses and the picture of this employment decreed by observers."[18] This observation underscores the necessity of paying close attention to what could be called intracultural sensory diversity—that is, the sense experience of subaltern classes, genders, and ethnicities. This can only be surmised by sensing between the lines of written sources. Classen has addressed this issue across a number of publications. In "The Senses," she writes:

> The sensory values propagated by the dominant social group are often internalized to a greater or lesser extent by all groups within a society. For example, members of the working classes will come to believe that, no matter how much they wash or what perfumes they use, they are somehow not as clean or as fragrant as members of the upper classes. Members of marginalized groups may challenge such sensory values, however, and propose alternative schemes whereby "clean-living" workers are contrasted with the "filthy" rich.[19]

Thus, it should never be assumed that a culture is reducible to a single sensory profile. Different groups within society may well value the senses differently from the dominant group and also use their senses differently.[20] The senses are made, not given, and therefore susceptible to contestation.

In my writings, I have consistently advocated for the adoption of a comparative approach to the study of sensibilities. One fine (if controversial) example of the deployment of the comparative method, and one which exercised a profound influence over my earliest writings on the senses, is Boman's *Hebrew Thought Compared with Greek*.[21] In this comparative study of the Semitic and Greek worldviews, Boman sought to elucidate the implications of the Hebrew and Greek languages for how people conceptualized and represented the world. In other words, he was interested in excavating "the sensory underpinnings of thought" in

---

[17] See Richard Leppert, *The Sight of Sound: Music, Representation and the History of the Body* (Berkeley: University of California Press, 1995), as regards musical instruments.

[18] Quoted in David Howes, "Introduction: On the History and Sociology of the Senses," in Howes, *History and Sociology*, 2.

[19] Constance Classen, "The Senses," in *Encyclopedia of European Social History from 1350 to 2000*, ed. Peter N. Stearns (New York: Scribner's Sons, 2001), 4:356–57.

[20] See Howes and Classen, *Ways of Sensing*, 65–92.

[21] For bibliographical references, see note 10.

the two cultures, as mediated by their respective languages.²² Boman noted that it is "astounding how far clear thinking depended for the Greeks upon the visual faculty" as exemplified by Euclid's geometry, Plato's doctrine of Ideas, and *theoria* (or theorizing) as a kind of "viewing," not to mention the institution of Greek theater.²³ Following Bruno Snell, Boman proclaims that the Greeks were "men of eyes" (*Augenmenschen*). "Quite as decided," he continues, "is the emphasis upon the significance of hearing and the word in its being spoken" in the Hebrew tradition. "Hear, O Israel" is the clarion call of the Hebrew tradition, and there is the well-known prohibition on graven images, which could be taken to suggest that vision is arrested in the Hebrew tradition. But Boman does not even make much of the latter point. Instead he points to evidence like the following: "True being for the Hebrews is the 'word', *dabhar*, which comprises all Hebrew realities: word, deed, and concrete object."²⁴ What is more, the word has "dynamic force" (i.e., it is not merely an expression of thought).²⁵ God calls or speaks the world into existence, and words, on account of their "dynamic force," impact the world. They do not simply represent it. Indeed, according to Boman, the Hebrew language is performative, or enactive, in orientation, rather than descriptive:

> In the entire Old Testament we do not find a single description of an objective "photographic" appearance.... Noah's ark is discussed in detail in Gen. 6.14 ff (P): "Make an ark of gopher wood; you shall make it with large rooms and caulk it inside and out with pitch.... Make a roof above for the ark ... and set the door of the ark in its side" ...
>
> It is striking in this description that it is not the appearance of the ark that is described but its construction. What interests the Israelite ... is how the ark was built and made.... It is impossible for us to form an intelligible image of the ark.²⁶

According to Boman, the radical antinomy between Greek and Hebrew thought is further manifest in contrasting conceptions of truth. For the Greeks, truth consisted in "that which is unveiled, ... that which is to be seen clearly" (objective, impersonal), whereas for the Israelites truth is "the completely certain, sure, steady, faithful" (subjective). On Boman's account, then, a penchant for logical thinking and a static worldview follow from the privileging of sight. By contrast, a stress on hearing leads to a "psychological understanding" of truth and a dynamic worldview or epistemology "directed towards events, living, history."²⁷

---

[22] Lucien Febvre, *The Problem of Unbelief in the Sixteenth Century: The Religion of Rabelais* (Cambridge, MA: Harvard University Press, 1982), 436.
[23] Boman, *Hebrew Thought Compared with Greek*, 200.
[24] Boman, *Hebrew Thought Compared with Greek*, 56.
[25] Boman, *Hebrew Thought Compared with Greek*, 58.
[26] Boman, *Hebrew Thought Compared with Greek*, 74–75.
[27] Boman, *Hebrew Thought Compared with Greek*, 202.

As a heuristic device, the "men of eyes" (Greek) versus "men of ears" (Hebrew) distinction evidently has great interpretive power. Boman's comparative approach throws many aspects of the two cultures into relief and facilitates their comprehension. But there are problems with his interpretation. The first is that his account obfuscates the issue of how Greek or Hebrew *women* may have perceived the world differently from Greek or Hebrew *men*. In other words, he does not pay sufficient attention to the issue of intracultural diversity.

A further problem with Boman's account is that it overemphasizes cross- or intercultural diversity. This is, in fact, a persistent problem with the comparative method—the tendency to polarize or dichotomize. James Barr called out Boman on this point in his influential critique of *Hebrew Thought Compared with Greek*,[28] and the debate over whether hearing or sight is the dominant sense in biblical epistemology has continued down to the present.

Yael Avrahami takes up this debate and recasts it in a number of highly illuminating ways.[29] The first thing to note is that her approach is thoroughly grounded in the anthropology of the senses. Her review of the tenets of sensory anthropology in the first chapter of *The Senses of Scripture* is, indeed, exemplary. Following from this propitious start, Avrahami takes "the 'sensorium' … as a cultural category" as her point of departure, instead of assuming a five-sense, "pentasensory" model. This led her to discover that the Israelites actually entertained a "septasensory" model of the sensorium, a model that included kinaesthesia (walking) and speech in addition to the canonical five senses.[30] Furthermore, she professes to have found "no evidence of a structural hierarchy of the senses": all of the senses are divine, or as she puts it "the sensorium is a divine creation."[31] This can be inferred from the mocking description of the sensory disability of idols, whose sense organs are fashioned by human hands. It is also evidenced by such affirmative pronouncements as "The hearing ear and the seeing eye—the Lord has made them both" (Prov 20:12).

Parenthetically, we find the same heterarchy, as it were, to the different interpretations of the scriptures that have congealed over time. The ostensible contradictions between the interpretations of the torah in different traditions within Judaism are not considered contradictory, because all are deemed to have been intended by God, the "Perfect Author." "These and these are equally law,"

---

[28] James Barr, *The Semantics of Biblical Language* (Oxford: Oxford University Press, 1961).
[29] Yael Avrahami, *The Senses of Scripture: Sensory Perception in the Hebrew Bible*, LHBOTS 545 (London: T&T Clark, 2012).
[30] On some accounts, the genitals and the heart are also numbered among the senses.
[31] Avrahami, *Senses of Scripture*, 225, 191. Nevertheless, some senses are more divine, or are invoked in more rhetorical contexts, than others: most notably sight, hearing, kinaesthesia, and speech (see 278).

as the saying goes. This "interstitial rationality," as the great comparative law scholar H. P. Glenn calls it, is attributable to the fact that the Hebrew tradition did not internalize the logic of writing but instead used writing as the means to continue a conversation without end.[32]

Avrahami's concluding chapter is dedicated to demonstrating the "centrality of sight" in the Hebrew Bible, which comes as a blow to those who argue for the supremacy of hearing. Her point, however, is that it is the very notion of a hierarchy of the senses, a Greek invention, that is the problem here. A hierarchy of the senses cannot be extended from the Hellenic to the Hebrew tradition without distorting the latter. Better to think in terms of heterarchy and focus on the "associative patterns" that are suggested by how the language of the senses is used in specific contexts, she argues. At the same time, Avrahami warns that "those who champion the superiority of sight claim[ing] it is a biological fact, which is only mirrored in the culture reflected in the biblical text," should not be so smug.[33] Seeing is a divine act, not simply a biological fact, as its narrativization, or metaphorical *construction*, throughout the Hebrew Bible attests. To suppose otherwise, to suppose that there can be a "natural history" of the senses, is a nonstarter. The senses are made, not given.

The emphasis on narration over biology or nature is one of the great strengths of Avrahami's account. Arguably, however, it can also be seen as a weakness because it deflects attention from enaction, the performance of sensation, due to its fixation on linguification. It is this idea of enaction that Classen and I have been trying to get at with the notion of "ways of sensing."[34] The latter notion shifts the focus of attention from text to technique and from sensory organ to sensory practice. It includes linguistic practice, but is not limited to it the way Avrahami considers herself to be limited to "go[ing] through language"—that is, to adducing linguistic evidence in support of all her propositions—given that language is "the major native data available," in her words.[35] Language can, however, always be supplemented by attending to the other sensory domains of a culture.

BIBLIOGRAPHY

Ankersmit, Frank. "Huizinga on Historical Experience." Pages 23–38 in *History and Sociology*. Vol. 2 of *Senses and Sensation: Critical and Primary Sources*. Edited by David Howes. London: Bloomsbury, 2018.

---

[32] See H. Patrick Glenn, *Legal Traditions of the World: Sustainable Diversity in Law*, 5th ed. (Oxford: Oxford University Press, 2014), 98–131.

[33] Avrahami, *Senses of Scripture*, 224. The "it" in this passage refers to the sensory dominance of sight.

[34] Howes and Classen, *Ways of Sensing*.

[35] Avrahami, *Senses of Scripture*, 43.

Avrahami, Yael. *The Senses of Scripture: Sensory Perception in the Hebrew Bible.* LHBOTS 545. London: T&T Clark, 2012.
Barr, James. *The Semantics of Biblical Language.* Oxford: Oxford University Press, 1961.
Boman, Thorleif. *Hebrew Thought Compared with Greek.* New York: Norton, 1970.
Classen, Constance. *The Color of Angels: Cosmology, Gender and the Aesthetic Imagination.* London: Routledge, 1998.
———. *The Deepest Sense: A Cultural History of Touch.* Studies in Sensory History. Urbana: University of Illinois Press, 2012.
———. *The Museum of the Senses: Experiencing Art and Collections.* Sensory Study Series. New York: Bloomsbury Academic, 2017.
———. "The Senses." Pages 4:355–64 in *Encyclopedia of European Social History from 1350 to 2000.* Edited by Peter N. Stearns. New York: Scribner's Sons, 2001.
Clifford, James, and George E. Marcus, eds. *Writing Culture: The Politics and Poetics of Ethnography.* Berkeley: University of California Press, 1986.
Cox, Rupert, Andrew Irving, and Chris Wright, eds. *Beyond Text? Critical Practices and Sensory Anthropology.* Manchester: Manchester University Press, 2016.
Elliott, Denielle, and Dara Culhane, eds. *A Different Kind of Ethnography: Imaginative Practices and Creative Methodologies.* Toronto: University of Toronto Press, 2017.
Febvre, Lucien. *The Problem of Unbelief in the Sixteenth Century: The Religion of Rabelais.* Cambridge, MA: Harvard University Press, 1982.
Geurts, Kathryn Linn. *Culture and the Senses: Bodily Ways of Knowing in an African Community.* Ethnographic Studies in Subjectivity 3. Berkeley: University of California Press, 2002.
Glenn, H. Patrick. *Legal Traditions of the World: Sustainable Diversity in Law.* 5th ed. Oxford: Oxford University Press, 2014.
Harvey, Susan Ashbrook. *Scenting Salvation: Ancient Christianity and the Olfactory Imagination.* Berkeley: University of California Press, 2006.
Howes, David. "Afterword: The Skinscape; Reflections on the Dermalogical Turn." *Body and Society* 24.1–2 (2018): 225–39.
———. "Introduction: On the History and Sociology of the Senses." Pages 1–20 in *History and Sociology.* Vol. 2 of *Senses and Sensation: Critical and Primary Sources.* Edited by David Howes. London: Bloomsbury, 2018.
———. *Sensual Relations: Engaging the Senses in Culture and Social Theory.* Ann Arbor: University of Michigan Press, 2003.
———, ed. *The Varieties of Sensory Experience: A Sourcebook in the Anthropology the Senses.* Toronto: University of Toronto Press, 1991.
Howes, David, and Constance Classen. *Ways of Sensing: Understanding the Senses in Society.* London: Routledge, 2014.
Herzfeld, Michael. *Anthropology: Theoretical Practice in Culture and Society.* Oxford: Blackwell, 2000.
Laplantine, François. *The Life of the Senses: Toward a Modal Anthropology.* London: Bloomsbury, 2015.

Leppert, Richard. *The Sight of Sound: Music, Representation and the History of the Body*. Berkeley: University of California Press, 1995.

McLuhan, Marshall, and Eric McLuhan. *Laws of Media: The New Science*. Toronto: University of Toronto Press, 1988.

Penfield, Wilder, and Theodore Rasmussen. *The Cerebral Cortex of Man: A Study of Localization of Function*. New York: Macmillan, 1950.

Pink, Sarah. *Doing Sensory Ethnography*. Los Angeles: Sage, 2009.

Ritchie, Ian. "The Nose Knows: Bodily Knowing in Isaiah 11:3." *JSOT* 87 (2000): 59–73.

Robben, Antonius C. G. M., and Jeffrey A. Sluka, eds. *Ethnographic Fieldwork: An Anthropological Reader*. Oxford: Blackwell: 2007.

Stoller, Paul. *Sensuous Scholarship*. Contemporary Ethnography. Philadelphia: University of Pennsylvania Press, 1997.

Wober, Mallory. "The Sensotype Hypothesis." Pages 31–42 in *The Varieties of Sensory Experience: A Sourcebook in the Anthropology the Senses*. Edited by David Howes. Toronto: University of Toronto Press, 1991.

Zimmer, Carl. "Mouseunculus: How the Brain Draws a Little You." Phenomena: A Science Salon. 24 July 2013. https://tinyurl.com/SBL2827a.

ANCIENT ISRAEL

EMPIRICISM OR RATIONALISM IN THE HEBREW BIBLE? SOME THOUGHTS ABOUT ANCIENT FOXES AND HEDGEHOGS

Jan Dietrich

THE HEDGEHOG AND THE FOX

"The fox knows many things but the hedgehog one important thing" (πόλλ' οἶδ' ἀλώπηξ, ἀλλ' ἐχῖνος ἓν μέγα).[1] Taking up this fragment from the Greek poet Archilochus, the English philosopher Isaiah Berlin once distinguished between the fox, which builds upon his many experiences and thereby gets to know a great plurality of things, and the hedgehog, which coins one decisive idea and interprets the world accordingly.[2] In the following, my aim is to find out whether the Hebrew Bible is populated mainly by foxes or hedgehogs.

Read as a symbol for epistemological systems, the fox represents empiricism, the idea that insight and knowledge are based on the senses. It is sensory experience that creates knowledge. Opinions, sentences, and judgments based on experience may be called a posteriori judgments. The hedgehog, however, represents rationalism, the idea that basic insights and truths may be gained by pure reason. Reason provides access to and reasons for knowledge beyond sensory experience. In epistemology, judgments based on reason independent of experience may be called a priori judgments.

LOOK OUT! FOXES ROAM THE ISRAELITE COUNTRY

Typically, most scholars believe to find foxes in the Hebrew Bible, maintaining that experience was the backbone to the ancient Hebrew "mindset," with tradition

---

[1] Isaiah Berlin, *The Hedgehog and the Fox: An Essay on Tolstoy's View of History* (London: Weidenfeld & Nicolson, 1967), 1. Berlin quotes fragment 201 in Martin L. West, ed., *Archilochos—Hipponax—Theognidea*, vol. 1 of *Iambi et elegi Graeci ante Alexandrum cantati*, 2nd ed. (Oxford: Clarendon, 1989), 78.

[2] Berlin, *Hedgehog and the Fox*.

and revelation close behind.³ Among these three, experience seems to be the most important. In the old days, aiming at a genuine theological anthropology, with obvious influence from dogmatics and mixing descriptive and normative aspects of anthropology, scholars regarded hearing as the main relational capacity. Much more so than seeing, hearing was regarded as ruling supreme. As a relational capacity, the hearing sense enables humans to listen to God and others and to respond accordingly. This is the main reason why Hans Walter Wolff, in his classic work *Anthropology of the Old Testament*, asserts that "the wisdom writings recognize the hearing as being the root of true humanity…. Thus the supreme importance of the ear and of speech for true human understanding is unmistakable."⁴

In classical research, the supremacy of hearing was not ascribed to humans in general; rather it was ascribed to ancient Israelite culture in particular. In this case, Greek and Hebrew thought were usually contrasted, with hearing being ascribed to ancient Hebrew culture and sight to ancient Greek culture. Each was a particular sensory mode for acquiring knowledge and viewing the world. It was especially Thorleif Boman who asserted that "we can conclude that for the Hebrew the most important of his senses for the experience of truth was his hearing (as well as various kinds of feeling), but for the Greek it had to be his sight; or perhaps inversely, because the Greeks were organized in a predominantly visual way and the Hebrews in a predominantly auditory way, each people's conception of truth was formed in increasingly different ways."⁵

Recent research on the senses, however, has turned the tables and has highlighted that sight played the supreme role in obtaining knowledge. In her recent book, *The Senses of Scripture*, Yael Avrahami aims to demonstrate the centrality of sight in Hebrew Bible perception, though in principle, she claims, like Bernd Janowski,⁶ that there is no hierarchy of the senses in general. Sight, hearing, kinaesthesia, speech, taste, olfactory, and touch are all expressed prominently in the Hebrew Bible.⁷ When looking at the senses from the angle of epistemology, however, sight emerges as superior to all others. Like previous researchers, Avrahami highlights terms, images, and metaphors from the field of sight to show that sight is superior to other senses in obtaining knowledge.⁸ For example, she points to the

---

³ See Annette Schellenberg, *Erkenntnis als Problem: Qohelet und die alttestamentliche Diskussion um das menschliche Erkennen*, OBO 188 (Fribourg: Universitätsverlag Fribourg; Göttingen: Vandenhoeck & Ruprecht, 2002), 18–21.

⁴ Hans Walter Wolff, *Anthropology of the Old Testament* (London: SCM, 1974), 74–75.

⁵ Thorleif Boman, *Hebrew Thought Compared with Greek* (New York: Norton 1970), 206.

⁶ See Bernd Janowski, *Arguing with God: A Theological Anthropology of the Psalms* (Louisville: Westminster John Knox, 2012), 96.

⁷ Yael Avrahami, *The Senses of Scripture: Sensory Perception in the Hebrew Bible*, LHBOTS 545 (London: T&T Clark, 2012).

⁸ Avrahami, *Senses of Scripture*, 223–76. For earlier studies, see Michael Carasik, *Theologies of the Mind in Biblical Israel*, StBibLit 85 (Frankfurt am Main: Lang, 2006),

fact that in legal disputes, witnesses of truth are mainly based on sight. Following David Daube's theory on public punishment in Deuteronomy, Avrahami highlights the general importance of sight in lawsuits and narratives that take up legal-like language. This metaphorical usage of sight, even beyond its concrete sensory aspect, becomes most obvious in Lev 5:1:

> When any of you sin in that you have heard a public adjuration to testify and—though able to testify as one who has seen or learned of the matter—does not speak up, you are subject to punishment.[9]

In this text, though the hearing of the adjuration is mentioned, it is sight that is used as the term for witnessing. Next to these juridical examples, Avrahami points to several other dimensions as well. Instead of advocating hearing as the supreme sense in biblical epistemology, she maintains that only sight was regarded as a form of first-hand learning. "The correlation between sight and thought in biblical perception is so self-evident that we do not need to expand on it.... This semantic correlation between sight and thought is based on a perception whereby sight is first-hand learning, and is based on personal experience."[10] Hearing, on the other hand, remains secondary to sight. While sight relies on personal experience, hearing's function is to pass this experience on: "So, if we accurately map the differences between sight and hearing within the semantic field of knowledge, sight means investigation and clarification, while hearing means learning."[11] In regard to an epistemology of the Hebrew Bible, this means that sight is superior to hearing and to the other senses; "if forced to choose a side in the age-old dispute of the supremacy of sight vs. hearing in biblical epistemology, one must choose sight."[12] Such a position leaves Athens and Jerusalem, Greece and Israel, on the same side and not in direct opposition, both championing sight.[13]

In highlighting the sense of sight when it comes to obtaining knowledge, Michael Carasik, in his book *Theologies of the Mind in Biblical Israel*, points to the biological fact that physical anthropology asserts the supremacy of sight over against hearing. "Indeed, it is a feature not merely of human but of primate evolution, dating back to the Eocene, 54–36 million years ago, when the primates

---

passim; George Savran, "Seeing Is Believing: On the Relative Priority of Visual and Verbal Perception of the Divine," *BibInt* 17 (2009): 320–61.

[9] Translation following Avrahami, *Senses of Scripture*, 235.
[10] Avrahami, *Senses of Scripture*, 248–49.
[11] Avrahami, *Senses of Scripture*, 250.
[12] Avrahami, *Senses of Scripture*, 274.
[13] Avrahami, *Senses of Scripture*, 278.

developed stereoscopic vision, greatly increasing their reliance on sight and reducing sensitivity to hearing and smell."[14] Looking at the terminology of sight in the Hebrew Bible, Carasik makes it clear that what he calls the "receptive mind" is based on sight and involved not only perception but also comprehension and observational knowledge. Among others, he gives the following example. In 2 Sam 7:2, David says to Nathan:

> Look, I live in a house of cedar, but the ark of God sits inside the tent-curtain.[15]

According to Carasik, in this as well as in other cases, "the command 'see!' must be taken as an instruction to the addressee not (merely) to look at something visible, but to comprehend a situation by forming an image of it in his or her mind.... It gives a dimension to ראה that שמע does not have."[16] Later in his book, Carasik highlights that, in Deuteronomy, seeing is equated with direct experience, especially with God, while hearing is not. All in all, sight seems to be highlighted in recent research as the main source of knowledge in the Hebrew Bible, thereby implicitly asserting ancient Israelite culture as essentially empirical: ancient Hebrew knowledge, wisdom, and worldview are all fundamentally based on sensory experience, especially sight. According to Bernd Janowski, it is sight that can "verify or correct what has been heard,"[17] and he quotes Ps 48:8–9 and Job 42:5–6 as case examples:

> As we have heard, so we have seen
> in the city of YHWH Sabaoth, in the city of our God:
> God establishes her forever! *Selah* (Ps 48:8–9)

> I had heard of you with my ears, but now my eye has seen you;
> therefore I retract and repent, with/as dust and ashes.[18] (Job 42:5–6)

As these examples show, recent research on anthropology and the senses highlights seeing as a knowledge-creating sense, next and above the other biblical

---

[14] Carasik, *Theologies of the Mind*, 33. For the importance of seeing according to metaphor theory and cognitive science, see George Lakoff and Mark Johnson, *Philosophy in the Flesh: The Embodied Mind and Its Challenge to Western Thought* (New York: Basic Books 1999), 238–39.

[15] The translation follows Carasik, *Theologies of the Mind*, 41.

[16] Carasik, *Theologies of the Mind*, 41.

[17] Janowski, *Arguing with God*, 88.

[18] Translation following Janowski, *Arguing with God*, 88. For Job, see also Savran, "Seeing Is Believing," 335–61.

senses.[19] What we have to bear in mind, though, according to these positions, is the implication that foxes roam in Israelite culture, more than hedgehogs.

I do not aim to add many new examples to support this thesis. Obviously, the senses do play a major role in obtaining knowledge, and it would be senseless to argue against the empirical basis of many ideas to be found in the biblical texts. Neither will I be trying to explore tradition and revelation as the other main strands of Israelite insight. Instead, since empiricism is usually contrasted with rationalism, in the second part of my paper, I will ask whether rationalism may be found in the Hebrew Bible as well.

Watch Out for the Hedgehog

The language of the biblical text may reflect a relationship between language and thought, and the text's content may reflect common assumptions of the given culture. However, the relationship between language and thought is a difficult one, and the so-called Sapir-Whorf hypothesis is widely criticized nowadays: language does not determine thought; if anything, it only influences thought. To conclude from the wide variety of sensory expressions in the Hebrew Bible that the Hebrew mind is thoroughly empirical, or that the main mode of acquiring insight is sight, is perhaps too dependent on theories of linguistic relativity.[20] So, let's try to find some rational way of thinking in the second part of this paper.

Concerning ancient Near Eastern studies, Marc Van De Mieroop, in his book *Philosophy before the Greeks*, has shown how weak the claim is that the ancient Babylonians were empiricists. The main items found in many Babylonian lists do not contain records of empirical findings. As Van de Mieroop states,

> The evidence that empirical observation led to the entries in the lists is so slim, however, that we can easily doubt it played a role at all. Those modern scholars who sought connections between law paragraphs and the hundreds of actually recorded cases have mostly drawn a blank. The historical omens at the heart of the argument that authentic observations were the basis of omen lists are so few

---

[19] However, I believe that hearing does play the main role in tradition-oriented wisdom literature. For Deut 4 see Stephen Geller, "Fiery Wisdom: Logos and Lexis in Deuteronomy 4," *Prooftexts* 14 (1994): 103–39; Ryan O'Dowd, *The Wisdom of Torah: Epistemology in Deuteronomy and the Wisdom Literature*, FRLANT 225 (Göttingen: Vandenhoeck & Ruprecht 2009), 93.

[20] See, e.g., Yael Avrahami, "The Study of Sensory Perception in the Hebrew Bible: Notes on Method," *HBAI* 5 (2016): 13: "Semantic analysis is a technique that enables the philological scholar to access the culturally distinctive patterns of thought implicit in the structure of a language." For a recent application of the Sapir-Whorf hypothesis on Sumerian language, see Sebastian Fink, *Benjamin Whorf, die Sumerer und der Einfluss der Sprache auf das Denken*, Philippika 70 (Wiesbaden: Harrassowitz, 2015).

in number and often so meaningless that they provide meagre support for the theory. Even in the case of lexical texts, from the beginning of the genre we see that the creativity of the lists far surpassed what appeared in other writings and what the compilers observed in reality. Rather than searching for an elusive core of real entries derived from empirical scholarship in all these lists, is it not more logical to regard them as the products of written creativity, fully composed by scholars who set out to investigate language, divination, and law? This work was purely rational and based on concepts the ancient scholars intuitively knew to be true and which they expanded through logical deduction.[21]

In the Hebrew Bible, we do not have hundreds of long lists with lexical entries or omen series, but we do have, for example, law collections. Here, as well, the most recent research points to the fact that many laws do not seem to be grounded on empirical observation but rather seem to be rational deductions by associative ways of thinking, and the research hints at the creative rational process laying behind conceptualizing the law codes as a whole.[22] This may not come as a surprise, given that a lot of scholars nowadays propose a close connection between wisdom and laws and that most laws and law codes were never enforced in reality but instead were intended as wisdom-like guidance.[23]

Therefore, it is no wonder that a similar position is adopted to Proverbs as well. Contrary to most scholars, Michael Fox, in his article "The Epistemology of the Book of Proverbs," asserts that empiricism, the wisdom of experience, is not the main epistemology to be found in Proverbs. Instead, empiricism seems to be "irrelevant to most of Proverbs."[24] Fox gives, among others, Prov 20:20 as a case example:

> He who curses his father or his mother—
> his lamp will be extinguished in deep darkness.[25]

Fox states that it would be extraordinary to see something like this happen. It might not be that simple, though, since the writers could be thinking of the normal observation that a good relationship to parents normally pays off; this proverb would just be a special extrapolation from a general life experience. Nevertheless, Fox seems to be right in assuming that behind Proverbs a general theory might rule that cannot simply be explained as stemming from sensible observations.

---

[21] Marc Van De Mieroop, *Philosophy before the Greeks: The Pursuit of Truth in Ancient Babylonia* (Princeton: Princeton University Press, 2016), 190.

[22] See, e.g., the new commentary by Eckart Otto, *Deuteronomium*, HThKAT (Freiburg: Herder, 2012–2016).

[23] See, e.g., Bernard S. Jackson, *Wisdom-Laws: A Study of the Mishpatim of Exodus 12:1–22:16* (Oxford: Oxford University Press, 2006).

[24] Michael Fox, "The Epistemology of the Book of Proverbs," *JBL* 126 (2007): 671.

[25] Translation following Fox, "Epistemology of the Book of Proverbs," 671.

Contrary to the general assumption, most proverbs, like most laws, were not "extracted from experiential data" but extrapolated by analogy and by following a "coherence theory of truth."[26] The general assumption that there is a close connection between deeds and consequences may not say something about what is but about what shall be. Similarly, many proverbs do not seem to follow experiential observation but an "ideal of harmony" and righteousness.[27] Let's take Prov 19:17 as a case example:

> He who is kind to the lowly lends to the Lord,
> and he will pay him the recompense of his hands.[28]

Here, the content does not stem from sensory experience but interprets the world by taking in a rationale that is used as a hermeneutic approach by which to view the world.

Logical deductions are often regarded as good examples for rationalism and the capability for analytical thinking.[29] Matitiahu Tsevat takes Ezek 14:12–23 as a case example and demonstrates that, in this text, a kind of syllogism is at work. In Ezek 14:12–23, two propositions rule: First, every land that sins against God will be destroyed. Second, Judah sinned against God. By application of rational reasoning, the logical conclusion follows that Judah had to be destroyed. By application of "pure reason," this kind of argumentation explains the empirical fact that the Babylonians conquered Judah, and it gives reasons as to why this fact was an inevitable outcome.[30]

Though "soft evidentialism" and empirical verification may often be part of Hebrew Bible reasoning, logical reasoning itself is still at work, as Jaco Gericke has shown in regard to 1 Kgs 18:27:

1. Belief in x as not אלהים is rational, given the absence of empirical verification.
2. Belief in x as אלהים is rational, given empirical verification.
3. There is not any empirical verification for Baal as אלהים.
4. There is empirical verification for Yhwh as אלהים.

---

[26] Fox, "Epistemology of the Book of Proverbs," 671, 675.

[27] Fox, "Epistemology of the Book of Proverbs," 677.

[28] Translation following Fox, "Epistemology of the Book of Proverbs," 680.

[29] Other examples may come from laws presenting a rationale over against emotions like in Deut 21:15–17.

[30] See Mattitiahu Tsevat, "An Aspect of Biblical Thought: Deductive Explanation," *Shnaton* 3 (1978): 53–58. Jaco Gericke rightly assumes that a "counterfactual view of causation" is presupposed in such discourse. Jaco Gericke, *The Hebrew Bible and Philosophy of Religion*, RBS 70 (Atlanta: Society of Biblical Literature, 2012), 385.

5. Therefore, a belief that Baal is אלהים is falsified.
6. Therefore, a belief that Yhwh is אלהים is verified.³¹

Furthermore, against normal experience, a kind of reversal logic seems to be applied in Jer 31:20a.³² The text reads:

> Is Ephraim a truly precious son to me? [Answer: No.]
> A child in whom I take delight? [Answer: No again.]
> How is it, then, that ever since I have disowned him,
> I still keep calling him to mind?³³

According to Edward Greenstein, the reversed syllogism at work here consists of the following reasoning:

1. Parents will keep calling to mind a favored/delightful child.
2. Ephraim is a far cry from being a favored/delightful child.
3. God the Parent keeps thinking of/is inclined to recognize Ephraim!³⁴

In these cases, Hebrew thinking may not be termed "pre-logical" in the sense of Lucien Lévy-Bruhl but logical indeed.

Counting, of course, has an empirical foundation, but in mathematics, it can be used totally independently of empirical data. While the Sumerian writing system was obviously invented for economic reasons—as a resource for counting goods—later on Mesopotamian maths could use pure reason when counting, without relying on particular empirical data. We do not know much about mathematics in ancient Israel and Syria, but the name of the God Meni, mentioned in Isa 65:11, obviously derives from the Hebrew verb מנה ("to count").³⁵ Carasik points to other roots like חשב, ערך, ספר, פלל, and תכן as well, showing that "the idea of manipulation of numbers as a metaphor for the activity of the mind is a general one."³⁶ The use of these roots as ways for calculation and thinking seems, in some instances, to go beyond mere empirical observations, like in Prov 16:1:

---

[31] Gericke, *Hebrew Bible and Philosophy of Religion*, 375.

[32] See Edward Greenstein, "Some Developments in the Study of Language and Some Implications for Interpreting Ancient Texts and Cultures," in *Semitic Linguistics: The State of the Art at the Turn of the Twenty-First Century*, ed. Shlomo Izre'el, IOS 20 (Leiden: Eisenbrauns, 2002), 452–53.

[33] Translation following Greenstein, "Some Developments in the Study of Language," 452.

[34] Greenstein, "Some Developments in the Study of Language," 453.

[35] See S. David Sperling, "Meni," *DDD*, 567; Carasik, *Theologies of the Mind*, 132.

[36] Carasik, *Theologies of the Mind*, 133.

The plans of the heart belong to man,
but the answer of the tongue is from the Lord.³⁷

Here, עָרַךְ plus לֵב pertain to planning and scheming. As several examples from this field of metaphorical usage show, "picturing the mind as something which does arithmetic, is ancient indeed."³⁸

Even Qohelet, who is supposed to be an empiricist to the core, does not solely rely on sensory experience.³⁹ Though Qohelet "seeks both to derive knowledge from experience and to validate ideas experientially,"⁴⁰ he moves well beyond experience when he deliberates on the limits of experience and wisdom in a totally new way. This way of thinking does not itself generate from sensory experience, but rather from a highly reflective way of thinking, that is, thinking about the limits of human thinking itself (second order thinking).⁴¹ In a way, Qohelet uses sensory experience as a *topos* to show the limits of empiricism and thinking in general. "So, when he finally advises against watching the wind and clouds rather than working (11.3–6), Qohelet is making an important point about the inadequacy of observation, the impossibility of genuine insight, and the need to get on with life all the same. If there is empiricism in Ecclesiastes, there is also seemingly a strong critique of empiricism."⁴²

As this example might show, we have to distinguish between the literal level and the writer's level, between the kind of expressions and metaphors the texts use and what the writers of the texts aim at. In other words, we may have to distinguish between, on the one hand, empiricism on the textual level, and, on the other hand, the way the biblical writers make use of the texts for introducing their own rationale. It is not enough, then, to describe what is to be found in the biblical texts themselves literally, but to excavate, on a meta-level, the author's deliberate and willful interest in making an argument and in affecting, controlling, and constructing the reader's mind. When the writers of the Hebrew texts show an interest in willfully directing the reader's mind in well-considered ways, we may speak of

---

³⁷ Translation ESV.
³⁸ Carasik, *Theologies of the Mind*, 133.
³⁹ On Qohelet's empirical epistemology, see especially Michael Fox, "Qohelet's Epistemology," *HUCA* 58 (1987): 137–55; Schellenberg, *Erkenntnis als Problem*, 161–200.
⁴⁰ Fox, "Qohelet's Epistemology," 137.
⁴¹ On these limits, see Schellenberg, *Erkenntnis als Problem*. On Qohelet in the context of second order thinking in the ancient Fertile Crescent, see Jan Dietrich, "Hebräisches Denken und die Frage nach den Ursprüngen des Denkens zweiter Ordnung im Alten Testament, Alten Ägypten und Alten Orient," in *Individualität und Selbstreflexion in den Literaturen des Alten Testaments*, ed. Andreas Wagner and Jürgen van Oorschot, VWGTh 48 (Leipzig: Evangelische Verlagsanstalt, 2017), 64–65.
⁴² Stuart Weeks, *An Introduction to the Study of Wisdom Literature* (London: T&T Clark, 2010), 114.

a highly developed thinking level, concealed behind the surface of the text. Especially in Deuteronomy, "there is hardly a paragraph that is not filled with discussion of thoughts and emotions," impacting the reader's mind as well as revealing "a complete system" that shows the writer's high standard in form of a "theoretic attitude" and second order considerations.[43]

According to the Exodus narrative, Dru Johnson, in his book *Biblical Knowing*, makes the point that the belief of the Israelites is more than brute seeing.[44] Throughout the story, pharaoh is seeing but not understanding. The brute facts of sensory experience do not make a believer. Instead, even on the literal level, Moses is called to interpret the facts, and this is also what is needed in Deuteronomy. When Avrahami maintains that sight is first-hand knowledge, then, she refers to the literal sense of what a text is stating. Concerning Deuteronomy, Avrahami compares Deut 11:2a, 7 with 4:9–10. Deuteronomy 11:2a, 7 reads as follows:

> Remember today that it was not your children (who have not known or seen the discipline of the Lord your God) ... for it is your own eyes that have seen every great deed that the Lord did.[45]

This text distinguishes between the generation who knows, because it has seen, and the following generations who have not seen and therefore do not have first-hand sensory knowledge. With Deut 4:9–10 as parallel, Avrahami then shows how later generations will achieve second-hand knowledge by hearing:

> But take care and watch yourselves closely, so as neither to forget the things that your eyes have seen nor to let them slip from your mind all the days of your life; make them known to your children and your children's children—how you once stood before the Lord your God at Horeb, when the Lord said to me "Assemble the people for me, and I will let them hear my words, so that they may learn to fear me as long as they live on the earth, and may teach their children so."[46]

The problem with this approach is that it does not distinguish between the literal sense of the text and the writer's means of using the text. On the face of it, it seems true that sight is regarded as first-hand sensory knowledge and that this sensory

---

[43] Carasik, *Theologies of the Mind*, 206–7. For the term *theoretic attitude*, see Merlin Donald, *Origins of the Modern Mind: Three Stages in the Evolution of Culture and Cognition* (Cambridge: Harvard University Press, 1991), passim. For second order thinking in Deuteronomy, see Dietrich, "Hebräisches Denken," 56–58.

[44] See Dru Johnson, *Biblical Knowing: A Scriptural Epistemology of Error* (Eugene: Cascade, 2013), 65–81.

[45] Translation following Avrahami, *Senses of Scripture*, 249.

[46] Translation following Avrahami, *Senses of Scripture*, 249–50.

knowledge, like the first-hand witness of truth, is the most important one in finding belief in God. As it happens, though, there are other levels of meaning to be aware of. In fact, several questions arise: Is Moses speaking to the old generation who was at Sinai and who saw God or to a new generation who was not there and therefore may come into the Holy Land? To move even farther away from the literal meaning of the text: Perhaps Moses is not speaking to a particular generation but to all generations and believers of faith who, in a way, all stood on mount Sinai and who saw God with their own eyes—though literally they did not—and who shall give their belief to the young ones as if a witness of truth? In all of these instances, the writers of the text seem to use sensory expressions as *topoi* in their rhetorical devices, and "the fact that Moses is *re*-interpreting this event, re-visiting it in Deuteronomy and re-explaining its significance, argues against the notion of brute seeing."[47]

The writers' own ways of thinking seem to be highly creative ones, constructing texts with the aim of implementing a rationale. This rationale uses "pure reason" to implement truth and belief, and the writers argue for their rationale by using sensory expressions. Following not the surface of the text, but the rationales of the ancient Hebrew writers, the Hebrew writers may not be thorough empiricists at heart but rational thinkers, telling about foxes but being hedgehogs themselves.

BIBLIOGRAPHY

Avrahami, Yael. *The Senses of Scripture: Sensory Perception in the Hebrew Bible.* LHBOTS 545. London: T&T Clark, 2012.

———. "The Study of Sensory Perception in the Hebrew Bible: Notes on Method." *HBAI* 5 (2016): 3–22.

Berlin, Isaiah. *The Hedgehog and the Fox: An Essay on Tolstoy's View of History.* London: Weidenfeld & Nicolson, 1967.

Boman, Thorleif. *Hebrew Thought Compared with Greek.* New York: Norton 1970.

Carasik, Michael. *Theologies of the Mind in Biblical Israel.* StBibLit 85. Frankfurt am Main: Lang, 2006.

Dietrich, Jan. "Hebräisches Denken und die Frage nach den Ursprüngen des Denkens zweiter Ordnung im Alten Testament, Alten Ägypten und Alten Orient." Pages 45–65 in *Individualität und Selbstreflexion in den Literaturen des Alten Testaments.* Edited by Andreas Wagner and Jürgen van Oorschot. VWGTh 48. Leipzig: Evangelische Verlagsanstalt, 2017.

Donald, Merlin. *Origins of the Modern Mind: Three Stages in the Evolution of Culture and Cognition.* Cambridge: Harvard University Press, 1991.

---

[47] Johnson, *Biblical Knowing*, 197. Emphasis by the author.

Fink, Sebastian. *Benjamin Whorf, die Sumerer und der Einfluss der Sprache auf das Denken*. Philippika 70. Wiesbaden: Harrassowitz, 2015.

Fox, Michael. "The Epistemology of the Book of Proverbs." *JBL* 126 (2007): 669–84.

———. "Qohelet's Epistemology." *HUCA* 58 (1987): 137–55.

Geller, Stephen. "Fiery Wisdom: Logos and Lexis in Deuteronomy 4." *Prooftexts* 14 (1994): 103–39.

Gericke, Jaco. *The Hebrew Bible and Philosophy of Religion*. RBS 70. Atlanta: Society of Biblical Literature, 2012.

Greenstein, Edward. "Some Developments in the Study of Language and Some Implications for Interpreting Ancient Texts and Cultures." Pages 441–79 in *Semitic Linguistics: The State of the Art at the Turn of the Twenty-First Century*. Edited by Shlomo Izre'el. IOS 20. Leiden: Eisenbrauns, 2002.

Jackson, Bernard S. *Wisdom-Laws: A Study of the Mishpatim of Exodus 12:1–22:16*. Oxford: Oxford University Press, 2006.

Janowski, Bernd. *Arguing with God: A Theological Anthropology of the Psalms*. Louisville: Westminster John Knox, 2012.

Johnson, Dru. *Biblical Knowing: A Scriptural Epistemology of Error*. Eugene: Cascade, 2013.

Lakoff, George, and Mark Johnson. *Philosophy in the Flesh: The Embodied Mind and Its Challenge to Western Thought*. New York: Basic Books 1999.

O'Dowd, Ryan. *The Wisdom of Torah: Epistemology in Deuteronomy and the Wisdom Literature*. FRLANT 225. Göttingen: Vandenhoeck & Ruprecht 2009.

Otto, Eckart. *Deuteronomium*. HThKAT. Freiburg: Herder, 2012–2016.

Savran, George. "Seeing Is Believing: On the Relative Priority of Visual and Verbal Perception of the Divine." *BibInt* 17 (2009): 320–61.

Schellenberg, Annette. *Erkenntnis als Problem: Qohelet und die alttestamentliche Diskussion um das menschliche Erkennen*. OBO 188. Fribourg: Universitätsverlag Fribourg; Göttingen: Vandenhoeck & Ruprecht, 2002.

Sperling, S. David. "Meni." *DDD*, 566–68.

Tsevat, Mattitiahu. "An Aspect of Biblical Thought: Deductive Explanation." *Shnaton* 3 (1978): 53–58.

Van De Mieroop, Marc. *Philosophy before the Greeks: The Pursuit of Truth in Ancient Babylonia*. Princeton: Princeton University Press, 2016.

Weeks, Stuart. *An Introduction to the Study of Wisdom Literature*. London: T&T Clark, 2010.

West, Martin L., ed. *Archilochos—Hipponax—Theognidea*. Vol. 1 of *Iambi et elegi Graeci ante Alexandrum cantata*. 2nd ed. Oxford: Clarendon, 1989.

Wolff, Hans Walter. *Anthropology of the Old Testament*. London: SCM, 1974.

MOVING AND THINKING: KINESTHESIS AND WISDOM IN THE BOOK OF PROVERBS

Greg Schmidt Goering

INTRODUCTION

Dated to the first millennium BCE, the book of Proverbs offers an example of ancient Israelite wisdom literature. Wisdom refers to a broad category of texts in the ancient Near East from the second and first millennia BCE. Anthological in form, Proverbs consists in collections of sayings, instructions, and poems about wisdom and how one can attain it. In brief, the wisdom tradition derived principles for living well from observations on nature and everyday life; these principles were distilled into pithy sayings and transmitted through oral and written instruction.

This essay is based on a chapter from my monograph in process, entitled *Wisdom in the Flesh: Disciplining the Senses and Forming the Self in the Book of Proverbs*. In it, I interpret wisdom instruction in the book of Proverbs as a bodily practice that aimed to discipline the senses. In the modern West, conventional thinking construes the senses as passive receptors for gathering data on the external world. In contrast, the sages of Proverbs viewed the senses as portals that mediated between a body's exterior and its interior—described variously as the heart, belly, or inner essence (נפש). As passageways between self and other, the senses required discipline in order for a person to have the right kinds of experiences, draw the correct inferences, and absorb and emanate wisdom rather than folly. Therefore, the sages developed strategies to educate the senses.

Out of this educational regimen emerged a *sensorium*—a cultural model that enumerates, ranks, and invests meaning in the senses. Like Pierre Bourdieu's habitus, the sensorium in Proverbs formed a system of lasting dispositions, or culturally patterned tendencies. Turning history into nature, the sensorium durably installed these dispositions in the body, placing them beyond the reach of conscious awareness.[1] The senses thus played a vital role in the practice of embodying the wisdom tradition's most cherished values. In this essay, I examine the sense of movement in Proverbs, in order to understand better the pedagogical strategies of the book and the nature of the wisdom it envisions.

MOVING IN PROVERBS

The book of Proverbs pays ample attention to movement. Verbs of moving—such as walk, tread, march, run, hasten, rush, descend, arrive, enter, cross, turn around, leave, turn aside, go straight, meander, totter, and stumble—occur frequently. In addition to these verbs, the foot appears prominently in the book as a means of locomotion.

We can enter this world of moving with an example from Prov 19:2:

בלא־דעת נפש לא־טוב   ואץ ברגלים חוטא:

A person without knowledge is not good,
and he who hastens with his feet misses (the way).

This verse offers a typical example of the basic unit of Hebrew poetry: a terse and balanced bicolon (or two line saying), each line in this saying containing only three words in Hebrew. A bicolon expresses a single idea in two related lines. This particular bicolon forms a proverb, or *mashal* in Hebrew, literally, a "comparison." To grasp the proverb's meaning, one must compare the two lines and determine their relation.[2] One way to interpret this proverb is to recognize an ABAB pattern on the grammatical level. In Hebrew, the first two words of each line form a grammatical subject: a person who lacks knowledge and one who moves quickly by means of his feet. The verb "hasten" (אוץ) always carries negative connotations in Proverbs.[3] The last word in each line forms a predicate. In the first line, "is not good" indicates a value judgment. In the second, "misses" is the basic verb in the Hebrew Bible for sinning; literally, it means "to miss the

---

[1] Pierre Bourdieu, *Outline of a Theory of Practice*, trans. Richard Nice, Cambridge Studies in Social and Cultural Anthropology 16 (Cambridge: Cambridge University Press, 1977).

[2] I do not suggest that there is only one possible meaning to a given proverb. Such sayings are always multivalent. I merely mean to indicate that each line does not communicate its own idea, but rather together two (sometimes three) lines point to a single, larger message. As James Kugel puts it, "The two halves [of a bicolon] are a single conceit"; James L. Kugel, *The Idea of Biblical Poetry: Parallelism and Its History* (Baltimore: Johns Hopkins, 1981), 10.

[3] See also Prov 21:5; 28:20; 29:20. Cf. the negative connotations of בהל ("hurry") in Prov 28:22.

mark," and here it implies a negative consequence.[4] In the context of moving too quickly with one's feet, perhaps "misses" means to err in navigation, that is, to miss the path on which one should walk. Recalling the essential idea of a proverb as comparison, the semantic similarities between the two lines emerge: hasty movements of the feet correlate to a lack of knowledge. This raises several questions: Why were the sages of Proverbs so interested in moving? What is the connection between moving one's feet and wisdom? And, finally, what role does movement play in the pedagogical program of Proverbs?

Before turning to other examples of movement in Proverbs, I address two matters: first, kinesthesia as a sense, and second the connection between moving and thinking.

THE SENSE OF MOVEMENT

In the modern West, we are unaccustomed to thinking of moving as a sense. Beholden to the Aristotelian sensorium—which is limited to seeing, hearing, smelling, tasting, and touching—we tend to forget that humans share other physical capacities defined as senses, such as balance, temperature, pain, proprioception, and kinesthesia (among others). Although scientists agree neither on the definition of sense nor on the enumeration of the senses, most would admit somewhere between ten and twenty-one senses, and, from a physiological point of view, they widely acknowledge kinesthesia as a sense.

More importantly, sensory anthropologists observe that sensoria vary from one culture to the next. For example, some cultures elaborate speaking or balance as a sense, though these are not part of our popular modern Western sensorium.[5] The Aristotelian model itself is not a natural sensorium but rather a cultural construct, which emphasizes exteroceptive senses.[6] Yael Avrahami argues that the sensorium in ancient Israel was sevenfold: in addition to the five senses that our modern Western culture acknowledges, ancient Israelites elaborated speaking and moving as senses.[7]

---

[4] BDB, s.v. "חטא."

[5] For a modern-day example of a culture that elaborates balance as a sense, see Kathryn Linn Geurts, *Culture and the Senses: Bodily Ways of Knowing in an African Community*, Ethnographic Studies in Subjectivity (Berkeley: University of California Press, 2002), 86–87, 98–107.

[6] On the sensory taxonomy exteroceptive, interoceptive, and proprioceptive, see Geurts, *Culture and the Senses*, 9.

[7] Yael Avrahami, *The Senses of Scripture: Sensory Perception in the Hebrew Bible*, LHBOTS 545 (London: T&T Clark International, 2012), 67–69. Avrahami bases her sevenfold sensorium on Pss 115 and 135, and Deut 4. Psalm 115:4–7, for example, polemicizes idols, who "have mouths, but do not speak, eyes, but do not see. They have ears, but do not hear, noses, but do not smell. They have hands, but do not feel, feet, but

Many definitions of kinesthesia, such as this one from Harvey Schiffman, combine what I would call the sense of movement and the sense of body position in space, or proprioception.

> Kinaesthesis refers to the sensory system that receives and processes information about the posture, location, and movement in space of the limbs and other mobile parts of the jointed skeleton.[8]

Proprioception and kinesthesia are often confused or combined, given that both senses depend in part upon the vestibular system, which provides information about the position of the body in space as well as how the body moves in its environment and relative to the force of gravity (up/down). For my study of Proverbs, I leave aside the proprioceptive sense and proceed with a narrower definition of kinesthesia as "the sensory awareness of one's body moving through space."[9]

Although kinesthesia involves the entire body, the Hebrew Bible elaborates the foot as the principle organ of movement. Pointing to the polemic against idols in Ps 115—"they have feet but do not walk"—Avrahami suggests that "the foot indicates the means of mobility ... in the Hebrew Bible."[10] She also asserts that the foot "bear[s] the metaphorical load of its related sensory experience, kinaesthesia."[11] In other words, the foot is more than a limb; it is an agent of moving. Citing Job 29:15, "I was eyes to the blind and I was feet to the lame," Avrahami observes, "The lame have feet, but what they do not have is (proper) walking."[12] An ancient Israelite definition of kinesthesia might well be "the sense of moving by means of the feet." For this reason, I attend especially to references to foot and footstep and to verbs that imply movement of the foot or movement of the person by means of the feet.

---

do not walk." Given the associative links between the various organs and activities in these passages, Avrahami argues that moving was elaborated as a sense in ancient Israel, alongside seeing, hearing, speaking, tasting, touching, and smelling.

[8] Harvey Richard Schiffman, "The Skin, Body, and Chemical Senses," in *Sensation and Perception*, ed. Richard L. Gregory and Andrew M. Colman (Essex, UK: Longman, 1995), 82–83.

[9] For a study that examines proprioception in conjunction with kinesthesia, see Nicole L. Tilford, *Sensing World, Sensing Wisdom: The Cognitive Foundation of Biblical Metaphors*, AIL 31 (Atlanta: SBL Press, 2017), esp. 149–72.

[10] Avrahami, *Senses of Scripture*, 118.

[11] Avrahami, *Senses of Scripture*, 119.

[12] Avrahami, *Senses of Scripture*, 120.

Moving and Thinking

Thanks to Descartes, we in the modern West tend to think of thinking in disembodied terms. The notion that thinking might be entwined with moving or with other bodily processes strikes us as odd. As Paul Stoller observes, "The underlying premise of this [Western] epistemology is fundamental: one can separate thought from feeling and action."[13] Despite the persistence of the Cartesian mind-body dualism, scholars in diverse fields such as dance movement theory, neuroscience, and philosophy have argued that thinking arises directly from the experience of the body in motion.

Ethnomusicologist and practitioner of traditional Japanese dance Tomie Hahn asks how one's body comes to know a certain dance movement.[14] She observes that the hand, for instance, knows without language, that it "thinks" without words. She recalls her dance teacher's instruction, "Know with your body."[15] As Hahn notes, her mentor's counsel points to a kind of knowledge distinct from the way knowledge is often construed in the Western intellectual tradition.[16] The dance instructor's knowledge is not one in which the mind first knows and then instructs the hand to do. As dance theorists have long maintained, "the body does not intellectualize theory before it learns—rather, theory arises from engagement in body practices."[17] What then, Hahn asks, can we learn from observing movement?[18] Or, for my study of Proverbs, what can we learn from observing instructions by sages to move in certain ways and not others?

Neuroscientist Rodolfo Llinás argues that mind (or what he calls "mindness state") results from "evolutionary processes that ... occurred in the brain as actively moving creatures developed from the primitive to the highly evolved."[19] A primary function of the brain is its capacity to predict moment-to-moment what is

---

[13] Paul Stoller, *The Taste of Ethnographic Things: The Senses in Anthropology* (Philadelphia: University of Pennsylvania Press, 1989), 7–8.

[14] Tomie Hahn, *Sensational Knowledge: Embodying Culture through Japanese Dance* (Middletown: Wesleyan University Press, 2007), xiv.

[15] Hahn, *Sensational Knowledge*, 1.

[16] Tomie Hahn, "Bodies as Fieldsites: Considering the Senses in Research and Performance" (paper presented to the University of Virginia Music Department Colloquium, Charlottesville, VA, 16 September 2016).

[17] Hahn, *Sensational Knowledge*, 2. Citing Cynthia J. Bull, "Sense, Meaning, and Perception in Three Dance Cultures," in *Meaning in Motion: New Cultural Studies of Dance*, ed. Jane Desmond (Durham: Duke University Press, 1997), 269–87; Susan Leigh Foster, "Dancing Bodies," in Desmond, *Meaning in Motion*, 235–57.

[18] Hahn, "Bodies as Fieldsites."

[19] Rodolfo R. Llinás, *I of the Vortex: From Neurons to Self* (Cambridge: MIT Press, 2001), ix.

likely to occur when an organism moves in its environment.[20] How did the brain develop such predictive capacity? Evolution embedded "properties of the external world" into the organizational structure of the nervous system, in what Llinás calls "an internal functional space."[21] As an organism moves in its environment, the internal functional space allows it to process the incoming sensory data about the external world and efficiently transform the signals into motor output in the external environment.[22] The internal "predictive image of an event to come that causes the creature to react or behave accordingly [is] the basis from which consciousness, in all living forms, is generated."[23] Llinás summarizes his view of this evolutionary process succinctly: "That which we call thinking is the evolutionary internalization of movement."[24] He writes, "Thinking ultimately represents movement, not just of body parts or of objects in the external world, but of perceptions and complex ideas as well."[25]

Finally, phenomenologist Maxine Sheets-Johnstone similarly connects moving and thinking. She rejects "the Cartesian assumption that minds think and bodies 'do.'"[26] "Thinking and moving are not separate happenings" but rather two facets of an intelligent body in motion.[27] *Animate forms* (by which she means "things that move") develop "a corporeal consciousness" through moving.[28] Animateness, she argues, "is the epistemological foundation of our learning to move ourselves with respect to objects.... *We literally discover ourselves in movement.*"[29] "A creature's corporeal consciousness," she writes, "is first and foremost a consciousness attuned to the movement and rest of its own body.... In effect, creatures know themselves ... in ways that are fundamentally and quintessentially

---

[20] Llinás, *I of the Vortex*, 18.

[21] Llinás, *I of the Vortex*, 64.

[22] Llinás, *I of the Vortex*, 64–65. "The nervous system has evolved to provide a plan, one composed of goal-oriented, mostly short-lived predictions verified by moment-to-moment sensory input. This allows a creature to move actively in a direction according to an internal reckoning—a transient sensorimotor image—of what may be outside" (18).

[23] Llinás, *I of the Vortex*, 55.

[24] Llinás, *I of the Vortex*, 35; see also 5, 55. "The brain's understanding of anything, whether factual or abstract, arises from our manipulations of the external world, by our moving within the world and thus from our sensory-derived experience of it" (58–59).

[25] Llinás, *I of the Vortex*, 62.

[26] Maxine Sheets-Johnstone, *The Primacy of Movement*, 2nd ed., Advances in Consciousness Research 82 (Amsterdam: Benjamins, 2011), xxxi.

[27] Sheets-Johnstone, *Primacy of Movement*, xxxi.

[28] Sheets-Johnstone, *Primacy of Movement*, 114. Sheets-Johnstone writes, "Consciousness is fundamentally a corporeal consciousness and the movement of organisms is fundamentally commensurate with their essentially tactile, proprioceptive, and/or kinesthetic sensitivities" (xxi).

[29] Sheets-Johnstone, *Primacy of Movement*, 117. Italics in original.

consistent with the bodies they are." Creatures know themselves, she observes, not by sight, by looking at their own bodies, but through kinesthesia, that is, by "sensing their bodies as animate forms in movement and at rest."[30]

Sheets-Johnstone finds this essential truth from evolutionary biology confirmed by Lois Bloom's research on infant-child psychology. Prior to acquisition of language or any symbolic mode of discourse, she observes, "thinking in movement is an infant's original mode of thinking.... As infants, we come to grasp objects, literally *and* epistemologically, through movement."[31]

KINESTHESIA AND THE PEDAGOGICAL STRATEGY OF PROVERBS

With these observations about the imbrication of thinking and moving, I turn to several passages from the book of Proverbs to see what role kinesthesia plays in the pedagogical aim of the sages to develop wisdom in their students.

Proverbs 7:1–27 (Lecture 10)[32]

In lecture 10 (Prov 7), a father warns his son about relations with another man's wife. At the center of the lecture, the father recounts a cautionary tale about a young man and the figure of the Strange Woman. In Proverbs, the Strange Woman is a literary construct of the sages presumably based on their own (mis)understanding of real women. She functions as a seductive and foolish foil for the sages' own teachings about wisdom. Despite the story-like quality of the cautionary tale and its history of allegorical interpretation, lecture 10 contains a plausible account of actual temptations imagined by the father.[33] We therefore cannot easily dismiss the kinesthetic references as mere metaphors. Hence, the chapter offers a profitable place to illustrate the sages' teachings about the significance of movement.

Although the chapter engages multiple senses, here I highlight the role kinesthesia plays in the pedagogical strategy of the lecture. In the cautionary tale we first encounter a young man described by the father as lacking sense (חסר־לב; 7:7).[34] The young man is on the move: crossing (עבר) through the market near the

---

[30] Sheets-Johnstone, *Primacy of Movement*, 62.

[31] Sheets-Johnstone, *Primacy of Movement*, xxv. Italics in original.

[32] In describing the passages treated here as "lectures," I follow the literary analysis of Michael Fox, who argues that Prov 1–9 consist of a series of ten lectures and five interludes; see Michael V. Fox, *Proverbs 1–9: A New Translation with Introduction and Commentary*, AB 18A (New York: Doubleday, 2000), 44–47.

[33] On the history of interpreting this passage allegorically, see Fox, *Proverbs 1–9*, 254–55.

[34] The Hebrew phrase means literally "lacking heart." In ancient Israel, the heart was thought to be the locus of thinking.

Strange Woman's corner, marching (צעד) on the road (דרך) that runs past her house. The verb "march" (צעד) marks the young man's movement as intentional,[35] and the Strange Woman's interruption of his movement (in 7:10) suggests that the goal of his journey is not her house.

The father describes the Strange Woman's habit of flitting about the city,[36] noting that "her feet do not stay in her house" (7:11). He further observes that she is "now in the streets, now in the squares" (פעם בחוץ פעם ברחבות). The word translated "now" (פעם) also has a concrete meaning "footstep," so we could read "a foot in the streets, a foot in the squares" (Prov 7:12).[37] The temporal sense of the term suggests her quick movements from one public place to the next, while the concrete sense highlights her uncontrolled footsteps.

The father's portrait of the Strange Woman thus far indicates her lack of kinesthetic self-control. Later in the tale, however, she tells the young man that she "came out" (יצא) to meet him, to "seek his face" (שחר). These verbs imply deliberate and energetic motion, suggesting she possesses some capacity to direct her steps. Overall, then, the Strange Woman's erratic movements result from a combination of her inability to control her feet and her intentional choice to move improperly.

The Strange Woman seduces the young man using kinesthetic means (among others). She invites the young man to her bed for a sexual rendezvous with the imperative "come!" (לכה), implying his own movements toward her house. With her flattery[38] she "turns him aside" (נטה) and "thrusts him aside" (נדח),[39] diverting him from the path on which he walked resolutely.

The young man responds kinetically and unthinkingly: he "follows her suddenly [הולך אחריה פתאם], he goes [בוא] like an ox to the slaughter, like a stag bounding to bonds,[40] like a bird rushing [מהר] to a trap." The similes emphasize the recklessness of the young man's movement. Quick movements generally have a negative valence in Proverbs, and in the case of the verb "rush" (מהר), harmful consequences always follow.[41]

---

[35] Fox argues that the verb צעד "suggests a bold and deliberate step" (*Proverbs 1–9*, 243).

[36] She is described literally as "boisterous" (המיה). Cf. the use of המה for bustling streets (Prov 1:21) and the commotion of a city (1 Kgs 1:41; Isa 22:2).

[37] פעם parallels אשר (step) in Ps 17:5 and רגל (foot) in Isa 26:6. Fox suggests we read v. 12 with double meaning (*Proverbs 1–9*, 245).

[38] Fox emends ברב "with much" to ברך "with soft" (*Proverbs 1–9*, 249).

[39] Fox suggests that both verbs mean "to deflect someone from the right path" and notes that נדח "retains the connotation of a physical shove" (*Proverbs 1–9*, 248).

[40] The Hebrew of this clause in the Masoretic Text makes no sense; see Fox's emendations (*Proverbs 1–9*, 249).

[41] See Prov 1:16; 6:18; 25:8.

The cautionary tale ends with the father's statement that the young man does not know (ולא־ידע) that his very life is at stake, until it is too late.[42] If thinking is the internalization of moving, as Llinás suggests, we ought to read the young man's perceptual failure as a result of his improper movement along the path onto which the Strange Woman deflected him. Indeed, in three of the four occurrences of the verb "rush" (מהר) in Proverbs, the sages associate faulty cognition with hurried movements.[43]

After the cautionary tale, the father again instructs his son[44] in proper movement: "Don't let your heart turn aside [שטה] to her ways; don't stray [תעה] in her paths" (7:25). Ancient Israelites understood the heart to be the locus of thinking and will, similar to the way we use the term "mind." Proverbs scholar Michael Fox, noting that the verb "stray in" (תעה ב) "means to wander or be lost *in* an area, rather than stray *into* an area," reads these two lines sequentially: "If you are attracted to her ways (25a), you will wander about in her crooked paths (25b)."[45] Progression is not, however, the only way to understand the poetry of verse 25, and Fox's interpretation follows his understanding of the Israelite philosophy of the body. Commenting on another passage (Prov 6:12–20), Fox suggests: "The eye is the point of entry to the will, whose organ is the heart; the hands and feet put the will into action, and the mouth gives expression to thought and will, and this utterance is received by the ears."[46] I would argue that all of the senses in ancient Israel, not only the eyes, form portals to the heart.[47] Moreover, in the present case, it is more than the sight of the Strange Woman that turns his heart to her ways. The young man's will is affected by touch—she grabs him and kisses him (7:13)—and by audition—she speaks flattering words to him (7:14–20, cf. 21). Rather than reading verse 25 as a progression, in which first the heart turns aside to the Strange Woman's ways and then the feet express the will by walking in her paths, we can recall Hahn's observation that the body does not first think and then do. Furthermore, we can understand the grammatical and semantic structure of the verse to suggest that the heart and the body operate in tandem. As

---

[42] Fox transposes 23a to the end of the verse (*Proverbs 1–9*, 239, 250).

[43] In addition to the present passage, in Prov 1:16, the sinners' feet run (רוץ) toward evil, and they rush (מהר) to shed blood. The proverb that follows in v. 17 may indicate that the sinners lack knowledge as a result of their hurried movements. In a list of things the Lord hates, Prov 6:18 includes: a mind that devises wicked plans, feet that run quickly (ממהרות לרוץ) toward evil, thus creating a parallel between the activity of mind and feet.

[44] This time in the plural, "sons"; cf. Prov 7:1.

[45] Fox, *Proverbs 1–9*, 250–51. Italics in original. See Gen 21:14; 37:15; Ps 107:4.

[46] Fox, *Proverbs 1–9*, 220.

[47] Elsewhere I have argued, for example, that in the case of flogging Israelite sages imagined the back to be a tactile portal to the heart; Greg Schmidt Goering, "Tactile Discipline: The Sense of Touch in the Book of Proverbs" (paper presented at the Annual Meeting of the Society of Biblical Literature, Chicago, IL, 18 November 2012).

Llinás argues, "The ... generation of movement and the generation of mind ... are ... different parts of the same process."[48]

Indeed, the father's reference to the "heart turning aside" (שטה) construes the very processes of thinking as kinesthetic. It is not just the son's foot that might wander about in the Strange Woman's path; his heart—that is, his mind—can also "turn aside" from the path it follows. Proverbs 2:2 suggests that the heart can "incline toward understanding," and Prov 2:10 imagines the process of attaining knowledge in kinesthetic terms: "wisdom will enter your heart" (תבוא חכמה בלבך). The cognitive and the kinesthetic coalesce. Thinking is moving.

In the case of the young man, the interrelated nature of moving and thinking forms a vicious cycle: he lacked knowledge (חסר־לב) to begin with and therefore walked unaware of the dangers that lurk in his environment. Due to his naiveté, the Strange Woman distracted him easily from his path. Moving on the path charted for him by her further obscured his knowledge: he failed to see that succumbing to her enticements would lead to his untimely death.

Proverbs 4:10–19 (Lecture 6)

The cautionary tale in Prov 7 illustrates the consequences of moving improperly. For instructions on proper movement, we can turn to two lectures in chapter 4.

In lecture 6 (Prov 4:10–19), the father characterizes his wisdom instruction as follows: "I guide you [הרתיך] in the way of wisdom; I lead you [הדרכתיך] in tracks of uprightness [במעגלי־ישר]" (4:11). Here, wisdom itself is a path (דרך), and through his instruction, the father claims to direct the son's movements in the way of wisdom.[49] If the son practices his instruction, the father assures: "When you walk [הלך], your step [צעדך] will not be impeded [צרר], and if you run [רוץ] you will not stumble [כשל]" (4:12). Traveling the path of wisdom will be smooth; one can walk easily and even run without tripping. Unlike the verbs "hasten" (אוץ) and "rush" (מהר), which always lead to harmful consequences, the verb "run" (רוץ) has a neutral valence. When "run" occurs adjacent to "rush," it has negative connotations.[50] When the verb appears alone, however, as it does here and in Prov 18:10, no negative connotations adhere: the righteous move swiftly without harmful consequences.

Verses 14–17 contrast the alternate path taken by wicked men. The father uses a series of kinetic terms to advise his son:

---

[48] Llinás, *I of the Vortex*, 5.

[49] Avrahami argues that Proverbs views wisdom as a verbal path one must walk (*Senses of Scripture*, xxx).

[50] See Prov 1:16; 6:18 and my comments above.

> In the pathway [ארח] of wicked men, do not enter [בוא],
> and do not proceed [אשר] in the way [דרך] of evil men.
> Avoid [פרע] it [i.e., the path], do not traverse [עבר ב] it;
> swerve away [שטה] from it, and pass on [עבר]. (4:14–15)

When in the course of his life the son encounters a path trod by the wicked, not only must he not travel on it; he also must not enter it; he must swerve so as to avoid even stepping on it.[51] This requires the development of self-control over his movements.

The final two verses of the lecture contrast the two paths in terms of light and darkness. While the pathway (ארח) of the righteous grows ever brighter, the way (דרך) of the wicked is obscured by darkness, such that "they know not [לא ידעו] on what they stumble [כשל]" (4:18–19).[52] In contrast to the father's promise that the one who travels the path of wisdom will not trip, even if he runs, here those who traverse the way of the wicked stumble, because they are unable to see obstacles in their way. Again we observe a close connection between moving and thinking: inappropriate movements lead to a lack of useful knowledge, which then causes kinesthetic problems (stumbling); appropriate movements, in contrast, lead to useful knowledge, which in turn helps one avoid kinesthetic missteps.

Proverbs 4:20–27 (Lecture 7)

Lecture 7 (Prov 4:20–27) encourages the son to proceed directly ahead on his path.

> Straighten [פלס] the course [מעגל] of your foot [רגלך],
> and all your ways [דרכיך] will be firm [כון].
> Do not turn aside [נטה] to the right or the left;
> turn away [סור] your foot [רגלך] from evil. (4:26–27)

Here the father gives the son clear instructions about controlling the movement of his foot. First, the son is instructed not to deviate from the path he is on, suggesting that, unlike the naïve youth in Prov 7, he is already on the path of wisdom. Second,

---

[51] Fox writes: "The path of the wicked is not somewhere off in the distance, far from the path of the righteous. Somehow, their path zigzags through the territory of life. You are in danger not only if you choose to seek it out; you may come upon it willy-nilly as it crosses or nears your own life course. When that happens, it is not enough just to continue on your way. You must actively 'shun' (*para'*) the evil path and 'veer aside' (*satah*) from it" (*Proverbs 1–9*, 180–81).

[52] In Proverbs, light represents knowledge (see, e.g., Prov 6:23). In the broader wisdom tradition, darkness serves as a metaphor for ignorance (see, e.g., Eccl 2:13–14; cf. Prov 2:13; Deut 28:29).

as in the previous passage (Prov 4:14–17), the son is told to steer his foot away from evil. Finally, the son is told to guide his foot, so that the tracks it makes will be straight.

This last instruction illustrates that paths do not simply exist; they must be reproduced as they are trod. As Sheets-Johnston observes: "Movement *creates* the qualities that it embodies and that we experience; thus it is erroneous to think that movement simply takes place *in* space.... On the contrary, we ... create space in the process of moving."[53] If the son manages to track straight ahead, the father promises that his "ways" will be firm (כון), suggesting the opposite experience of stumbling.[54]

As Fox rightly observes, lecture 7 "seeks to shape the student's moral self-image by framing it in physiological terms."[55] In addition to the instructions regarding the foot, cited above, the father exhorts his son:

> Incline your *ear* to my sayings ...
> let them not escape your *eyes*;
> keep them within your *heart* ...
> With all vigilance, guard your *heart* ...
> Remove from yourself crookedness of *mouth*,
> and distortion of *lips* put far from you.
> Let your *eyes* look directly to the front,
> and let your *eyeballs* peer straight ahead. (Prov 4:20–25)

The father's instruction includes at least five or six individual body parts, in addition to the foot. Fox continues his observation: "Although the imagery is of body organs, only the act of looking straight ahead (v. 25) could receive actual physical expression."[56] I would argue that the teachings to straighten the course one's foot plots, not deviate to the right or left, and turn one's foot away from evil, *all* imply

---

[53] Sheets-Johnstone, *Primacy of Movement*, 124. Italics in original. Among the "four primary qualitative structures of movement," Sheets-Johnstone describes "the linear quality with both the felt linear contour of our moving body and the linear paths we sense ourselves describing in the process of moving" (123). Or consider Fox's observation: "One's life course, as understood here, is not laid out in advance; rather, one must level or 'pave' it himself as he moves along, removing obstacles to moral progress" (*Proverbs 1–9*, 188). Given that fools meander (see, e.g., Prov 5:6 and my discussion below), we might assume they have no path. Nonetheless, the sages speak of the path of the wicked (e.g., Prov 2:12–15). Insofar as people tread the same foolish path, it too gets reproduced.

[54] Note, e.g., that the sages construe the verb "be firm" (כון) in opposition to the verb "be shaken" (מוט) in Prov 12:3. Cf. Prov 3:23, where walking on one's way securely is paired with "not stumbling" (נגף).

[55] Fox, *Proverbs 1–9*, 188.

[56] Fox, *Proverbs 1–9*, 188–89.

physical expression.⁵⁷ They aim to develop in the son self-control over his foot. The teachings regarding body parts, then, do more than depict metaphorically the proper moral disposition, as Fox argues. They instruct the son in the correct physical comportment of the various body parts, which in turn leads to the desired moral comportment.

Proverbs 5:1–23 (Lecture 8)

The final two passages I discuss provide counter examples for the father's kinesthetic instruction.

Lecture 8 (Prov 5:1–23) illustrates the Strange Woman's improper movements, both intentional and unintentional (as we observed in lecture 10). The father warns that "her feet [רגליה] descend [ירד] to Death, her steps [צעדיה] grasp [תמך] Sheol" (Prov 5:5).⁵⁸ The verb "grasp" (תמך) indicates controlled movement, suggesting that she marches purposefully toward Sheol, the abode of the dead, rather than without kinesthetic control, as we observed in Prov 7:15. In the next verse, the father adds that: "She does not straighten [פלס] the pathway [ארח] of life; her tracks [מעגלתיה] meander [נוע]" (Prov 5:6). The winding nature of her course indicates that she also suffers from an inability to control her movements. Translations interpret the last clause of verse 6 "she knows not" (לא תדע) to mean either that she does not know that her tracks meander or that she meanders for lack of knowledge.⁵⁹ Given the connection we have observed between moving and thinking, I propose that we read "knows not" in an absolute sense and interpret the clause to mean that she lacks knowledge *because* she moves improperly, whether deliberately or for want of self-control.⁶⁰

---

⁵⁷ Perhaps even inclining the ear, twisting the mouth, and contorting the lips were thought of as physical expressions.

⁵⁸ On 5:5, Fox observes: "Elsewhere *tamak* 'hold fast' is used of feet staying on the path only in Ps 17:5, where it is the opposite of tottering. Here the use of *tamak* suggests that the woman is deliberately proceeding with firm, secure strides to Sheol. Eventually, she too will fall, but for now she sticks to her path" (*Proverbs 1–9*, 192).

⁵⁹ The NRSV and Fox follow the former interpretation (*Proverbs 1–9*, 189). This reading assumes an unexpressed direct object "it," referring back to her meandering. The NJPS follows the latter interpretation. This latter reading construes cause and effect as follows: she lacks knowledge; therefore she wanders.

⁶⁰ For the use of ידע in the absolute sense to mean "have knowledge," see Isa 1:3, "An ox knows [ידע] its owner, and the donkey its master's crib, but Israel does not know [לא ידע], my people do not understand"; Isa 56:10, "The watchmen are blind, all of them, they perceive nothing [לא ידעו]. They are all dumb dogs that cannot bark"; and Eccl 9:11, "The race is not to the swift, nor the battle to the strong, nor bread to the wise, nor riches to the intelligent, nor favor to those who know [לידעים]."

Proverbs 1:8–19 (Lecture 1)

Finally, in Lecture 1 (Prov 1:8–19), a group of male sinners, like the Strange Woman in Lecture 10, provides a counter-example to the development of kinesthetic self-control.[61] Here the father cautions his son not to succumb to invitations from criminal elements to join them in wrongdoing. The father quotes the hypothetical words of the sinners, "Go with us" (לכה אתנו; 1:11). After describing in the sinners' own words the immoral acts they intend to commit, the father, mirroring the sinners' invitation, warns his son: "Don't go on the way with them" (אל־תלך בדרך אתם; 1:15). The added phrase "on the way" (בדרך) stresses the kinetic element inherent in the son's decision: he would be stepping onto the road down which the sinners go. The father's next directive builds upon the momentous decision about which path to take and emphasizes the need for kinesthetic control: "hold back your foot from their path" (מנע רגלך מנתיבתם; 1:15). The following motive clause invokes the dangerous movements of the sinners: "for their feet [רגליהם] run [רוץ] toward evil, and they rush [מהר] to shed blood" (1:16). Construing "their feet" (רגליהם) as the grammatical subject of "run" (ירוצו) heightens the sinners' lack of kinesthetic control: the sinners' feet, having a mind of their own, hasten toward evil.[62] Warning that the sinners' uncontrolled movements will result in their own harm, the father stresses the negative consequences of all those who travel these "pathways" (ארחות; 1:19).[63] The improper movements of the sinners obscure their knowledge: they fail to realize that the blood they hurry to shed is their own (1:18).[64]

---

[61] The term "sinners" (חטאים) derives from the same root as the verb "miss" (חטא) in Prov 19:2.

[62] See the nearly identical wording of Isa 59:7: רגליהם לרע ירצו וימהרו לשפך דם נקי. On the verb-subject disagreement in Prov 1:6a, see Fox, *Proverbs 1–9*, 88. To mitigate the gender disagreement, we could interpret the first clause as an adverbial accusative: "*They* (the sinners) run toward evil *by means of their feet*." If we permit the gender disagreement, we might also construe via ellipsis "their feet" as the subject of the verb "rush" in v. 16b. Recall Prov 6:18 "feet that hurriedly run [ממהרות לרוץ] toward evil" and the discussion above. Here in Prov 1:16, as in 6:18, the verbs "run" (רוץ) and "rush" (מהר) appear together. While "rush" always has negative connotations in Proverbs, "run" is neutral, and its valence depends on other factors. Clearly in the context of the sinners' quick movements toward evil and in parallel with "rush," the verb "run" here has negative connotations.

[63] The "pathways" of the sinners here may be understood in a double sense. It refers more abstractly to the life course chosen by the sinners and more concretely to the physical path the sinners take on their way to attack innocents. Thus Fox, *Proverbs 1–9*, 87.

[64] This passage fits with the idea of a deed-consequence nexus, first proposed by Klaus Koch, "Gibt es ein Vergeltungsdogma im Alten Testament?," *ZTK* 52 (1955): 1–42; Koch, "Is There a Doctrine of Retribution in the Old Testament?," in *Theodicy in the Old Testament*, ed. James L. Crenshaw (Philadelphia: Fortress, 1983), 57–87. The sinners think

CONCLUSION

What does this exploration of moving and thinking in Proverbs teach us about the role of kinesthesia in the pedagogical strategy of the book? I close with four brief observations.

First, the vignettes about the Strange Woman and the male sinners have been frequently allegorized. Here I have considered references to movement concretely to discern what such an approach might teach us about the nature of wisdom in Proverbs. By examining the body in motion, not as a metaphor but as cognition itself, we perceive that wisdom in Proverbs results from kinesthetic processes. To be sure, the book sometimes portrays moving on a path as a metaphor for journeying through life. Yet I would caution against viewing these instances as mere metaphors. Metaphors have consequences, and a metaphor's source domain matters greatly for interpretation.[65]

Second, theories about moving and thinking help us understand why the sages attended so amply to kinesthesia. As the original mode of thinking for animate forms, moving brings about corporeal consciousness or self-awareness. By moving through space, the body becomes an object for inquiry, for understanding who one is. So, too, moving in Proverbs provides the opportunity for the son to refine his sense of self. Skillfully navigating one's environment, straightening the track one's foot takes, and actively avoiding the path of death are in themselves forms of wisdom.[66]

The connection between moving and thinking in Proverbs can also be observed in the motricity of the mind itself. The book construes mental processes kinetically: the heart can turn away from the path it treads (7:25), it can incline toward understanding (2:2), and wisdom itself is kinetic, entering the heart of the son (2:10). Moving leads to cognition, and cognition itself is moving.

Third, the eye and the ear have long been acknowledged as physical organs for the acquisition of knowledge in Proverbs.[67] Alongside these celebrated organs

---

they are going to commit evil (רע) against an innocent person but fail to realize the evil toward which they run is the harm that will befall them! While Koch's thesis has been influential, scholars have also critiqued its applicability to Proverbs; see, e.g., Peter Hatton, "A Cautionary Tale: The Acts-Consequence 'Construct,'" *JSOT* 35 (2011): 375–84.

[65] On cognitive metaphor theory, see George Lakoff and Mark Johnson, *Philosophy in the Flesh: The Embodied Mind and Its Challenge to Western Thought* (New York: Basic Books, 1999); Lakoff and Johnson, *Metaphors We Live By* (Chicago: University of Chicago Press, 1980).

[66] The idea that Proverbs construes a sense such as kinesthesia as a form of wisdom is not without parallel; the book explicitly identifies the sense of taste with wisdom: Prov 11:22; 26:16; 31:18.

[67] About "the pupil of the eye" in Prov 7:2, Fox writes: "As the organ of sight, it is the physical medium of knowledge, alongside the ear" (*Proverbs 1–9*, 239).

we must also include the lowly foot as a medium for obtaining wisdom. The foot does more than enact the will of the heart; it also shapes the will. A foot that treads the path of life exercises kinesthetic self-control and thereby enhances the will to behave in an upright manner.

Finally, moving properly enhances wisdom, while moving improperly diminishes it. For this reason, the sages engaged in a regimen of kinesthetic training, steering the student's foot away from deadly paths and onto the path of life. This regimen sought to create in the student the ability to govern the movements of his own feet. Such kinesthetic control required the development of kinesthetic awareness, the awareness of whether one's movements were proper or not. Part of the training regimen, therefore, included instruction in kinesthetic feedback. The sages described what it was like to walk the path of life versus the path of death. If the student sensed that his path inscribed a smooth, level, linear projection without stumbling blocks, he knew he was on the right path. If his foot meandered, moved with great difficulty, or tripped over obstacles, he knew he was on the wrong path. Such kinesthetic awareness is itself a kind of wisdom.

Bibliography

Avrahami, Yael. *The Senses of Scripture: Sensory Perception in the Hebrew Bible*. LHBOTS 545. London: T&T Clark International, 2012.

Bourdieu, Pierre. *Outline of a Theory of Practice*. Translated by Richard Nice. Cambridge Studies in Social and Cultural Anthropology 16. Cambridge: Cambridge University Press, 1977.

Bull, Cynthia J. "Sense, Meaning, and Perception in Three Dance Cultures." Pages 269–87 in *Meaning in Motion: New Cultural Studies of Dance*. Edited by Jane Desmond. Durham: Duke University Press, 1997.

Foster, Susan Leigh. "Dancing Bodies." Pages 235–57 in *Meaning in Motion: New Cultural Studies of Dance*. Edited by Jane Desmond. Durham: Duke University Press, 1997.

Fox, Michael V. *Proverbs 1–9: A New Translation with Introduction and Commentary*. AB 18A. New York: Doubleday, 2000.

Geurts, Kathryn Linn. *Culture and the Senses: Bodily Ways of Knowing in an African Community*. Ethnographic Studies in Subjectivity. Berkeley: University of California Press, 2002.

Goering, Greg Schmidt. "Tactile Discipline: The Sense of Touch in the Book of Proverbs." Paper presented at the Annual Meeting of the Society of Biblical Literature. Chicago, IL, 18 November 2012.

Hahn, Tomie. "Bodies as Fieldsites: Considering the Senses in Research and Performance." Paper presented to the University of Virginia Music Department Colloquium. Charlottesville, VA, 16 September 2016.

———. *Sensational Knowledge: Embodying Culture through Japanese Dance*. Middletown: Wesleyan University Press, 2007.

Hatton, Peter. "A Cautionary Tale: The Acts-Consequence 'Construct.'" *JSOT* 35 (2011): 375–84.
Koch, Klaus. "Gibt es ein Vergeltungsdogma im Alten Testament?" *ZTK* 52 (1955): 1–42.
———. "Is There a Doctrine of Retribution in the Old Testament?" Pages 57–87 in *Theodicy in the Old Testament*. Edited by James L. Crenshaw. Philadelphia: Fortress, 1983.
Kugel, James L. *The Idea of Biblical Poetry: Parallelism and Its History*. Baltimore: Johns Hopkins, 1981.
Lakoff, George, and Mark Johnson. *Metaphors We Live By*. Chicago: University of Chicago Press, 1980.
———. *Philosophy in the Flesh: The Embodied Mind and Its Challenge to Western Thought*. New York: Basic Books, 1999.
Llinás, Rodolfo R. *I of the Vortex: From Neurons to Self*. Cambridge: MIT Press, 2001.
Schiffman, Harvey Richard. "The Skin, Body, and Chemical Senses." Pages 70–96 in *Sensation and Perception*. Edited by Richard L. Gregory and Andrew M. Colman. Essex: Longman, 1995.
Sheets-Johnstone, Maxine. *The Primacy of Movement*. 2nd ed. Advances in Consciousness Research 82. Amsterdam: Benjamins, 2011.
Stoller, Paul. *The Taste of Ethnographic Things: The Senses in Anthropology*. Philadelphia: University of Pennsylvania Press, 1989.
Tilford, Nicole L. *Sensing World, Sensing Wisdom: The Cognitive Foundation of Biblical Metaphors*. AIL 31. Atlanta: SBL Press, 2017.

ON THE SENSE OF BALANCE IN THE HEBREW BIBLE

Thomas Krüger

In this article I would like to draw attention to some passages in the Hebrew Bible that are related to the sense of balance. Within the limits of this paper, it is not possible to provide more than a brief and preliminary overview, which may inspire further, more detailed and more in-depth research.

By sense of balance (or equilibrium) I mean the sense(s) that help(s) people determine whether they sit, stand, or walk in an upright position. There are overlaps, but also differences, between the sense of balance (equilibrioception), the sense of movement (kinesthesia), and the sense of position (or position and movement: proprioception), each of which respectively covers a wider range of sense functions than the sense of balance.[1]

It can be assumed that the ancient Hebrews were able to sit, to stand, and to walk in an upright position. Perhaps they would also have acknowledged the existence of something like a sense of balance, even if probably they would not have called it a sense.[2] To my knowledge, there is no word for sense in the Hebrew

---

[1] My impression is that the terms *kinesthesia* and *proprioception* are not uniformly used in the academic literature on the physiology of the senses; see, e.g., *Encyclopaedia Britannica*, "Human sensory reception," https://www.britannica.com/science/human-sensory-reception; Frédérique de Vignemont, "Bodily Awareness," in *The Stanford Encyclopedia of Philosophy*, ed. Edward N. Zalta, spring 2018 ed., plato.stanford.edu/archives/spr2018/entries/bodily-awareness/. Phenomenologically, the distinction between balance, movement, and bodily posture appears to be plausible and comprehensible; see, e.g., Mădălina Diaconu, *Phänomenologie der Sinne*, Grundwissen Philosophie (Stuttgart: Reclam, 2013).

[2] For instructive comparative cases, see Kathryn Linn Geurts, *Culture and the Senses: Bodily Ways of Knowing in an African Community* (Berkeley: University of California Press, 2002), esp. 71–84, 144–65; Geurts, "Consciousness as 'Feeling in the Body': A West African Theory of Embodiment, Emotion and the Making of the Mind," in *Empire of the Senses*, ed. David Howes (Oxford: Berg, 2005), 164–78. See also Yael Avrahami, *The Senses of Scripture: Sensory Perception in the Hebrew Bible*, LHBOTS 545 (London: T&T Clark, 2012), 75–84, Nicole L. Tilford, *Sensing World, Sensing Wisdom: The Cognitive*

Bible, like modern Hebrew חוש or טעם, maybe with the exception of Prov 31:18 (where the verb טעם may mean "perceive" or "sense") and Job 20:2 (where the noun חוש may mean "perception" or "sense").[3]

Since there is no term for "balance" in the Hebrew Bible, we have to look for descriptions of the phenomenon in the biblical texts. When we do so, it turns out that there are far more instances of someone failing to maintain balance than of someone maintaining balance without problems. If a person loses balance, they have trouble standing upright or walking straightforward. They start to sway or stagger, to reel or totter. Subsequently they may fall over, or they may regain their equilibrium.

Why People Lose Balance

In the Hebrew Bible, the loss of balance may be caused by drunkenness or dizziness, by being on a ship in heavy swell or riding in a swaying cart, by stumbling or slipping, or by being pushed or overthrown by a snare. Two of these reasons are often mentioned together: drunkenness and heavy swell. In Prov 23:33–34 a teacher cautions his pupils against drinking too much wine by describing the annoying side effects of drunkenness:

> Your eyes will see strange things,
> and your mind utter perverse things.
> You will be like one who lies down in the midst of the sea,
> like one who lies on the top of a mast.
> (NRSV)

A drunken person feels like a sailor in a crow's nest. He stands on shaky ground. Everything around him sways to and fro. He becomes dizzy and loses his balance. He has trouble standing upright and walking straightforward. But in the case of the sailor in a storm everything around him actually sways to and fro, whereas the swaying is only an illusion in the case of the drunk person. He is not thrown out of balance by a swaying environment, but by a breakdown of his sense of equilibrium under the influence of alcohol, which affects not only his sense of balance but also his sense of sight ("your eyes will see strange things") and his mind ("your mind [lit., 'heart'] will utter perverse things").

Foundation of Biblical Metaphors, AIL 31 (Atlanta: SBL Press, 2017), 149–72, and Greg Schmidt-Goering's article in this volume.

[3] Prov 31:18: "She perceives [טעם] that her merchandise is profitable" (NRSV). In Job 20:2 חוש stands in parallel to שעפים ("disquieting thoughts") and thus may mean "feel (pain)" (*CDCH*, s.v. "חוש II"; cf. NJPS) rather than "be agitated" (NRSV) or "disturbed" (NIV), lit., "hasten" (ESV; *CDCH*, s.v. "חוש I").

In Prov 23 drunkenness is compared to seasickness; in Ps 107 seasickness is compared to drunkenness. (Perhaps the difference is because the teacher in Prov 23 thinks that his pupils have no personal experience with drunkenness and that it is easier for them to imagine seasickness, whereas the author of Ps 107 thought that his readers were more acquainted with drinking than with seafaring.)

> Some went down to the sea in ships,
> doing business on the mighty waters;
> they saw the deeds of Yahweh,
> his wondrous works in the deep.
> For he commanded and raised the stormy wind,
> which lifted up the waves of the sea.
> They mounted up to heaven,
> they went down to the depths;
> their courage [נפש] melted away in their calamity;
> they reeled [חגג] and staggered [נוע] like drunkards,
> and were at their wits' end [lit., and their wisdom was ruined].
> (Ps 107:23–27, NRSV [modified])

Isaiah accuses priests and prophets of "reeling" (שגה) with wine and "staggering" (תעה) with strong drink, even when they have a vision or give judgment, and vomiting on all tables and in all places (Isa 28:7–8). As in many other cases, it is not clear whether these reproaches are meant literally or figuratively or both. The same is true of Hab 2:15–16:

> Alas for you who make your neighbors drink,
> pouring out your wrath until they are drunk,
> in order to gaze on their nakedness!
> You will be sated with contempt instead of glory.
> Drink, you yourself, and stagger [רעל N][4]!
> The cup in Yahweh's right hand will come around to you,
> and shame will come upon your glory!
> (NRSV [modified])

This text takes it for granted that drunk people do not shy away from showing their nakedness and that they stagger—and that both, showing oneself naked and staggering, are dishonorable and degrading behaviors. The accused person humiliated others and therefore will be humiliated by Yahweh in recompense for his evildoing.

---

[4] Reading (with the ancient versions) והרעל (*CDCH*, s.v. "רעל I," N: "stagger, reel") instead of והערל (*CDCH*, s.v. "ערל," N: "show the foreskin, i.e. expose oneself, or perh. act as one uncircumcised"); cf. *BHQ*.

Habakkuk 2:15–16 is not the only instance in the Hebrew Bible where Yahweh punishes people by making them drunk and stagger (Isa 19:13–14; 51:17–23; Jer 25:15–28; Zech 12:2–3; Ps 60:3–5; cf. Job 12:24–25) or just by making them stagger (Isa 29:9–10; 1 Kgs 14:15; Deut 32:35) or stumble (Isa 8:14–15; Jer 20:11; 23:12; 46:6; 50:32; Hos 4:5). In these instances, staggering probably has not only the connotation of humiliation, but also of weakness. When Lev 25:35 speaks about a person who "becomes poor" (ימוך, from מוך) and "whose hand totters" (ומטה ידו, from מוט), it means that the person is too weak to maintain "a minimum of economic independence."[5] Accordingly, the participle כושל ("stumbling") sometimes "denotes someone who cannot walk because he has fallen or is exhausted (Isa 5:27; Ps 105:37; Job 4:4; 2 Chr 28:15)." It "can also refer to someone weak with age (Sir 42:8; 1QSa 2:7)."[6] Likewise, it is a sign that an image of a deity is weak, if one needs "to fasten it with nails so that it will not totter" (לא ימוט: Isa 41:7; cf. Isa 40:20).[7]

Besides seasickness and drunkenness, the Hebrew Bible mentions bearing a heavy load as a cause of losing one's balance. Thus Isa 24:19–20 describes how

> The earth is utterly broken,
> the earth is torn asunder,
> the earth is violently shaken [מוט התמוטטה].
> The earth staggers [נוע תנוע] like a drunkard,
> it sways [והתנודדה, from נוד] like a hut;
> its transgression lies heavy upon it,
> and it falls, and will not rise again.
> (NRSV)

Lamentations 5:13 reports that "boys stagger [כשל] under loads of wood" (NRSV). Perhaps another instance is Amos 2:13, if the Hebrew verb עוק H in this context means "make sway."[8] Then Yahweh says here:

> I will make it sway [מעיק] under you,
> just as a cart makes sway [תעיק] [those sitting on it?] when it is full of sheaves.

Proverbs 5:18–23 mentions love as another cause of staggering, if one translates the verb שגה here as "stagger" (which is one of the attested meanings of the verb in Classical Hebrew):

---

[5] Arnulf Baumann, "מוט," *TDOT* 8:154.

[6] Christoph Barth, "כשל," *TDOT* 7:355.

[7] Baumann, "מוט," 8:156.

[8] Other possible meanings are "press," "hinder/be hindered," "roar/cause a roar," and "split/make a furrow," see *DCH*, s.v. עוק.

> Let your fountain be blessed,
> and rejoice in the wife of your youth,
> a lovely deer,
> a graceful doe.
> May her breasts satisfy you at all times;
> may you stagger [שגה] always by her love.
> Why should you stagger [שגה], my son, by another woman
> and embrace the bosom of an adulteress?
> For human ways are under the eyes of Yahweh,
> and he examines all their paths.
> The iniquities of the wicked ensnare them,
> and they are caught in the toils of their sin.
> They die for lack of discipline,
> and because of their great folly they stagger [שגה].

If this translation is correct, the passage shows that the weakness connoted by staggering is not always assessed as bad.

More tangible causes for losing one's balance in the Hebrew Bible are being struck or thrusted (1 Kgs 14:15; Job 12:15; Amos 9:5); stumbling over an obstacle, maybe a hump, a stone, or a corpse (Jer 31:9; 46:12; Nah 3:3); running into a trap (Job 18:7–10); or slipping on greasy ground (Jer 23:12).

"PROPER" AND "FIGURATIVE" MEANINGS

Frequently it is said that the foot, gait, or step of a person, or their knees, hips, or loins, stagger or stumble or slip (מוט, מעד, כשל, etc.),[9] as for instance in Ps 73:2:

> my feet had almost stumbled [נטה Gp];
> my steps had nearly slipped [שפך Gp].
> (NRSV)

Should this manner of speaking be understood as pars pro toto, the foot representing the whole person? Or is the foot here envisaged as some kind of organ for the sense of balance (like the seeing eye or the hearing ear)?

In view of the Hebrew texts and considering basic theoretical questions of semantics, it appears difficult and problematic to distinguish between a "proper" manner of speaking about balance in the Hebrew Bible and a "figurative" or "metaphorical" one.[10] However, in the majority of cases, it is possible to distinguish texts where it is more or less evident that they talk about balance and its problems in a bodily sense from texts that envisage a broader view of the phenomenon.

---

[9] See Barth, "כשל," 7:354.
[10] Barth, "כשל," 7:357–58.

There is also a reasonably clear difference between texts that talk about human beings or animals, on the one hand, and those that talk about things like the earth, mountains, a city, a hut, or a wall.

Manners of speaking about balance:

	regarding living beings	regarding inanimate things
in a bodily sense		
in a broader sense		

But even this distinction can be questioned, because it is far from clear that the ancient Hebrews would have agreed with our distinctions between animate and inanimate beings—not to mention that they may have had different conceptions of the body. With these reservations in mind, I shall now briefly and by way of example discuss the different manners of speaking about balance in the Hebrew Bible.

When "boys stagger [כשל] under loads of wood" (Lam 5:13 NRSV), the expression refers fairly unambiguously to problems of living beings who have balance in a bodily sense. The same appears to be true in principle for the following passage from a prophetic oracle:

> [God] will raise a signal for a nation far away,
> and whistle for a people at the ends of the earth;
> Here they come, swiftly, speedily!
> None of them is weary, none stumbles [כשל],
> none slumbers or sleeps,
> not a loincloth is loose,
> not a sandal-thong broken;
> their arrows are sharp,
> all their bows bent,
> their horses' hoofs seem like flint,
> and their wheels like the whirlwind.
> (Isa 5:26–28 NRSV)

The text sets before the eyes of the readers an image of a strong and well equipped army marching in combat column. None of the soldiers are tired or stumble or sleep in a literary sense. However, the text's rhetoric is obviously hyperbolic, and the concrete image illustrates the more abstract notion of an unshakeable and irresistible army.

When speakers of psalms utter their confidence that they will not be shaken (Psa 16:8; 30:7; 62:3, 7), their fear that they will stumble (Ps 38:18), or their hope that their enemies will stumble (Ps 27:2; Jer 20:11), they probably do not refer to tumbling and stumbling in a physical sense, or at least not only in a physical sense but also in a broader sense. In the words of Christoph Barth, the notion of "drastic disaster on the way" can refer more narrowly to concrete "disaster on the road" or more broadly to "disaster in life."[11]

The latter is quite obviously true for the way of speaking about the stumbling or the not stumbling of righteous or wicked people, or wise and foolish people, as the following examples from Prov 4 may illustrate:

> I have taught you the way of wisdom;
> I have led you in the paths of uprightness.
> When you walk, your step will not be hampered;
> and if you run, you will not stumble [כשל].
> (Prov 4:11–12 NRSV)

> The way of the wicked is like deep darkness;
> they do not know what they stumble over [כשל].
> (Prov 4:19 NRSV)

Even here, a concrete bodily understanding of tumbling and stumbling cannot be excluded completely. Traveling by foot was probably more dangerous in ancient times than today, and injuries caused by stumbling and falling were more threatening for the ancient Hebrews than for us. Nevertheless, it appears quite evident that a broader understanding is more appropriate in this context.

"Disaster on the road" or "in life" can refer to calamity or failure, as in the above examples or in Prov 10:30:

> The righteous will never be removed [lit., "will not stagger," בל־ימוט],
> but the wicked will not remain [or "abide," לא ישכנו־ארץ] in the land.
> (NRSV)

However, tumbling, stumbling, or falling on one's way can also symbolize moral weakness or mistakes, as in the following instances: "I have trusted in Yahweh without wavering [or 'I will not waver,' לא אמעד]" (Ps 26:1 NRSV). More clearly:

> My feet had almost stumbled [or: slipped: נטה Gp];
> my steps had nearly slipped [שפך Dp].
> For I was envious of the arrogant;
> I saw the prosperity of the wicked.
> (Ps 73:2–3 NRSV)

---

[11] Barth, "כָּשַׁל," 7:358.

> Like a muddied spring or a polluted fountain
> are the righteous who give way [lit., "stagger," מט] before the wicked.
> (Prov 25:26 NRSV)

> But my people have forgotten me,
> they burn offerings to a delusion;
> they have stumbled in their ways, in the ancient roads,
> and have gone into bypaths, not the highway.
> (Jer 18:15 NRSV)

The loss of balance—in a narrower or in a broader sense—can affect not only an individual being but also a collective (see Amos 8:12) like Israel and/or Judah and/or Jerusalem (1 Kgs 14:5; Isa 3:8; 8:14; 51:17, 22), cities (Amos 4:8), kingdoms (Ps 46:7), Egypt (Isa 19:13), one or more other nations (Ps 60:5; Jer 18:15; 25:16; Zech 12:2), or the whole world (Ps 99:1).

Examples of inanimate beings tumbling and/or stumbling in a bodily sense are a cart (Amos 2:13), a hut (Isa 24:20), Mount Zion (Ps 125:1), and the city of God (Ps 46:6). In the latter two instances one may ask whether the meaning is concrete and bodily or broader and more abstract.

The same is true for the following examples speaking of the balance or imbalance of the earth:

> [God] has established the world;
> it shall never be moved [or "shaken," מוט N].
> (Ps 93:1 NRSV)

> [He] set the earth on its foundations,
> so that it shall never be shaken [מוט N].
> (Ps 104:5 NRSV)

> [He] looks on the earth and it trembles [רעד],
> [he] touches the mountains and they smoke.
> (Ps 104:32 NRSV)

It appears that according to Ps 104 the earth will never "be shaken" (מוט N), but it may "tremble" (רעד). In Ps 104 it is only God who is able to make the earth tremble, whereas in Ps 75 God leaves open who makes the earth totter:

> When the earth totters [מוג N], with all its inhabitants,
> it is I who keep its pillars steady [תכן D].
> (Ps 75:4 NRSV)

The three psalms agree that the stability of the world is the work of God.

Complementary to the picture of God as guarantor of the stability of a well-ordered world is the picture of God as the one who throws an unjust and corrupted world off balance, as in the following examples:

> The earth reeled [געש] and rocked [רעש];
> the foundations of the heavens trembled [רגז] and quaked [געש HtD],
> because he was angry.
> (2 Sam 22:8 = Ps 18:8 NRSV)

> You have caused the land to quake [רעש H];
> you have torn it open;
> repair the cracks in it, for it is tottering [מוט].
> (Ps 60:4 NRSV)

> The pillars of heaven tremble [or "shake," רפף Lp],
> and are astounded at his rebuke.
> (Job 26:11 NRSV)

> Yahweh is king; let the peoples tremble [רגז]!
> He sits enthroned upon the cherubim;
> let the earth quake [or "shake," נוט]!
> (Ps 99:1 NRSV)

According to Ps 46, the city of God is an island of stability in a world out of balance:

> God is our refuge and strength,
> a very present help in trouble.
> Therefore we will not fear,
> though the earth should change [מור H],[12]
> though the mountains shake [מוט] in the heart of the sea;
> though its waters roar and foam,
> though the mountains tremble [רעש] with its tumult …
> There is a river whose streams make glad the city of God,
> the holy habitation of the Most High.
> God is in the midst of the city;
> it shall not be moved [or "shaken," מוט N];
> God will help it when the morning dawns.
> The nations are in an uproar,
> the kingdoms totter [מוט];
> he utters his voice,

---

[12] Reading והמור (or והמר) instead of והמיר (*CDCH*, s.v. "מור I," H: "change, alter") one could also translate "though the earth should quake/shake" (*CDCH*, s.v. "מור II," N); cf. NJPS: "though the earth reels."

the earth melts.
Yahweh of hosts is with us;
the God of Jacob is our refuge.
(Ps 46:1–7 NRSV)

Isaiah 54 takes the view that God is more stable than the world:

For the mountains may depart [מוש]
and the hills be removed [or "stagger," מוט],
but my steadfast love shall not depart [מוש] from you,
and my covenant of peace shall not be removed [or "stagger," מוט],
says Yahweh, who has compassion on you.
(Isa 54:10 NRSV)

Here the notion of imbalance refers to an abstract entity, Yahweh's covenant of peace, like truth in Isa 59:

Justice is turned back,
and righteousness stands at a distance;
for truth stumbles [כשל] in the public square,
and uprightness cannot enter.
(Isa 59:14 NRSV)

Conclusion

This brief and preliminary review of the sense of balance in the Hebrew Bible brings me to the following conclusion: the sense of balance is a matter of some consequence for the worldview of the Hebrew Bible. In the culture expressed or construed by this corpus of writings, balance and stability are highly valued. For individual humans, it was important not to tumble or stumble (see above), or not to fall if they did stumble (Ps 37:23–24), or to stand up again if they have fallen (Prov 24:16). Ideally, righteous, wise, and pious people should not tumble and stumble, whereas the wicked and the enemies should do so (Prov 10:30). If other people stumble and fall down, solidarity demanded that the righteous help them stand up again (Lev 25:35; Isa 35:3; Job 4:4; 12:5).

Also in the broader view of the world, stability and balance were fundamental for a good order and well-being. When the gods do not care for justice, "all the foundations of the earth are shaken" (Ps 82:5 NRSV). In view of such disturbances of balance and stability, Yahweh is expected to secure or restore equilibrium. However, there are also texts that see the world as stable but deeply corrupted. From this point of view, the only hope may be that God will shake the earth and throw the corrupt structures out of balance.

BIBLIOGRAPHY

Avrahami, Yael. *The Senses of Scripture: Sensory Perception in the Hebrew Bible*. LHBOTS 545. London: T&T Clark, 2012.
Barth, Christoph. "בשל." *TDOT* 7:353–60.
Baumann, Arnulf. "מוט." *TDOT* 8:152–58.
Diaconu, Mădălina. *Phänomenologie der Sinne*. Grundwissen Philosophie. Stuttgart: Reclam, 2013.
Geurts, Kathryn Linn. "Consciousness as 'Feeling in the Body': A West African Theory of Embodiment, Emotion and the Making of the Mind." Pages 164–78 in *Empire of the Senses*. Edited by David Howes. Oxford: Berg, 2005.
———. *Culture and the Senses: Bodily Ways of Knowing in an African Community*. Berkeley: University of California Press, 2002.
Tilford, Nicole L. *Sensing World, Sensing Wisdom: The Cognitive Foundation of Biblical Metaphors.* AIL 31. Atlanta: SBL Press, 2017
Vignemont, Frédérique de. "Bodily Awareness." In *The Stanford Encyclopedia of Philosophy*. Edited by Edward N. Zalta. Spring 2018 ed. plato.stanford.edu/archives/spr2018/entries/bodily-awareness/

TASTING METAPHOR IN ANCIENT ISRAEL

Pierre Van Hecke

Whoever browses through the references to the senses in the Hebrew Bible will notice their frequent metaphorical use. The following examples illustrate some of these nonliteral uses of the different senses:

(1) Gen 2:19
ויבא אל־האדם לראות מה־יקרא־לו
and [God] brought them to the man to *see* what he would call them.[1]

(2) 1 Kgs 3:9
ונתת לעבדך לב שמע לשפט את־עמך
Give your servant therefore *a listening heart*[2] to govern your people.

(3) Ps 34:9
טעמו וראו כי־טוב יהוה
O *taste* and *see* that the LORD is good.

Even though these verses are easy enough to understand for English speakers, the sensory verbs are all used in a figurative, nonliteral way, a linguistic phenomenon which is as common as it is fascinating. God is able to *hear* which names Adam gives to the animals but is not able to *see* this name-giving. Similarly, Solomon is not praying for a heart that can literally *hear*; rather, he is praying for an understanding mind. Finally, God's goodness is not something that can be literally *seen* and even less *tasted* with the senses, though in the Bible God's goodness may find expression in observable events and God is sometimes portrayed as the provider of food (e.g., Ps 145:15).

I wish to thank Thomas Krüger and Annette Schellenberg, the organizers of the Sounding Sensory Profiles Conference (Vienna, March 2017), for their kind invitation and for fostering this important conference and academic exchange.

[1] All biblical quotations are taken from the NRSV unless mentioned otherwise. Italics by P. Van Hecke.

[2] NRSV: "an understanding mind."

Metaphors, especially sensory metaphors, are thus ubiquitous in the biblical writings. In this contribution, I wish to highlight one particular group of metaphors, namely, those metaphors that, like Ps 34:9 mentioned above, make use of the sense of taste. The question I wish to raise is what these metaphors mean in their contexts. Does it make any difference to *taste* God's goodness rather than to *see* it? What does Job mean when he describes his situation as saltless or tasteless as the white of an egg (Job 6:6)? Why does the psalmist speak about God's word as if it is as sweet as honey to the palate? In order to answer these questions, it is important to first briefly reflect on the way metaphors function in our speech and our thinking. Subsequently, I will turn to the characteristic of the gustatory sense that plays a role in metaphorical uses, after which a systematic analysis of these metaphorical uses in the Hebrew Bible will be presented.

1. The Functioning of Metaphor

Ever since Aristotle, much thinking and writing has been devoted to the phenomenon of metaphor.[3] This is not without reason, since metaphors constitute a peculiar linguistic phenomenon. In a metaphor, a word (or several words) is used not in its literal meaning; rather a word is used figuratively in a context in which it usually does not feature. As shown in the examples above, this is a very common feature of language, but why do people turn to this kind of language use? Why are words used outside of their common, literal meanings? Does this not lead to unwanted confusion and lack of precision? The difficulty Bible translations sometimes seem to encounter in dealing with metaphor illustrates the point: translators regularly avoid taking over the metaphor for fear that it might confuse the readers. While the sensory metaphors from Ps 34:9 quoted above are translated literally as "taste and see" in most English translations, the JPS translation (1917), for example, decides to render the first verb more cognitively as "*consider* (and see)." The French Louis Segond translation, to give another example, apparently opines that a different sense would fit the context better and translates "sentez et voyez," the first verb meaning either "to feel" or "to smell." Both translations consider the metaphor of tasting or savoring God's goodness to be conceptually problematic.

What this demonstrates is that metaphors make readers (including translators) think. And that is precisely their function. Rather than a phenomenon of language, metaphors are firstly a matter of human thinking, as scholars have repeated throughout the centuries. To quote George Lakoff and Mark Johnson, who revived the scholarly attention to this function: "The essence of metaphor is understanding

---

[3] Aristotle, *Poet.* 21.1457b6–7; 22.1458a21–23; *Rhet.* 3.2, passim. See John T. Kirkby, "Aristotle on Metaphor," *AJP* 118 (1997): 517–54.

and experiencing one kind of thing in terms of another."[4] This is what happens in Ps 34: the authors use the common human knowledge of taste to understand and explain what the experience of God's goodness could be like. Lakoff and Johnson also pointed to another aspect of metaphor, namely, that it is not limited to or specific of poetic language; our daily language is replete with examples of this thought pattern. Take the following examples:

> I *see* what you mean.
> This *sheds a new light* on the whole issue.
> The investigators *remain in the dark*.

These three sentences describe the (in)ability to understand or to know something using the sense of vision. Just as one is able to see objects or events with the eyes, it is possible to *see* what someone means. The reason why we use this type of language is that our experiences of seeing are more directly accessible and more easily put into words than our cognitive activity; we hence use our knowledge of the former to think analogically about the latter. And we do so in quite a consistent way. As light is a necessary condition for seeing, we use concepts of light and darkness to speak metaphorically about our thoughts. New elements leading to new *insights* are conceptualized as *shedding new light*, whereas our inability to understand certain aspects is consistently described as *remaining in the dark*. Examples such as these demonstrate that metaphors are not isolated instances of word use but are conceptually related. Cognitive metaphor theory argues that in metaphor our knowledge of one conceptual domain—the source domain—is used to gain insight into a different, nonrelated domain—the target domain—since the latter is less directly accessible to our understanding.[5] Aspects of the source domain are subsequently mapped onto the target domain in order to gain a better understanding of the latter. In our latter example, the elements of *light* and *darkness* from the source domain of VISION are mapped onto the target domain of KNOWLEDGE, specifically describing the resources facilitating knowledge and the obstacles standing in its way.

Understanding this mapping operation involves interpretation, especially when dealing with less frequently used metaphors or with metaphors taken from a language and culture that is not ours. To return to our example of Ps 34, it is not immediately clear what *tasting* God's goodness precisely means or if that *tasting* is any different from *seeing* divine goodness. Interpreting and understanding metaphors involves a number of steps. First, it is necessary to have a solid knowledge of the source domain of the metaphor. That is why the specific characteristics of

---

[4] George Lakoff and Mark Johnson, *Metaphors We Live By* (Chicago: University of Chicago Press, 1980), 5.

[5] Lakoff and Johnson, *Metaphors We Live By*, 14–21.

the gustatory sense will be analyzed in the next paragraph, as a precondition to understanding what it means, for example, that Job regards his life as *tasteless*. It is important to stress here that not all aspects of the source domain are transferred to the target domain in a metaphor.[6] In more technical terms: each metaphorical conceptualization is partial or selective.[7] An example will make this clear. When God is described metaphorically as a shepherd, many aspects of the source domain of PASTORALISM are mapped onto God's activities, for instance, the knowledge that the shepherd is responsible for the well-being of the flock by providing them with food and physical care and the knowledge that shepherds are expected to protect the flock from external threats, like robbers or wild animals. These pastoral activities are easily transferred to God as a shepherd. When speaking of God, however, other aspects of the pastoral business remain completely out of sight, for example, the knowledge that shepherds eventually try to make a living by tending their flocks and therefore regularly sell or slaughter animals. It is clear that this—central—aspect of animal husbandry is not mapped onto God's dealings with people. To have knowledge of the source domain and to know which elements of it are mapped or transferred is therefore crucial for the interpretation of metaphor. A thorough acquaintance with the target domain is also necessary: in order to assess whether the selling of sheep is a characteristic that is metaphorically applicable to God, it is necessary to know how God is conceptualized elsewhere in the Hebrew Bible. Technically speaking, metaphors should comply with what Lakoff termed the invariance principle, which states that mappings from the source domain can only be accepted when they do not violate the basic structure of the target domain.[8]

2. THE METAPHORICAL USE OF TASTE

On the basis of these insights, we can ask how the source domain of TASTE is used metaphorically in the Hebrew Bible. The first question should pertain to the characteristics of the source domain, in other words, to what is typical of the gustatory sense. As with all senses, a distinction should be made between the perception itself and the intentional direction of the sensory attention. For a number of senses, our languages' vocabulary makes a distinction between both aspects, for example, the distinction between *seeing* and *watching* or between *hearing* and *listening*. The second verb of each pair expresses the intentional use of the sense: watching is directing the attention in order to see something, whereas listening is wanting

---

[6] As the ancients knew: "Omnis comparatio claudicat nisi in puncto comparationis" ("Every comparison limps, except in the point of comparison").

[7] Lakoff and Johnson, *Metaphors We Live By*, 52–55.

[8] George Lakoff, "The Invariance Hypothesis: Is Abstract Reason Based on Image-Schemas?," *Cognitive Linguistics* 1 (1990): 39–74.

to hear. Both aspects do not coincide, however: one can listen without hearing, and hear something without consciously having listened. For the sense of taste, the issue is more complicated: the verb "to taste" can, on the one hand, express the sheer perception ("He couldn't taste anything because he had a cold.") and, on the other hand, the intentional aspect of it ("I tasted the soup and thought it was too salty."). The verb, moreover, also means "to have a taste," as in "the cake tastes delicious."

Hebrew, too, only has one verb to express both aspects of tasting, namely, טעם. This immediately raises an interpretational question in the case of Ps 34:9: does the psalmist invite the reader to experience that God is good (perception) or to test this goodness carefully (intention)? The fact that the following verb (ראה) expresses both the perceptive "to see" and the intentional "to watch"[9] does not help to solve the issue. The following object clause leaves little doubt, however, that the former meaning is intended: the reader is called to taste and see *that* God is good, not *whether* God is good. Also, in Prov 31:18, the verb טעם has the meaning of "experiencing." In this well-known Song of the Valiant Woman, the protagonist is said to "*taste* that her business profit is good," meaning that she perceives or experiences that such is the case, as most translations render the verb.[10] In other cases, however, the verb has the meaning of intentional tasting, as one can read, for example, in Job 12:11: "Does not the ear test words as the palate tastes food?"

The sense of taste is distinct from the other senses on a number of important points, which also affects the way it is used metaphorically.[11] First, an important characteristic of the gustatory sense is that the taste stimuli—like the olfactory stimuli, for that matter—are activated by direct contact with the molecules of the perceived object itself. Whereas vision and hearing only perceive waves emitted by the object, tasting and smelling involves parts of the perceived object entering the body and coming into contact with the gustatory and olfactory receptor neurons. The direct consequence thereof is that the taste of an object is a strongly individual property of that object. This is precisely the reason why a top chef will personally taste each dish that leaves the kitchen. Using the correct ingredients and faithfully following the recipe will not guarantee that the taste will be precisely as the cook had in mind. Only tasting the dish and adding ingredients "to

---

[9] See also Pierre Van Hecke, "The Verbs ראה and שמע in the Book of Qohelet: A Cognitive-Semantic Perspective," in *The Language of Qohelet in Its Context: Essays in Honor of Prof. A. Schoors on the Occasion of His Seventieth Birthday*, ed. Angelika Berlejung and Pierre Van Hecke, OLA 164 (Leuven: Peeters, 2007), 203–20.

[10] NRSV: "She perceives that her merchandise is profitable"; NIV: "She sees that her trading is profitable."

[11] An excellent description of the following aspects of the gustatory sense can be found in Priscilla Parkhurst Ferguson, "The Senses of Taste," *AHR* 116 (2011): 371–84.

taste" can do so.¹² A second characteristic of the sense of taste is intimately connected with the previous: as with the tactile sense, taste implies direct physical contact with the perceived object. One cannot taste something from a distance, one has to touch it and even bring it inside the body. In this, the sense of taste is the most proximal of senses, in contrast to the more distal senses of audition and particularly of vision.¹³ A third characteristic of taste is that it is directly related to the vital intake of food, for which it has the function of judging whether or not the food is suited for consumption, which can be a matter of life or death. Finally, gustatory and olfactory stimuli are very difficult to describe or define in words. For the properties of visual stimuli (e.g., shape and color), we have a large vocabulary at our disposal, but for the description of taste we only have terms for a number of basic tastes, such as sweet, salt, sour, and bitter; for anything beyond that, we only have recourse to descriptions and comparisons. Whoever wishes to compare the taste of a strawberry to that of a raspberry will not get much further than saying that the first, well, tastes like strawberry and the second like raspberry. Or just read any wine-tasting notes: "Medium bodied, quite soft and silky, with almost, but not quite high pitched fruits. The freshness works here, with all the gentle tannins, strong floral, earthy, tobacco notes and sweet, red cherry and red plum in the finish."¹⁴

The sense of taste thus has a number of properties, which each can play a role when the sense of taste is used as the source domain of metaphorical conceptualizations. It is remarkable that taste metaphors have come to conceptualize different aspects in the course of the centuries; when reading metaphors from distant cultures and periods, it is therefore of the highest importance to pay close attention to which exact aspect is transferred. In contemporary language use, one can speak about *having good taste* in order to point to a well-educated and sophisticated esthetical judgment. This way of speaking has only come into use in the eighteenth century, however.¹⁵ The metaphor is based on the fact that the sense of taste is able to perceive very subtle differences in taste and that this capacity to distinguish these differences can and should be trained. The metaphor of *good*

---

¹² This is also the reason why the food industry adds different kinds of (synthetic) flavorings to prepared food: only the addition of these substances will guarantee that, e.g., their strawberry-flavored yogurt will always taste the same. Whoever eats fresh strawberries knows that their taste is strongly dependent on sunshine and precipitation.

¹³ Johan de Joode, *Metaphorical Landscapes and the Theology of the Book of Job: An Analysis of Job's Spatial Metaphors*, VTSup 179 (Leiden: Brill, 2018), 154.

¹⁴ "1995 Château Brane-Cantenac Margaux Wine Tasting Note," The Wine Cellar Insider, https://www.thewinecellarinsider.com/wine-tasting-note/?vintage=1995&wine=Ch%E2teau%20Brane-Cantenac.

¹⁵ Roland Mortier, "Taste," in *Encyclopedia of the Enlightenment*, ed. Michel Delon, trans. Philip Stewart and Gwen Wells, vol. 2 (London: Routledge, 2002), 1306–11.

taste adopts these characteristics: it is the capacity to make subtle esthetical distinctions, which can only be acquired by initiation and exercise in a specific social milieu.

A different common metaphorical use of the sense of taste can be found in the expression "this is just a matter of taste." Here it is not so much the subtlety of a judgment, but rather its subjectivity (and more negatively, its relativity) that is highlighted. This conceptualization goes back to the fact that, more than the other senses, tasting is a very direct and individual way of perceiving that causes strong (often negative) reactions due to its relation to food ingestion. The aversion for certain tastes in humans is much stronger than the aversion for certain sounds or colors, and it is often very individual. It therefore is no coincidence that subjective value judgments are described in terms of taste and not in terms of other senses. It is virtually inconceivable that the expression "this is just a matter of audition" would ever acquire the meaning "this is just a matter of taste" in contemporary English.

However common both metaphorical expressions are for speakers of English (and many other European languages for that matter), they are not as universal as one might think; in the Hebrew Bible, for example, they are not attested. When the biblical writings mention taste metaphorically, other aspects of the source domain are mapped. The challenge for readers is not to allow contemporary understandings of these metaphors to spill over into the interpretation of biblical texts.

3. Metaphors of Taste in the Hebrew Bible[16]

3.1. The Verb טעם "Taste"

A survey of taste metaphors in the Hebrew Bible should start with the verb טעם, even though it does not occur all that often with a metaphorical meaning.[17] As remarked above, the verb may point both to the perception of taste and to testing by taste. With the former meaning, the verb only occurs in Ps 34:9 ("Taste and see that the Lord is good.") and Prov 31:18 ("She tastes that her merchandise is profitable."). In what sense is perceiving conceptualized as tasting here, however?

---

[16] Excellent treatments of (aspects of) this topic can be found in: Yael Avrahami, *The Senses of Scripture: Sensory Perception in the Hebrew Bible*, LHBOTS 545 (London: T&T Clark, 2012); Tova Forti, "Bee's Honey: From Realia to Metaphor in Biblical Wisdom Literature," *VT* 56 (2006): 327–41; Greg Schmidt Goering, "Honey and Wormwood: Taste and the Embodiment of Wisdom in the Book of Proverbs," *HBAI* 5 (2016): 23–41.

[17] The verb is used literally in 2 Sam 19:36, and with the meaning of "eating just a little" (often negatively: "you should not taste/eat anything") in 1 Sam 14:24, 29, 34; 2 Sam 3:35; Jonah 3:7. The metaphorical use is limited to Job 12:11; 34:3; Ps 34:9; and Prov 31:18.

Which aspects of tasting are transferred metaphorically here? Three elements seem to play a role. First, the sense of taste is capable of discerning subtle variations in taste and hence perception very accurately. Probably this is the element of the source domain of TASTE that is transferred metaphorically here: tasting God's goodness means to perceive the full richness (the palate, one could say) of this goodness. A second aspect of the sense of taste that plays a role here is the proximity that is a condition for any tasting. Taste is not experienced at a distance; it is a direct appreciation. For this reason, some commentators have made a distinction between the tasting and the seeing of God's goodness in Ps 34:9:[18] tasting involves the immediate experience, while seeing points to the more distant insight or understanding of this goodness.[19] Bernard of Clairvaux explains the succession of tasting and seeing in the following way: *Nisi gustaveris, non videbis*: if one does not experience spiritually, one will not acquire insight either.[20] Finally, since both Ps 34:9 and Prov 31:18 deal with positive experiences, one could suppose that the tasting also implies "experiencing with pleasure, with approval." When the strong woman in Proverbs tastes that her business is profitable, this not only means she perceives this to be the case, but also that she is pleased to note this. Similarly, the call to taste God's goodness, undoubtedly involves the invitation to do so with pleasure.

In two other cases of the verb טעם (in the almost parallel verses Job 12:11 and 34:3), the focus is on intentional testing: the ear tests words, as the palate tastes food. Even though the second phrase is strictly speaking literal, it is clear that taste is used as a comparison for the critical assessment of words.[21] Again it is the sense of taste that is invoked here as a comparison, which has everything to do with its capacity for making subtle gustatory distinctions.

---

[18] Note that on the basis of several biblical verses, Mitchell Dahood interprets the imperative וראו as a form of ירא *II*, cognate to רוה, with the meaning of "to drink deeply," precisely continuing the taste metaphor. Mitchell Dahood, *Psalms I:1–50*, AB 16 (Garden City: Doubleday, 1966), 206. In his recent NICOT-commentary, Rolf Jacobson reads Ps 34:9 metonymically: "probably a reference to sacrificial meals that worshippers would share as part of the thanksgiving ritual." Nancy deClaissé-Walford, Rolf Jacobson, and Beth LaNeel Tanner, *The Book of Psalms*, NICOT (Grand Rapids: Eerdmans, 2014), 326.

[19] See Franz Delitzsch, *Biblischer Commentar über die Psalmen*, 3rd ed. (Leipzig: Dörffling und Franke, 1873), 285.

[20] Delitzsch, *Biblischer Commentar über die Psalmen*, 285.

[21] Contemporary metaphor theory has repeated the insight already formulated by Aristotle, namely, that metaphor and simile (as an explicit figurative comparison) do not differ fundamentally. Even though their linguistic form may be different, the conceptual operation underlying both is the same.

3.2. The Noun טעם "Taste"

The verb's latter meaning comes to the fore most clearly in the cognate טעם. In its literal meaning of "taste," the word rarely occurs in the Hebrew Bible (Exod 16:31; Num 11:8) but it did develop a number of interesting metaphorical meanings. The term is used most frequently with the meaning of "judgment" or "reason," as is the case, for example, in 1 Sam 25:33, where David praises Abigail for her judicious intervention (טעם) by which she not only saved the lives of her fellow kinsmen but also protected David from shedding blood. Conversely, a beautiful woman without reason (טעם) is depicted very negatively in Prov 11:22. The meaning of "judgment" for the word טעם occurs most clearly in Job 12:20 and Ps 119:66: in the former verse God is said to take away the טעם of the elderly and the speech of the advisors, whereas in the latter the psalmist prays that God would grant good טעם and insight. The context of both verses leaves little doubt that the term refers here to discriminatory power or reason. In the Hebrew Bible, *good taste* therefore has nothing to do with aesthetic judgment or an eye for beauty, but everything to do with discernment and judicious action.[22]

This meaning has also led to an expression used twice in the Hebrew Bible, namely, in 1 Sam 21:14 and Ps 34:1. In both verses, David is said to have gone out of his mind in order to escape from imprisonment.[23] The expression used in both cases is that David "changed his טעם," which clearly means that he had lost his senses. It is not entirely clear how this expression should be interpreted. Does it mean that David changed his reason (his discriminatory power understood as taste), in other words, that he gave the impression to have lost his mind? Or did he rather alter the way in which he was "tasted" or perceived by others? Given the fact that the word טעם is never used elsewhere in Hebrew to refer to the perception others have of somebody, the meaning of the expression seems to be that David willingly changed or perverted his reason, by "feigning madness," as the NRSV translates it.

In Jonah 3:7, the word טעם has an even more specific meaning, namely, as the official "judgment" (and hence "decision") of Nineveh's kings and nobles. Probably, the word here adopted even the very specific meaning of "decree," which the word has quite frequently in Aramaic (e.g., Dan 3:10) and Akkadian, but which is very far from what is semantically possible with the English word "taste." In itself, the semantic development from "taste" to "judicious power," and

---

[22] See de Joode's analysis of the metaphor KNOWING OR DISCERNING IS TASTING (*Metaphorical Landscapes and the Theology of the Book of Job*, 157). See also Prov 26:16: "answer sensibly."

[23] In 1 Samuel, the story is set in the court of Achish, the king of Gath, whereas the heading of Ps 34 makes mention of King Abimelech. Possibly, the two names refer to the same person, so that only one story is alluded to.

subsequently from "judgment" to "decree," is easy to follow, however. It is likely that the meaning of the word in Jonah 3:7 is influenced by the potential of the cognate noun in Aramaic, or even in Akkadian, given the setting of the story in Nineveh. Moreover, Stephen A. Kaufman has argued that this meaning in Aramaic itself is a calque from Akkadian, where the meaning "taste" for the word *ṭēmu* has not been attested.[24]

Finally, a completely different meaning of the word טעם can be found in Jer 48:11. In metaphorical terms, it is said that Moab (in contrast to Judah and Israel) has never gone into exile. The imagery used is that Moab has been able to rest like wine on its dregs without having been poured from one vessel to another. As a result, Moab has been able to retain its own "taste" and "smell"; it has, in other words, retained its identity.[25] This seems to be the only instance in which people are said to (metaphorically) have a taste and a smell; the imagery fits with the wider wine metaphor of the verse,[26] however, and therefore probably never has been an independent expression or an independent conceptualization of identity as taste or smell.

3.3. Specific Tastes

Besides the verb and noun of the root טעם, the Hebrew Bible contains a number of metaphors that use specific tastes as their source domain, in particular the tastes "sweet" and "bitter." As in many other languages, sweet tastes always have positive meaning when used metaphorically. This language use is based on the fact that sweet tastes often go together with high-calorie foods and that humans are therefore programmed to like sweet foods.[27] The figurative comparison in Prov 24:13–14 is therefore easy to understand: "My child, eat honey, for it is good, and the drippings of the honeycomb are sweet to your taste. Know that wisdom is such

---

[24] Stephen A. Kaufman, *The Akkadian Influences on Aramaic*, AS 19 (Chicago: University of Chicago Press, 1974), s.v; see *CAD* 19:85–97.

[25] Possibly, this resting on the dregs could be a metaphorical conceptualization of Moab's self-indulgence, as in Zeph 1:12. Additionally, it has been suggested that the metaphor should be interpreted as pointing to the danger that wine that is kept for too long turns into vinegar, in other words that Moab will ultimately be ruined. The context does not seem to warrant this interpretation, however. The description of Moab as ripe wine seems to be quite positive in this verse; it is only in the next verse 12 that Moab's ruin is described, including the metaphorical emptying and smashing of its wine-jars. For this discussion, see Georg Fischer, *Jeremia 26–52*, HThKAT (Freiburg im Breisgau: Herder, 2005), 510.

[26] This metaphor is extended in vv. 32–33 of the same chapter.

[27] Adam Drewnowski et al., "Sweetness and Food Preference," *Journal of Nutrition* 142 (2012): 1142–48. It should be noted that foods tended to be much less sweet until very recently with the advent of added sweeteners.

to your soul."[28] Not only wisdom, but also the pleasing and wise words of people, and even the word of God, are described as sweet, or as the long Psalm of the Law has it: "How sweet are your words to my taste [PVH: "my palate"], sweeter than honey to my mouth!" (Ps 119:103) This image is extended even further in Ezekiel's inaugural vision, in which he receives God's word in a scroll as sweet food:[29]

> [1] He said to me, O mortal, eat what is offered to you; eat this scroll, and go, speak to the house of Israel. [2] So I opened my mouth, and he gave me the scroll to eat. [3] He said to me, Mortal, eat this scroll that I give you and fill your stomach with it. Then I ate it; and in my mouth it was as sweet as honey. (Ezek 3:1–3)

Also, the attraction of evil is described as sweet, as in Job 20:12–15 in which the taste metaphor is again extended and combined with the closely related metaphor of digestion:[30]

> [12] Though wickedness is sweet in their mouth, though they hide it under their tongues, [13] though they are loath to let it go, and hold it in their mouths, [14] yet their food is turned in their stomachs; it is the venom of asps within them. [15] They swallow down riches and vomit them up again; God casts them out of their bellies.

When evil tastes sweet, and hence presents itself as positive, the sense of discrimination is impaired, and one is unaware of the danger. Doing evil is subsequently conceptualized as eating evil, by which the offenders ultimately poison themselves.

Next to the sweet taste, the latter text also mentions bitterness. In this Joban verse, as often in the Hebrew Bible (e.g., Gen 27:34; 1 Sam 15:32; Ruth 1:20), the taste of bitterness conceptualizes negative experiences, a language use that is common cross-linguistically.[31] The Hebrew Bible speaks about bitterness in two other ways. On the one hand, bitterness can express embitterment and anger: in 2 Sam 17:8, David and his men are said to be "enraged [מרי נפש; lit., "bitter of mind"], like a bear robbed of her cubs in the field."[32] On the other hand, deeds may be described as bitter, meaning that they are morally reprehensible. An example may be found in Jer 2:19: "Your wickedness will punish you, and your

---

[28] See Forti, "Bee's Honey," 335; Schmidt Goering, "Honey and Wormwood," 28.
[29] Compare with Jer 15:16a: "Your words were found, and I ate them."
[30] Forti, "Bee's Honey," 339; de Joode, *Metaphorical Landscapes and the Theology of the Book of Job*, 161.
[31] Compare English "bitter memories, the bitter end."
[32] See also Judg 18:25; 1 Sam 22:2; Job 3:20; Prov 31:6; Hab 1:6.

apostasies will convict you. Know and see that it is evil and bitter for you to forsake the LORD your God."[33] This ethical meaning is most explicit in the prophet Isaiah: "Ah, you who call evil good and good evil, who put darkness for light and light for darkness, who put bitter for sweet and sweet for bitter" (Isa 5:20). Good and evil are not only described with light metaphors, as often in biblical literature, but also with the taste metaphors under consideration here.

Differently than in the New Testament,[34] the Hebrew Bible hardly makes use of the taste of salt as a metaphorical source domain. The only case can be found in an intriguing verse in the book of Job: "Can that which is tasteless be eaten without salt, or is there any flavor in the juice of mallows?" (Job 6:6). The verse is not without its interpretational difficulties, the first being that the final word group ריר חלמות, translated here as "the juice of mallows," is a *hapax legomenon* in the Hebrew Bible, with only the word ריר having one other occurrence, namely, in the already mentioned verse 1 Sam 21:14, where it refers to the spittle or saliva that David let run down his beard. It is clear, then, that the ריר חלמות should refer to a tasteless, slimy substance and is therefore either interpreted as the juice of a particular plant or as the white of an egg.[35] In the first part of Job 6:6, Job's "food" is described as תפל. Although the etymology of the word is difficult, it is clear that the term refers to food without taste.[36] In these words, Job describes the unpalatable fate that has befallen him. As he explains in the following verse: "My appetite refuses to touch them; they are like food that is loathsome to me" (Job 6:7). With this metaphor, Job tries to explain to his friends that he justifiably resists his fate. Had he been given a tastier dish, he would not have complained, he argues. In his own words: "Does the wild ass bray over its grass, or the ox low over its fodder?" (Job 6:5). Instead of this grass and fodder, Job has been given poison to drink (Job 6:4), and hence his resistance is legitimate in his view. With complex taste and food metaphors, Job thus describes how critical and grim his situation has become: it is poison, rather than good food, and insipid and unpalatable at that.[37]

---

[33] Similarly, in Ps 64:4 "bitter words"; Prov 5:4.

[34] Most famous in this regard is of course Jesus's word in Matt 5:13 "You are the salt of the earth," but see also Mark 9:50; Luke 14:34 and Col 4:6.

[35] See *HAL*, s.v. "חלמות" (Anchusa officinalis); BDB, s.v. "חלמות" (following the targum and rabbinical sources, white of an egg).

[36] See Johannes Marböck, "תפל," *ThWAT* 8:729. It is particularly difficult to establish whether the instances of the roots תפל and טפל referring to plastering and whitewashing should be regarded as semantically related to the cases dealing with insipid or worthless activities under investigation here. It is interesting to note that in the Talmud, the term is used to refer to unsalted meat or fish (which is also its meaning in Modern Hebrew), but it is very well possible that this later usage is based precisely on the Job verse discussed here (see Marböck, "תפל," 8:729; Jastrow, s.v. "תפל").

[37] Hanneke van Loon, *Metaphors in the Discussion on Suffering in Job 3–31: Visions of Hope and Consolation*, BIS 165 (Leiden: Brill, 2018), 82.

Not only human experiences as Job's can be tasteless; the acts of people can also be described in these terms. With the same root תפל as in Job 6:6 the deeds of the prophets in Samaria are portrayed in Jer 23:13: "In the prophets of Samaria I saw a disgusting thing [תפלה]: they prophesied by Baal and led my people Israel astray." Rather than positing a more general meaning like "unseemliness" (JPS 17) or "an offensive thing" (NAS), it seems better to view this instance as a metaphorical use of "tastelessness." When people lose their taste, in other words, their sense of discrimination, they tend to do unsavory things. This is exactly what Job does not do at the beginning of the book, illustrating his righteousness: in spite of all his suffering he—literally translated—"gave no tasteless thing to God" (Job 1:22); in other words, he did not make unsavory reproaches to God, usually translated in a paraphrasing way: "he did not charge God with wrongdoing."

3.4. Taste and Disgust

The most negative gustatory experience is that of disgust. Even though, in English, the term *disgust* may refer to any feeling of revulsion to unpleasant experiences, its etymology (*dis-gust*) is clearly related to the sense of taste. Also, from an evolutionary perspective, it has been argued that the emotion of disgust developed from the gustatory aversive response to potentially poisonous or contaminating food.[38]

In Hebrew, I will argue, terms for gustatory aversion have come to be used metaphorically for moral or social disgust. Admittedly, it is not always easy to determine whether a term had a more general meaning of aversion, which included aversion to contaminated food, or whether it referred prototypically to gustatory revulsion and subsequently acquired a broader application to include disgust towards many different objects and acts. For the correct understanding of individual texts, the issue may only be of limited importance, but when it comes to understanding the overall religious conceptualizations of the Hebrew Bible, including the metaphors of taste under investigation here, the matter is worthy of some attention.

In his commentary on Prov 13:19 ("A desire realized is sweet to the soul, but to turn away from evil is an abomination to fools"), William McKane argues that the expression "pleasurable to a *nepeš*" (or "sweet to the soul," NRSV) "is a metaphor which has its basis in the sensation of tasting appetizing food."[39] Indeed, it

---

[38] William Ian Miller, *The Anatomy of Disgust* (Cambridge: Harvard University Press, 1998); Daniel Kelly, *Yuck! The Nature and Moral Significance of Disgust*, Life and Mind (Cambridge: MIT Press, 2011); Rachel S. Herz and Alden Hinds, "Stealing Is Not Gross: Language Distinguishes Visceral Disgust from Moral Violations," *The American Journal of Psychology* 126 (2013): 275–86.

[39] William McKane, *Proverbs: A New Approach*, OTL (London: SCM, 1970).

could be argued that the verb ערב, meaning "to be pleasurable," has a basic meaning of "to be tasty," especially when one considers that several of the verb's occurrences deal with food offerings that do not please God, in other words, are not to his taste (Jer 6:20; Hos 9:4; Mal 3:4). Also, the related adjective ערב is used in Prov 20:17 in a context of (metaphorical) eating: "Bread gained by deceit is sweet [ערב], but afterward the mouth will be full of gravel." On the other hand, the verb is also used for the pleasure one finds in a good night's rest (Jer 31:26; Prov 3:24) or the pleasure lovers find in their beloved (Ezek 16:37, see also the adjective in Song 2:14 speaking about the voice of the beloved). All in all, then, the case for a gustatory origin of the verb ערב is not impossible to make, but conclusive arguments are lacking, as is often the case in Hebrew semantics. The case is stronger, in my opinion, for the frequent word תועבה, found in the second half of Prov 13:19 quoted above and usually translated as "abomination." Being an important term in the Hebrew Bible, תועבה has been discussed extensively in the scholarly literature, most recently in the elaborate article by Carly L. Crouch.[40] It is usually acknowledged that the term has both a cultic meaning, which is to be found primarily in Deuteronomy and in Ezekiel, and a moral one, mainly used in the book of Proverbs.[41] Scholars debate which of the two meanings is to be considered the most fundamental, with one having subsequently given rise to the other meaning: Richard John Clifford sees a transfer of ritual language to ethical issues in Proverbs, while authors ever since Paul Humbert have argued that the cultic language was adopted from the earlier sapiential and ethical meaning of the term.[42] In her article, Crouch argues that any attempts to reconcile both aspects of the term remain unsuccessful, as do any attempts to classify all the noun's instances as either religious or ethical. In her opinion, what is common to all instances of the term is that they are "used in texts that are concerned with boundary delineation, boundary transgression and boundary protection."[43] She therefore

---

[40] Carly L. Crouch, "What Makes a Thing Abominable? Observations on the Language of Boundaries and Identity Formation from a Social Scientific Perspective," *VT* 65 (2015): 516–41.

[41] Ruth E. Clements, "The Concept of Abomination in the Book of Proverbs," in *Texts, Temples and Traditions: A Tribute to Menahem Haran*, ed. Michael V. Fox et al. (Winona Lake, IN: Eisenbrauns, 1996), 211–25.

[42] Richard John Clifford, *Proverbs: A Commentary*, OTL (Louisville: Westminster John Knox, 1999), 121. Paul Humbert, "Le substantif *to ʿēbā* et le verbe *tʿb* dans l'Ancien Testament," *ZAW* 72 (1960): 224: "Pourrait-on supposer que la formule aurait été empruntée à la vieille tradition sapientiale d'Israël par le Deutéronome, mais que ce dernier l'aurait infléchie dans un sens plus théologique et polémique?"

[43] Crouch, "What Makes a Thing Abominable?," 519.

sides with Saul Olyan's suggestion that the term relates to the "violation of a socially constructed boundary."[44] While this is an adequate description of the referential meaning of the term or its contexts, it does not explain the term's sense or semantics: the lexeme תועבה does not in itself convey the meaning of a boundary or border. In my opinion, the lexeme is semantically close to the English "disgust": prototypically related to the gustatory sense, תועבה metaphorically developed a broad range of meanings, including ethical, religious, and social disgust vis-à-vis unacceptable behavior and objects. First, the term occurs a number of times in the context of meals, both human meals and food offerings for the gods. Genesis 43:32 describes how the Egyptians would not eat with the Hebrews, because that was a תועבה to them, while in Exod 8:22 Moses explains that the offerings of the Israelites would be a תועבה to the Egyptians.[45] Moreover, in most cases, the term is used as a classification or value judgment of an act or a person, hence the frequent expression "X is a תועבה to Y."[46] The term rarely designates a concrete object directly. It does so, however, in Deut 14:3, where the Israelites are forbidden to *eat* a תועבה, the context making clear that unclean animals are being referred to. This could be a first indication that the term is prototypically related to the sense of taste. Admittedly, however, the term is used in so many different contexts that this argument alone is only quite weak.

It is interesting to note, however, that in the Septuagint the term is predominantly translated as βδέλυγμα/βδέλυγμος, a typical Septuagint word related to the verb βδελύσσομαι, which has as its primary meaning "to feel a loathing for food,"[47] having acquired also the more general meaning of "to abhor." Also related nouns display the same relation to the sense of taste: LSJ notes that βδελυγμία can mean both "nausea, sickness" and "filth, nastiness," while βδελυρία is listed as meaning both "beastly, coarse, or objectionable behaviour" and again "disgust, nausea."[48] This type of polysemy is common in many languages and is conceptually very well explainable as the extensive recent literature on disgust has made clear: revulsion against what is immoral or even against what

---

[44] Saul Olyan, "'And with a Male You Shall Not Lie the Lying Down of a Woman': On the Meaning and Significance of Leviticus 18:22 and 20:13," *Journal of the History of Sexuality* 5 (1994): 180 n. 3, as quoted in Crouch, "What Makes a Thing Abominable?," 520.

[45] As some have argued, this disgust of the Egyptians vis-à-vis burnt offerings might also have been the reason for the destruction of the Jewish Elephantine Temple as described in TAD A4.7–8, and the only partial restauration of its cult (excluding burnt offerings) granted in TAD A4.9. Porten et al. have argued, however, that this exclusion of burnt offerings indicates that the latter was reserved for the Jerusalem temple. See Bezalel Porten et al., *The Elephantine Papyri in English: Three Millennia of Cross-Cultural Continuity and Change*, DMOA 22 (Leiden: Brill, 1996), 149 no.12.

[46] See *DCH* 8, s.v. "תועבה."

[47] LSJ, s.v. "βδελύσσομαι."

[48] LSJ, s.v. "βδελύσσομαι."

is unfamiliar to a person is often conceptualized in terms of physical disgust and can even go together with feelings of bodily nausea or sickness.[49] In my opinion, it is quite possible that the term תועבה displays a similar polysemy, even though in the biblical corpus the metaphorical (primarily cultic and ethical) meanings of the term are quantitatively predominant.

The etymology of the term, finally, can help in establishing its meaning, even though one should exercise great caution in using etymological arguments in lexical semantic questions.[50] In his study on the noun's etymology (the verb תעב being denominative), Humbert argues that it morphologically derives from the weak root יעב.[51] Discarding previous attempts to explain the root, Humbert relates יעב to the hollow root עוב/עיב (pointing as examples of a similar variation to roots like יטב/טוב). In his opinion, this root is in its turn related to Arabic ʿāba: meaning "to be stained by a mistake." From a meaning of "stain" or "dirt," the root then developed the meaning of "disgust" (as the reaction to dirt or filth) as we encounter it in the Hebrew noun.[52] The conceptualization of immoral behavior as "staining" is quite common in Biblical Hebrew,[53] so that this possibility is not to be discarded a priori. The semantic link between staining and disgust is not so convincing, however, since the strongest physical reactions of disgust are not evoked by filth or stains, which are perceived visually, but by taste or smell. It is better therefore, in my opinion, to relate the noun תועבה to the root ġb(b). If, as

---

[49] See the literature mentioned in n. 41.

[50] James Barr, "Etymology and the Old Testament," in *Language and Meaning: Studies in Hebrew Language and Biblical Exegesis*, ed. James Barr, OtSt 19 (Leiden: Brill, 1974), 1–28.

[51] Paul Humbert, "L'étymologie du substantif *toʿēbā*," in *Verbannung und Heimkehr: Beiträge zur Geschichte und Theologie Israels im 6. und 5. Jahrhundert v. Chr., Wilhelm Rudolph zum 70. Geburtstage, dargebracht von Kollegen, Freunden und Schülern*, ed. Arnulf Kuschke (Tübingen: Mohr, 1961), 157–60. The noun is a feminine *taqtel*-formation of a *pe-waw* root, see Joüon Muraoka §88r. Compare with תוכחה, תולדות, and possibly תועלה. Humbert does not examine this root יעב any further, and for a good reason. It is not attested in Hebrew, nor in any of the closest cognate languages. Arabic does have a cognate root *wʿb*, but its meaning of "to gather" and "to exterminate" does not seem to allow for any semantic connections with the noun תועבה under investigation here. Since Hebrew *ayin* can represent Proto-Semitic *ġayin* as well, the Arabic root *wġb* could also be taken into consideration, but its meaning of "to be mean, stupid, weak" is not very helpful for the interpretation of תועבה, in my opinion.

[52] Humbert, "L'étymologie du substantif *toʿēbā*," 159: "Ce substantif désigne ce qui présente une tare, un défaut, un vice, ce qui passe pour impur … et inspire, à ce titre, dégoût, horreur, aversion, blâme et interdiction."

[53] See Joseph Lam, *Patterns of Sin in the Hebrew Bible: Metaphor, Culture, and the Making of a Religious Concept* (New York: Oxford University Press, 2016), 179–206.

Humbert suggests, the noun derives from a biradical hollow stem עב, it is morphologically very well possible to relate it to the said root ġb(b) given the fact Hebrew ayin can represent two different Proto-Semitic phonemes, namely, ʿayin (ʿ) and ġayin (ġ), which languages like Arabic have retained. In Arabic, the root ġb is said of food that "became altered (for the worse) in its odor" or that "became stinking," and hence it also acquired the meaning of something becoming "very corrupt."[54] It is not inconceivable, in my opinion, that the Hebrew noun תועבה has semantically developed from this meaning: it then refers to objects and acts that elicit the same reaction of disgust and revulsion as food turned bad, in other words, to something detestable. Objects and acts are often described as being a תועבה to God; also, in this case, the emotions of disgust (through taste or smell) can be implied; it suffices to point to the fact that, conversely, acceptable offerings are frequently described as ריח ניחח "a pleasing odor" to God.[55]

4. Conclusion

Taking together all the metaphorical expressions treated above, it becomes clear that they are strongly interrelated. Many aspects of the sense of taste are used metaphorically in the Hebrew Bible, and these metaphors display inner consistency.[56] On the one hand, the gustatory sense is used to conceptualize very direct and personal experiences: when one tastes something, whether literally or figuratively, one has acquired a very immediate, unmediated experience of the object of tasting. It is completely consistent with the latter conceptualization that the pleasing tastes sweet and salt are said of positive experiences, while bitterness and insipidity are attributed to negative ones. The sense of taste is also used to conceptualize the human sense of discrimination: whoever is able to make fine gustatory distinctions, metaphorically speaking, has a sound judgment. It is remarkable that in Hebrew even a decision or decree can be understood in terms of tasting.

This survey has far from exhausted the topic of taste metaphors in the Hebrew Bible. In the present contribution, the focus has been on the experience of taste itself and its metaphorical usages, but other aspects are worth pursuing. For example, nothing has been said about the tasting organs, which are also occasionally used metaphorically in the Hebrew Bible, for example, in the already mentioned

---

[54] Lane 6, s.v. "غب."

[55] See Gen 8:21, and a subsequent forty-two occurrences in the books of Exodus, Leviticus, Numbers, and Ezekiel.

[56] On consistency between metaphors, see Lakoff and Johnson, *Metaphors We Live By*, 41–45 and 94–95.

sixth chapter of Job: "Is there any wrong on my tongue? Cannot my palate[57] discern calamity?" (Job 6:30). Another aspect that has not been analyzed in the present contribution is the link between (metaphorical) tasting and eating, while Avrahami has pointed out that a sharp semantic distinction between both cannot be made.[58] As she has made clear, moreover, several texts point to the intimate relationship between what one metaphorically tastes and consumes through the mouth, on the one hand, and what leaves the mouth as speech, on the other, Ezek 3:1 being a prime example: "O mortal, eat what is offered to you; eat this scroll, and go, speak to the house of Israel."[59] Future research will have to elaborate on these aspects.

When studying all these metaphors, it is striking how similar some of them are to expressions in English or other contemporary languages. Since tasting is a common human experience, it should not come as a surprise that different, even unrelated, languages metaphorically make use of our sense of taste in comparable ways. On the other hand, the precise meaning and interpretation of the taste metaphors can be remarkably different in Biblical Hebrew and in, for example, English. It is important, therefore, to be aware of the fact that biblical expressions may have meanings that are significantly different from what our contemporary linguistic feeling may make us believe. *Taste* has much less the connotation of a subjective or arbitrary value judgment than it has in contemporary Western languages. I hope this contribution has at least given a sense of the flavors biblical metaphors may have.

BIBLIOGRAPHY

"1995 Château Brane-Cantenac Margaux Wine Tasting Note." The Wine Cellar Insider. https://www.thewinecellarinsider.com/wine-tasting-note/?vintage=1995&wine=Ch%E2teau%20Brane-Cantenac.

Avrahami, Yael. *The Senses of Scripture: Sensory Perception in the Hebrew Bible.* LHBOTS 545. London: T&T Clark, 2012.

---

[57] NRSV reads: "Cannot my *taste* discern calamity?" The Hebrew term חך used here, refers to the body part, however, and not to the sense of taste.

[58] Avrahami, *Senses of Scripture*, 93.

[59] I am less convinced, however, by the "*semantic proximity* between eating and speech" (italics by P. Van Hecke) for which Avrahami finds an indication in "the metaphoric use of adjectives from the field of taste to describe the content of speech" (*Senses of Scripture*, 94). The taste of words is their quality as perceived by the hearer, not by the speaker. In that sense perceiving is akin to tasting and eating, as discussed above, and that perception can be sweet, bitter, tasteless, and the like. Whether what is perceived is the result of previous speech production does not seem to play a role in qualifying it as having a particular taste, in my opinion. Also, other experiences than words can be described in taste terms.

Barr, James. "Etymology and the Old Testament." Pages 1–28 in *Language and Meaning: Studies in Hebrew Language and Biblical Exegesis*. Edited by James Barr. OtSt 19. Leiden: Brill, 1974.
Clements, Ruth E. "The Concept of Abomination in the Book of Proverbs." Pages 211–25 in *Texts, Temples and Traditions: A Tribute to Menahem Haran*. Edited by Michael V. Fox et al. Winona Lake, IN: Eisenbrauns, 1996.
Clifford, Richard John. *Proverbs: A Commentary*. OTL. Louisville: Westminster John Knox, 1999.
Crouch, Carly L. "What Makes a Thing Abominable? Observations on the Language of Boundaries and Identity Formation from a Social Scientific Perspective." *VT* 65 (2015): 516–41.
Dahood, Mitchell. *Psalms I: 1–50*. AB 16. Garden City: Doubleday, 1966.
DeClaissé-Walford, Nancy, Rolf Jacobson, and Beth LaNeel Tanner. *The Book of Psalms*. NICOT. Grand Rapids: Eerdmans, 2014.
de Joode, Johan. *Metaphorical Landscapes and the Theology of the Book of Job: An Analysis of Job's Spatial Metaphors*. VTSup 179. Leiden: Brill, 2018.
Delitzsch, Franz. *Biblischer Commentar über die Psalmen*. 3rd ed. Leipzig: Dörffling und Franke, 1873.
Drewnowski, Adam, Julie A. Mennella, Susan L. Johnson, and France Bellisle. "Sweetness and Food Preference." *Journal of Nutrition* 142 (2012): 1142–48.
Ferguson, Priscilla Parkhurst. "The Senses of Taste." *AHR* 116 (2011): 371–84.
Fischer, Georg. *Jeremia 26–52*. HThKAT. Freiburg im Breisgau: Herder, 2005.
Forti, Tova. "Bee's Honey: From Realia to Metaphor in Biblical Wisdom Literature." *VT* 56 (2006): 327–41.
Herz, Rachel S., and Alden Hinds. "Stealing Is Not Gross: Language Distinguishes Visceral Disgust from Moral Violations." *The American Journal of Psychology* 126 (2013): 275–86.
Humbert, Paul. "L'étymologie du substantif *toʿēbā*." Pages 157–60 in *Verbannung und Heimkehr: Beiträge zur Geschichte und Theologie Israels im 6. und 5. Jahrhundert v. Chr., Wilhelm Rudolph zum 70. Geburtstage, dargebracht von Kollegen, Freunden und Schülern*. Edited by Arnulf Kuschke. Tübingen: Mohr, 1961.
———. "Le substantif *toʿēbā* et le verbe *tʿb* dans l'Ancien Testament." *ZAW* 72 (1960): 217–37.
Kaufman, Stephen A. *The Akkadian Influences on Aramaic*. AS 19. Chicago: University of Chicago Press, 1974.
Kelly, Daniel. *Yuck! The Nature and Moral Significance of Disgust*. Life and Mind. Cambridge: MIT Press, 2011.
Kirkby, John T. "Aristotle on Metaphor." *AJP* 118 (1997): 517–54.
Lakoff, George. "The Invariance Hypothesis: Is Abstract Reason Based on Image-Schemas?" *Cognitive Linguistics* 1 (1990): 39–74.
Lakoff, George, and Mark Johnson. *Metaphors We Live By*. Chicago: University of Chicago Press, 1980.
Lam, Joseph. *Patterns of Sin in the Hebrew Bible: Metaphor, Culture, and the Making of a Religious Concept*. New York: Oxford University Press, 2016.
Marböck, Johannes. "תפל." *ThWAT* 8:728–32.
McKane, William. *Proverbs: A New Approach*. OTL. London: SCM, 1970.

Miller, William Ian. *The Anatomy of Disgust*. Cambridge: Harvard University Press, 1998.
Mortier, Roland. "Taste." Pages 1306–11 in *Encyclopedia of the Enlightenment*. Edited by Michel Delon. Translated by Philip Stewart and Gwen Wells. Vol. 2. London: Routledge, 2002.
Olyan, Saul. "'And with a Male You Shall Not Lie the Lying Down of a Woman': On the Meaning and Significance of Leviticus 18:22 and 20:13." *Journal of the History of Sexuality* 5 (1994): 179–206.
Porten, Bezalel, et al. *The Elephantine Papyri in English: Three Millennia of Cross-Cultural Continuity and Change*. DMOA 22. Leiden: Brill, 1996
Schmidt Goering, Greg. "Honey and Wormwood: Taste and the Embodiment of Wisdom in the Book of Proverbs." *HBAI* 5 (2016): 23–41.
Van Hecke, Pierre. "The Verbs ראה and שמע in the Book of Qohelet: A Cognitive-Semantic Perspective." Pages 203–20 in *The Language of Qohelet in Its Context: Essays in Honor of Prof. A. Schoors on the Occasion of His Seventieth Birthday*. Edited by Angelika Berlejung and Pierre Van Hecke. OLA 164. Leuven: Peeters, 2007.
van Loon, Hanneke. *Metaphors in the Discussion on Suffering in Job 3–31: Visions of Hope and Consolation*. BIS 165. Leiden: Brill, 2018.

FECES: THE PRIMARY DISGUST ELICITOR IN THE HEBREW BIBLE AND IN THE ANCIENT NEAR EAST

Thomas Staubli

Feces are the main elicitors of disgust across all cultures.[1] Feelings of disgust are primarily triggered by the senses. Feces stink and appeal to the sense of smell.[2] As they leave the bowels, feces also cause characteristic noises that may evoke disgust but also a range of other emotions.[3] However, since Darwin, disgust has

---

[1] Valerie Curtis and Adam Biran, "Dirt, Disgust, and Disease: Is Hygiene in Our Genes?," *Perspectives in Biology and Medicine* 44 (2001): 17–31; Lisa S. Elwood and Bunmi O. Olatunji, "A Cross-Cultural Perspective on Disgust," in *Disgust and its Disorders: Theory, Assessment, and Treatment*, ed. Bunmi O. Olatunji and Dean McKay (Washington DC: American Psychological Association, 2009), 99–122.

[2] The fear of being "stinky" (באש), attested in the Bible, illustrates the strong effect of olfaction. For example, Jacob complains to Simeon and Levi that they made him stinky with their violent action against the inhabitants of the country (Gen 34:30). The Hebrew people complain to Moses and Aaron that they made the people stinky to Pharaoh and his officials (Exod 5:21). The Israelites under Saul were stinky to the Philistines (1 Sam 13:4). The Ammonites see that they are stinky to David, and so they prepare for war (2 Sam 10:6). Wife and siblings turn away from the stinky Job (Job 19:17). It is striking that the Bible does not refer to others as stinky, but rather self-critically brings up the issue of the danger of being stinky to others. Isaiah, in particular, criticizes Israel as a vineyard, which has produced stench instead of grapes for God, the vineyard's owner (Isa 5:2, 4; cf. 30:5; 34:3). That is how he explains why YHWH is disgusted and turns away from Israel, leaving it to destruction. The goal of Israel should be to smell good, to spread a fragrance that attracts God. That aspect was emphasized in early Christianity, where prayers, gifts for the poor, and one's whole life could be interpreted as fragrant offerings (Rev 5:8; 8:3–4; Phil 4:18; Eph 5:2).

[3] The fart does not appear to have been mentioned in the Bible. Perhaps Isaiah is concerned with this when he writes, that his belly (מעה) will sound like a lyre if he thinks about Moab (Isa 16:11). But Josephus Flavius certainly directs our attention to the human sound whose scale of meaning can range from embarrassment to contempt, from humorous intent to obscene disrespect. He reports that under Cumanus (48–52 CE), a Roman security official on the roof of the pillared hall pulled back his garment and, cowering down after an

been thought to be related primarily to the sense of taste. Disgust prompts the individual to avoid the ingestion of human and animal waste products (feces, vomit, menstruum, sweat, etc.).[4] Disgust has been understood as an emotion acquired by the omnivorous *Homo sapiens* in order to protect against disease.[5] Furthermore, magical behaviors also play a role; that is, disgust presumes that even brief contact with a contagion results in permanent contamination (Frazer's law of contagion) and that an object that appears similar to a contagion will often be perceived as contagious (Frazer's law of similarity).[6]

Man's feelings of disgust are not innate. They appear in the course of a child's development, mainly between the third and seventh year; they are gendered, and it is not clear exactly how they arise.[7] It seems that we learn from our role models.[8] Moreover, disgust is not only triggered by bodily excretions and body parts, spoiled food, and nonhuman creatures, but also by people who are different from one's own in-group and by violations of the in-group's moral or social norms, as for instance, in the case of modern moral vegetarianism.[9] Translated back to the Darwinian paradigm: not only our physical body, but also the social body wants to protect itself from dangerous external influences. Thus, disgust, functioning as

---

indecent manner, turned his breech to the Jews and uttered a sound corresponding to such a posture. A popular uprising, with tens of thousands of deaths, was the result of that sound, called the first Judean war against Rome (*B.J.* 2.224).

[4] Charles Darwin, *The Expression of the Emotions in Man and Animals* (Chicago: University of Chicago Press, 1965), 256; András Angyal, "Digust and Related Aversions," *Journal of Abnormal and Social Psychology* 36 (1941): 393–412; Paul Rozin and April E. Fallon, "A Perspective on Disgust," *Psychological Review* 94 (1987): 23–41. William I. Miller, *The Anatomy of Disgust* (Cambridge: Harvard University Press, 1997), 86, followed by Martha C. Nussbaum, *Hiding from Humanity: Disgust, Shame, and the Law* (Princeton: Princeton University Press, 2004), 92, places smell and touch before taste in a sensory hierarchy of disgust.

[5] Paul Rozin, Jonathan Haidt, and Clark R. McCauley, "Disgust," in *Handbook of Emotions*, ed. M. Lewis and J. Haviland, 2nd ed. (New York: Guilford, 2000), 637–53.

[6] Paul Rozin, Linda Millman, and Carol Nemeroff, "Operation of the Laws of Sympathetic Magic in Disgust and Other Domains," *Journal of Personality and Social Psychology* 50 (1986): 707.

[7] April E. Fallon, Paul Rozin, and Patricia Pliner, "The Child's Conception of Food: The Development of Food Rejections with Special Reference to Disgust and Contamination Sensitivity," *Child Development* 55 (1984): 566–75.

[8] Susan Mineka and Michael Cook, "Mechanisms Involved in the Observational Conditioning of Fear," *Journal of Experimental Psychology General* 122 (1993): 23–38.

[9] Jonathan Haidt et al., "Body, Psyche, and Culture: The Relationship between Disgust and Morality," *Psychology and Developing Societies* 9 (1997): 107–31; Daniel M. T. Fessler et al., "Disgust Sensitivity and Meat Consumption: A Test of an Emotivist Account of Moral Vegetarianism," *Appetite* 41 (2003): 31–41.

a guardian of the body and the social group, belongs to the so-called other-condemning moral emotions.[10] In contrast to contempt and anger, which are also other-condemning moral emotions, disgust is a sensory-somatic emotion: "The look, feel, taste or smell of something determines its disgust value, not its functional or dynamic properties."[11]

In short, disgust is a complex, culturally and ethically constructed emotion. As a sensory-somatic emotion, it is of special interest for the cultural study of the impact of senses. The purpose of this article is to discuss some aspects of the cultural construction of disgust in the ancient Near East (including the Hebrew Bible) with a focus on feces, the primary elicitor of disgust. Observations will mainly derive from textual and visual evidence from the Levant and its neighborhood.[12]

The result is fascinating: (1) while it is evident that great efforts have been made in Levantine documents to render human feces invisible, the prevalent disgust of feces still prompted the construction of (2) Egyptian funerary spells that sought to prevent the ingestion of feces in the afterworld, (3) prophetic actions and speeches from Mesopotamia and the Levant that evoked or otherwise made feces visible, and (4) priestly speeches in the Hebrew Bible where foreign gods and their laws were made disgusting with a rhetoric of shit.

1. THE UNSIGHTLY ONE: MAKING FECES INVISIBLE

Unfortunately, an archeology of latrines is lacking at the moment. Certainly, only a tiny upper class was able to afford houses with a cool upper room that could contain a latrine, as it was the case in the palace of the Moabite king Eglon (Judg 3:24). But we know nothing about the toilet-custom of the simple people. We only can suspect that they had special places for voiding outside the houses (cf. the

---

[10] Other types of moral emotions include self-conscious moral emotions (shame, embarrassment, and guilt), other-suffering moral emotions (compassion), and other-praising moral emotions (gratitude and elevation). Jonathan Haidt, "The Moral Emotions," in *Handbook of Affective Sciences*, ed. Richard J. Davidson, Klaus R. Scherer, and H. Hill Goldsmith (Oxford: Oxford University Press, 2003), 852–70. For a critique, see, e.g., David Pizarro, Yoel Inbar, and Chelsea Helion, "On Disgust and Moral Judgment," *Emotion Review* 3 (2011): 267–68.

[11] Colin MacGinn, *The Meaning of Disgust* (Oxford: Oxford University Press, 2011), 44. Note that the sense of hearing seems to be free of disgust triggers.

[12] Analysis of ancient feces focuses primarily on pollen analysis, paleobotanical observations, and parasitological questions. As far as I can see, a thorough analysis of archeological evidence of human feces in respect to emotional and sensory aspects of the organization of human social life is missing, but it is beyond of the scope of this paper. Parts of the paper are further developed in chapter 42 of Thomas Staubli, "Von Ausscheidungen und Ekel," in *Menschenbilder der Bibel*, ed. Thomas Staubli and Silvia Schroer (Ostfildern: Patmos Verlag 2014), 264–69.

expression "pissing at the wall," משתין בקיר, for a male in 1 Sam 25:22, 34; 1 Kgs 14:10). In any case, during a war there weren't such privileges like an upper room, even for a king. In En-Gedi, a cave is still being shown to tourists, where King Saul reportedly defecated (lit., "covered his feet"[13]) while David, who was hidden in that cave with some of his guerilla friends, secretly cut off a corner of Saul's garment (see 1 Sam 24:5). The fact that Saul went into a cave to relieve himself indicates that defecation required separation from the group and a secluded location. The War Law of Deuteronomy specifies that defecation must happen in a marked area[14] outside the camp and that every soldier has to carry a spike/dibble in his baggage so that he may bury his excrements in a hole (Deut 23:13–15). The ruling is based on the argument that God, traveling with and protecting his people, is not to see "anything unseemly/untoward/indecent" (ערות דבר) among Israelites or he would turn away from them.

This general custom does not seem to have prevailed among the Israelites, for Josephus Flavius, himself a Jewish priest, mentions as a peculiarity of the Essenes that they are forbidden to defecate on Shabbat and that

> on other days they dig a small pit, a foot deep, with a paddle (which kind of hatchet is given them when they are first admitted among them); and covering themselves round with their garment, that they may not affront the Divine rays of light, they ease themselves into that pit, after which they put the earth that was dug out again into the pit; and even this they do only in the more lonely places, which they choose out for this purpose; and although this easement of the body be natural, yet it is a rule with them to wash themselves after it, as if it were a defilement to them. (*B.J.* 2.148–149)[15]

Living in a state of spiritual war with the sons of the darkness, the sons of the light evidently followed a rigid form of the Deuteronomic War Law during their lifetime.

Still another view is hold by the Temple Scroll (11QT 46:13–16): "You shall make for them latrines outside the city where they shall go out, north-west of the city. These shall be roofed houses with holes in them into which the filth shall go down. It shall be far enough not to be visible from the city, (at) three thousand cubits."[16] The text conforms with the Essenite practice insofar as the distance of

---

[13] את־רגליו (*hiphil*) סכך; The cowering for defecation makes the long garment cover the feet. The text thus presupposes that the king wore a long, lined garment (כתנת) of the upper class and not a skirt (מד) like the warriors.

[14] יד; see Jeffrey H. Tigay, *Deuteronomy* (Philadelphia: Jewish Publication Society of America, 1996), 214.

[15] Flavius Josephus, *The Works of Flavius Josephus*, trans. William Whiston (Auburn: John E. Beardsley, 1895).

[16] Géza Vermès, *The Dead Sea Scrolls in English*, 3rd ed. (Harmondsworth: Penguin Books, 1990), 144.

three thousand cubits is more than the Temple Scroll allows an individual to walk on Shabbat. Thus, the text indirectly bans defecation on Shabbat. The fixed installation differs from the custom of the Essenes, but both practices share aspects of the Deuteronomic War Law: the Temple Scroll designates a marked area, while the Essene practice promotes the digging of a hole. Despite the differences, I am hesitant to follow Baumgarten's conclusion that the two quoted instances speak about totally different groups. The texts serve different functions—one is intended to describe an actual group from an outside perspective (Josephus's *Bellum judaicum*) while the other is intended to prescribe group behavior from an inside perspective (Temple Scroll). They could, therefore, reflect the same group in different ways.[17]

In sum, Saul's reported behavior suggests that urination and defecation happened in separate places. However, private latrines, that is, distinct buildings for this purpose, were a privilege of the upper class alone. The Deuteronomic Law and, probably based on it the laws of the Essenes, demand that feces are made invisible by defecating in a specially dug pit or in latrines outside the city.

The disgusting effect of feces on humans—bad smell or taste; ugly form, color, and consistency; or disgusting sound—is never mentioned explicitly. Rather, the emotion of disgust (triggered by feces) is projected on God.[18] These texts convey a fear that God could turn away or that the divine rays of light could be affronted. This fear, I believe, is a reflex of human disgust. We are afraid to soil with our feces, and we turn away from the feces of the others. So, too, does God.

2. Strategies to Avoid Scatophagy and Other Acts Disgusting for Gods in Egypt

Feces as disgust elicitor in Egypt is known primarily from the spells in the Book of the Dead, where scatophagy (eating excrement) is mentioned several times as an atrocity or abomination (*bwt*). In order to understand what exactly the Egyptians feared and what the spell's function was, it is necessary to interpret the spells in a larger context.

The overall picture of *bwt* in Egypt is based on texts from different periods. As Paul John Frandsen, who studied the subject in a series of papers, noted, the

---

[17] Albert I. Baumgarten, "The Temple Scroll, Toilet Practices, and the Essenes," *Jewish History* 10 (1996): 9–20.

[18] For the use of חראים (dung): 2 Kgs 6:25; 18:27; Isa 36:12; צאה (filth): Deut 23:24; 2 Kgs 18:27; Isa 4:4; 28:8; 36:12; Ezek 4:12; Prov 30:12; סחי (scum): Lam 3:45; מאוס (garbage): Lam 3:45; and טיט (mire of the streets, mud): 2 Sam 22:43; Isa 57:20; Jer 38:6; Mic 7:10; Zech 9:3; 10:5.

number of occurrences of *bwt* in Egyptian material is too scarce to allow a thorough reconstruction of a diachronic history of the term.[19] Nevertheless some insight is possible, and some tendencies can be highlighted.

According to Frandsen, *bwt* is an ontological category, part of a matrix in which there is a border in space (*h3w*) between "that which is" (*ntt*), the created, differentiated world (cosmos), and "that which is not" (*jwtt*), the uncreated, undifferentiated realm (chaos).[20] In the cultic realm, this border is architectonically realized and manifest in the temple wall. The wall separates humankind in a cultic realm from the feces of the creator, generated during creation, which is *bwt* for them.[21] *Bwt* also indicates the fear to do something forbidden/taboo in human acts. The ethical aspect became more and more important in the course of the Egyptian history.

With this Egyptological background in mind, Nili Shupak reexamined how Jewish commentaries reflect on the three items listed in the Bible as abominations to the Egyptians: eating with Hebrews (Gen 43:32); shepherds (Gen 46:34); the offerings of the Hebrews (Exod 8:22).[22] For Shupak, *bwt* represents the forbidden, that which is evil and the negative. She categorizes the occurrences of *bwt* into four different groups: forbidden food, prohibitions related to moral and social behavior, prohibitions associated with the worship of a deity, and other miscellaneous prohibitions According to Shupak, to eat with the Hebrews was prohibited for an upper-class Egyptian for two of these reasons: first, there was a social distance between Joseph as part of the kings' court and his family as shepherds that required separate dishes; second, the mutton was holy for Amun, Chnum, and others gods and therefore was *bwt* to be eaten in Egypt.

As can be seen from this very short summary of the interpretations of Frandsen and Shupak, *bwt* is a complex category, because it is strongly bound to social sensitivities and theological aspects. Furthermore, the theological dimensions do not imply an unambiguous, stringent list of objects and behaviors which are *bwt*.

---

[19] Paul John Frandsen, "On the Avoidance of Certain Forms of Loud Voices and Access to the Sacred," in part 2 of *Egyptian Religion: The Last Thousand Years; Studies Dedicated to the Memory of Jan Quaegebeur*, ed. Willy Clarysse, Antoon Schoors, and Harco Willems (Leuven: Peeters, 1998), 975.

[20] Paul John Frandsen, "Durkheim's Dichotomy Sacred: Profane and the Egyptian Category *bwt*," in vol. 1 of *Millions of Jubilees: Studies in Honor of David P. Silverman*, ed. Zahi Hawass and Jennifer Houser Wegner (Cairo: Conseil suprême des antiquités de l'Égypte, 2010), 149–74.

[21] For this aspect, see Paul John Frandsen, "Faeces of the Creator or the Temptations of the Dead," in *Ancient Egyptian Demonology: Studies in the Boundaries between the Demonic and the Divine in Egyptian Magic*, ed. P. Kousoulis (Leuven: Peters, 2011), 25–62.

[22] Nili Shupak, "The Abomination of Egypt: New Light on an Old Problem" [Hebrew], in *Marbeh Hokmah: Studies in the Bible and the Ancient Near East in Loving Memory of Victor Avigdor Huowitz*, ed. Shamir Yona et al. (Beer-Sheva: Gen-Gurion University of the Negev Press, 2015), 271–94*.

On the contrary: what is *bwt* for one god may be pleasant to another. Osiris, the Lord of Silence, for example, required silence in his realm. The restriction applied to funerary areas as attested since the Middle Kingdom and to different kinds of sanctuaries in later periods. Silence was important to such a degree that it became strongly associated with the Egyptian ideas of holiness, wisdom, and a good behavior, as attested in biographical texts.[23] On the other hand, joyful noise was required in the realm of Mut and Hathor. The pacification of the lion-like Mut into the cat-like Bastet was at the core of a series of celebrations in the cult of Egypt's goddess. According to a hymn to Hathor from the Graeco-Roman era, the nourishment of Hathor is music and dance. Therefore, mourning (*snm*), hunger, thirst, and lament (*št3*) are taboo (*bwt*) on the goddess' feast of drunkenness, which occurred on the twentieth day of the first month of inundation.[24] Any behavior connected with fasting, including castigating oneself, is an abhorrence for the goddess.

The Egyptians were afraid of displeasing a deity and being persecuted by the furious sun eye as a rebel of the gods. While dying was part of the natural life cycle and a chance for an eternal life in the West as an Osiris, being killed by the gods as a rebel was the definite end and therefore the Egyptians' main fear. This cardinal anxiety is reflected in the spells of the Book of the Dead and therefore the main source for our understanding of what *bwt* means for the Egyptians, what they avoid in life and what they hope to avoid in the afterworld.[25]

The Book of the Dead—similar to the Hebrew Bible—is a corpus of wisdom, teachings, and insight that grew over centuries and was transmitted in a more or less canonized form. It therefore provides information about the very core taboos of Egyptian culture. However, the following observations on abominations in the Book of the Dead, based on Thomas George Allen's translation,[26] are only a first

---

[23] Frandsen, "Avoidance of Certain Forms," 975–1000. This view comes close to biblical concepts, depicting God as revealing himself in a hush rather than in a storm, earthquake, or fire (1 Kgs 19:12) and maybe presupposing a "sanctuary of silence"—see Israel Knohl, *Sanctuary of Silence: The Priestly Torah and the Holiness School* (Minneapolis: Fortress, 1995)—and praising the ability to keep silent, be it by prudence (Prov 17:27; 23:9; 30:32–33), by slyness (Prov 12:16, 23), by solidarity (Prov 11:13; 20:19; 25:9–10), or by respect (Prov 11:12).

[24] Paul John Frandsen, "On Fear of Death and the Three *bwts* Connected with Hathor," in *Gold of Praise: Studies on Ancient Egypt in Honor of Edward F. Wente*, ed. Emily Teeter and John A. Larson (Chicago: Oriental Institute of the University of Chicago, 1999), 131–48.

[25] This is not to deny that there are other important sources for understanding the Egyptian feeling of disgust, e.g., medical texts referring to the disgust of the heart; see Heinrich Joachim, *Papyros Ebers: Das älteste Buch über Heilkunde* (Berlin: de Gruyter, 1890), 182–84.

[26] Thomas George Allen, *The Book of the Dead or Going Forth by Day: Ideas of the Ancient Egyptians Concerning the Hereafter as Expressed in Their Own Terms*, SAOC 37 (Chicago: The University of Chicago Press, 1974).

attempt to sketch out some general ideas about the concept.[27] Allen has the word *abomination*[28] in his translation eighty times, often more than one time in a sentence. An analysis of the relevant passages shows different types and aspects of abominations that bother the Egyptians at death's door. It goes without saying that the fear of the dead in the spells is in fact the fear of the living who have to die one day. Thus, the abominations of the dead are (also) abominations of the living under the condition of eternity. The following abominations are mentioned in the Book of the Dead.

2.1. Abominations, Representing a General Fear

Some spells express a general fear by designating it as an abomination. Thus, "being punished" is an abomination (Spell 137 A T11) and the "executioners" in the netherworld are abominations (Spell 144e S). The dead assert that they have "committed no abomination against the Gods" (Spell 29A). Different amulets cover the body of the dead in order to protect them from evil in the afterlife. The papyrus-amulet of feldspar, for instance, is an important gift for the dead that is designed to protect them against injury in the afterlife. The spells express this specific function of the amulet with the words: "Injury is (its) abomination" (Spell 160 S1). The secret knowledge of the spells is so constitutive for the dead's persistence in the afterlife that the Egyptians fear the revelation of the precious magic by enemies. Therefore, to let anyone see "the roll great of mystery" is an abomination too (Spell 162 T5).

2.2. The Abomination of the Second Death

The general fear in ancient societies was not the fear of biological death, but of social or cosmic death.[29] That is, people were afraid of not being provided with a funeral and offerings by the surviving family and not being accepted by the gods in the netherworld. It is this "second" death that is referred to when the dead recite: "Dying is my abomination" (Spell 85b) or "to die again" (Spell 109b S2). The

---

[27] As far as I can see a thorough study of the subject is lacking.

[28] Mainly the translation for *bwt*. "Der Abscheu, das Widerliche"; cf. *Wb* 1:453; Rainer Hannig, *Großes Handwörterbuch Ägyptisch-Deutsch (2800–950 v. Chr.): Die Sprache der Pharaonen*, 5th ed. (Mainz: von Zabern, 2009), 267. The corresponding verb *bwj* is cognate with the Semitic root *עבי, attested with the meaning "to refuse" in many Semitic languages; see Gábor Takács, *Etymological Dictionary of Egyptian*, vol. 2 (Leiden: Brill, 2009), 183–84.

[29] Hans-Peter Hasenfratz, *Die Toten Lebenden: Eine religionsphänomenologische Studie zum sozialen Tod in archaischen Gesellschaften; Zugleich ein kritischer Beitrag zur sogenannten Strafopfertheorie*, BZRGG 24 (Leiden: Brill, 1982).

dead fear the executioners of the netherworld. The god's slaughtering-block (Spell 28a S1) and losing the breast (Spell 28b S2) are abominations. As cosmic beings, the dead want to rest in a transfigured state. To see again the "land of the east" (of sunrise, of dying again and going back to earthly life) is therefore another abomination to the dead (Spell 176 S). The same horror springs from the vision of sleeping eternally in the netherworld. "The sleep that clings to thee" is the abomination of Osiris (Spell 168e S54). What the dead want is to live quietly and comfortably in the afterworld as transfigured beings.

2.3. The Abomination to Eat Dung, to Drink Urine, and to Walk Upside Down

Another cardinal abomination of the Book of the Dead is scatophagy, that is, eating dung (Spell 82b S), touching it (Spells 51 S; 52a S; 102b S; 124b S; 189a.d.f and i S), and drinking urine (Spells 53b S1; 116 T; 178f S2). Typically, the two horrors are combined with a third one, the fear of walking upside down (Spell 51; cf. Spell 189).[30] The trinity is already attested in the Pyramid Texts (Spells 210; 409) and in the Coffin Texts (Spells 173, 216, 581, and 1011).[31] The three horrors are abominations of a "world [in] reverse,"[32] where everything is upside down. If the dead have to walk on their hands, they risk coming in contact with urine and dung on the street. At least in the Coffin Texts it seems that dung and urine are also symbols of death; in divine comparisons the fear of ingesting urine and dung or even touching them is associated with the gods' distance from death.[33] The disgusting effect is not based on the fecal matter as such[34] but on its impact on

---

[30] The recapping verse in Spell 53b S1 reads: "My abomination is my abomination; I will not eat dung, I will not drink urine, (nor) walk upside down."

[31] Doris Topmann, *Die "Abscheu"-Sprüche der altägyptischen Sargtexte: Untersuchungen zu Textemen und Dialogstrukturen*, Göttinger Orientforschungen 4/39 (Wiesbaden: Harrassowitz, 2002), 206.

[32] Jan Zandee, *Death as an Enemy according to Ancient Egyptian Conceptions*, SHR 5 (Leiden: Brill, 1960), 73–78, followed by Erik Hornung, *Altägyptische Höllenvorstellungen*, ASAW 59.3 (Berlin: Akademieverlag, 1968), 13 and 15–16; Gerald E. Kadish emphasizes the aspect that the death is tested and has to prove that he belongs to the world of order of *m3'.t*. Gerald E. Kadish, "The Scatophagous Egyptian," *JSSEA* 9 (1979): 203–17. Similar Paul J. Frandsen, "BWT: Divine Kingship and Grammar," in *Linguistik, Philologie, Religion*, vol. 3 of *Akten des vierten internationalen Ägyptologenkongresses, München 1985*, ed. Sylvia Schoske (Hamburg: Buske, 1989), 151–58.

[33] Topmann, "'Abscheu'-Sprüche," 54–55.

[34] As part of the created, "natural" world, excrements have even the potential to be divine. Alexandra von Lieven has shown that the Egyptians used a kind of adobe mixed with animal dung for the production of models of divine figures. They also mummified dung of dogs or the Apis bull. Dung of cows was used for many things, e.g., to build beehives. This has been reflected on a mythological level. Very rarely the use of human dung

gods, including the transfigured dead. They should be far from excrements, symbolizing dissolution and caducity.

The "swallower of the ass," an "abomination of Osiris," is perhaps a cognate of the abomination to eat feces (Spell 40 P1 and S1). This is probably a continuation of the personification of excrements as demonic beings attested in the Coffin Texts.[35]

The noble Egyptian who equipped his tomb or his sarcophagus with spells wanted to eat "bread of white wheat" and drink beer "of red barley" (Spell 52b S2) and stretch his intestines when he joined the ferryboat of the sky (Spell 53b S2). This latter phrase may indicate that the noble Egyptians defecated normally on the boat into the water of the Nile. The wish to eat bread and to drink bear in the afterworld implies that hunger and thirst are seen as an abomination (Spell 178g S).

Another spell combines dung and lies, both abominations of the gods that should not be offered to the deceased (Spell 17 S5). This brings us to the next category of abomination, which may be labeled "moral" abominations.

2.4. The Abomination of Not Being Righteous

"To tell lies" is the abomination of "the son of a righteous man" found in a spell for not letting seat and throne be taken away from the dead (Spell 47 S var.). To be "seated at the right hand of the Father," the privilege of the son of God still quoted in the apostolic credo of the Christian church, was the longing of the Egyptian dead. Therefore, lies are an abomination (Spell 178n S). As righteous individuals, the dead were incarnations of Thot. "Falsehood" (Spells 182a S1; 183b S1; 184b S2) and "lying" (Spell 182a S1 variant) are Thoth's abominations.

In a more general way every kind of sin is an abomination. Thus, the dead may recite: "Sin is my *abomination*." The statement is paralleled by the statements like "god is my soul," "I created authority," and "I am lord of light" (Spells 85a S1–2; 153c S2). The association of righteousness and light does not come as a surprise, since the rising light all over the ancient Near East was strongly connected with jurisdiction. Those who carry the light of the night in its boat are the baboons. Hence Spell 126 reads: "O ye baboons ... whose *abomination* is sin, remove my evil, blot out my sins."

---

for divination by a scarab is attested and the funerary gift of the dung of cattle in *qaab*-bowls. Von Lieven thinks that, as a general rule, the divine status of a being makes its dung potentially a positive *materia magica*. Alexandra von Lieven, "'Where There Is Dirt There Is System': Zur Ambiguität der Bewertung von körperlichen Ausscheidungen in der ägyptischen Kultur," *Studien zur Altägyptischen Kultur* 40 (2011): 287–300.

[35] Topmann, "'Abscheu'-Sprüche," 56–59.

2.5. Other Abominations

Besides the hitherto mentioned cardinal abominations, several abominations are mentioned that are difficult to systematize and sometimes also difficult to understand from a modern Western point of view. An enemy and therefore an abomination of the dead is the crocodile. The crocodile is residing in the water, which is covering all the land during the flood. Therefore the flood as well is an abomination of the dead (Spell 130b S6). In another spell the dead recites that the abomination of the crocodiles of the four cardinal directions are in his belly (Spell 32b). In other words, the abomination of an abomination is a magic resource for the dead.

Further spells mention food-abominations of the gods. The eating of a mouse by a snake is "the abomination of Re" (Spell 33 S), as the mouse is holy for Re. "Pig-abomination for Horus's sake by the gods" is explained by an attack of Horus by Seth in the shape of a black boar. In order to save Horus the gods are asked to abominate the pig which originally was even part of offerings for the Horus child (Spell 112a S1).

"Shu's Mutilator" is the abomination of the cutter of heads, who wants to put incoherence into the speech of the blessed (Spell 90 S2). "Storm is Osiris NN.'s abomination" (Spell 130b S2). "Carnage" is the abomination of Sokar (Spell 168b S9)—probably another variant meant to express the horror of the second death (see above 2.2.). Finally, the dead wishes to linger on in the presence of the god's face. The godly aspect of the resting face in Egypt is Hathor. "She likes to enter, (but) to come forth is [her] abomination" (Spell 186Ba S1).

2.6. Facit

To conclude, it seems to me that nothing in ancient Egypt is disgusting per se. Rather everything has the potential to be divine, including feces. In other words, for the Egyptians disgust exists only as contextually limited feeling. It is a relative feeling. Disgust, as a feeling of strong aversion triggered by our senses, is linked to a deity according to the formula: xy is *bwt* for DN (including a human once he is dead, that is, transfigured, that is, an Osiris). As the deity represents a specific aspect of the civilized world we may translate the formula into our world and language with: xy is disgusting in a specific context/realm/time/place/et cetera.

In the realm of the living, feces do not seem to be *bwt* because they are a natural part of life and special places were reserved for defecation.[36] However, for

---

[36] A pertinent study on sanitation in ancient Egypt, however, is lacking. Some material is listed in Nabil I. Ebeid, *Egyptian Medicine in the Days of the Pharaohs* (Cairo: The General Egyptian Book Organization 1999).

the dead, feces represent a danger because a mummy lies in the earth and is therefore in a position that could force him to eat dung. That is why magical protection is needed for this eventuality.

3. Fecal Disgust: Connecting Factor for Prophetic Action and Teaching

That feces are elicitors of disgust does not prejudge a solely negative symbolism —on the contrary. For intellectuals and artistic or sexually liminal persons who served as cathartic instances in their own society, the daily need to defecate, the feelings of disgust feces elicited, and the above illustrated wish to eliminate feces made all feces a perfect starting point from which to teach a lesson. Babylonian (3.1), Judean (3.2) and Greek (3.3) examples illustrate this aspect.

3.1. Kurgarrû

An early example is the Old-Babylonian *kurgarrû*, a male or hermaphrodite prostitute, musician, jester, and prophet.[37] Probably this guy is to be identified with a

---

[37] *Kurgarrû* together with *assinnu* are part of the cultic servants of Ishtar. In lexical lists *kurgarrû* is identified with Sumerian *pi-li-pi-li*, probably an onomatopoetic word and maybe belonging to *pi.lá*, "to be dirty/different." In some contexts he plays a sexually ambivalent role as in the Inanna-cult-rites of exchange of garments—see Brigitte Groneberg, "Die sumerisch-akkadische Inanna/Ištar: Hermaphroditos?," *WO* 17 (1986): 34 n. 54—and on tablet IV, 56 of the Erra Epic: "Whose masculinity Ištar has turned to femininity to make the people reverent"; see Wilfried G. Lambert, "Prostitution," in *Außenseiter und Randgruppen: Beiträge zu einer Sozialgeschichte des Alten Orients*, ed. Volkert Haas, Xenia 32 (Konstanz: Universitätsverlag, 1992), 148. He belongs to the representatives of ecstatic prophecy; cf. Eckart Frahm, "Prophetie," *RlA* 11 (2006): 8 with sources. In a Balag he is associated with a potter, a *kalû*-singer, and a shepherd; see Walther Sallaberger and Miguel Civil, *Der babylonische Töpfer und seine Gefäße: Nach Urkunden altsumerischer bis altbabylonischer Zeit sowie lexikalischen und literarischen Zeugnissen*, Mesopotamian History and Environment 2/3 (Gent: University of Gent, 1996), 15. Later, in Neo-Assyrian times the *kurgarrû* imitate the wars of the king with loud music in a ritual ceremony; see Michael Haul, *Stele und Legende: Untersuchungen zu den keilschriftlichen Erzählwerken über die Könige von Akkade*, Göttinger Beiträge zum Alten Orient 4 (Göttingen: Universitätsverlag, 2009), 203 n. 42. As a performer of cultic games, he is already mentioned in the texts of Ebla (Gu-ga-ar, Gu-gàr, Gu-ga-lum); see Alfonso Archi et al., *The Prosopography of Ebla: Lettera G* 47 (2011), http://www.sagas.unifi.it/upload/sub/eblaweb/dbase_prosopografia/g.pdf. According to the myth, "Ishtar's Descent to the Netherworld," the *kurgarrû* was created by a god and therefore had supernatural powers. Different than normal human beings—and probably as a consequence of his transgender nature—he could transgress the border between life and death without danger. Furthermore, Ea, god of the art of incantation, equipped him with the "water of life" and the "herb of life" in order to cure people.

figure found on an old Babylonian terracotta plaque (fig. 1): a naked male, crouching, defecating, playing the lute, and flanked by a barking dog and a pig (?), smelling his feces.[38]

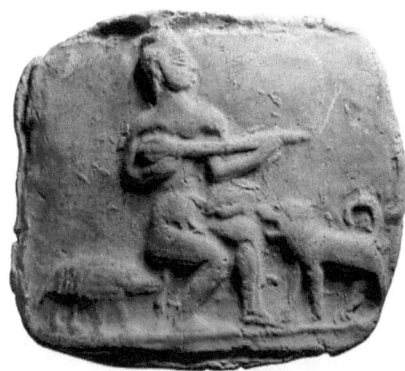 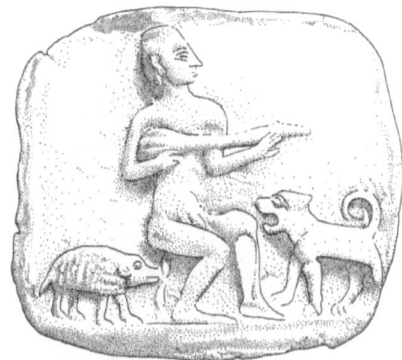

Fig. 1a–b. Defecating lute player with dog and pig (?). Old Babylonian terracotta plaque, probably from Nippur,[39] Eighteenth–Sixteenth century BCE. Courtesy of BIBLE+ORIENT Museum, Fribourg, Switzerland, VFig 2002.7.

He also is told to play music and to perform together with specialists of music as *maḫḫû* and *zabbu*. He plays his part in exorcistic rituals as he is able to convoke the congregation (of the gods). In other words, *kurgarrû* was a kind of shaman. People took fright of him, on the one hand, because of his sexual ambiguity and, on the other hand, because of his magic power. While in the second millennium BCE *kurgarrû* was a rather respected person in the midst of a series of similar ritual specialists, it seems that in late Babylonian times he was rather feared and object of curses; see Stefan M. Maul, "*Kurgarrû* und *assinnu* und ihr Stand in der babylonischen Gesellschaft," in Haas, *Außenseiter und Randgruppen*, 159–72. But his shamanistic nature should not be understood in a clerical way. Rather *kurgarrû* was more of a juggler comparable to some figures of the commedia dell'arte; see Dietz Otto Edzard, "Zur Ritualtafel der sog. 'Love Lyrics,'" in *Language, Literature, and History, Philological and Historical Studies Presented to Erica Reiner*, ed. Francesca Rochberg-Halton, AOS 67 (New Haven: American Oriental Society, 1987), 57–69; Felix Blocher, "Gaukler im Alten Orient," in Haas, *Außenseiter und Randgruppen*, 79–111.

[38] In a first attempt this image has been interpreted as a bucolic scene, see Leon Legrain, *Terracottas from Nippur*, PBS 16 (Philadelphia: University of Pennsylvania Press, 1930), 19. But a more precise iconographic analysis points to an urban context: Marie-Thérèse Barrelet, *Figurines et reliefs en terre cuite de la Mésopotamie antique*, Bibliothèque archéologique et historique 85 (Paris: Geuthner, 1968); Dominique Parayre, "Les suidés dans le monde syro-mésopotamien aux époques historiques," *Topoi Suppl* 2 (2000): 169 with n. 144 and fig. 23.

[39] Parallels for this piece are attested in Nippur: in the temple of Bêl, see Bruno Meissner, *Babylonien und Assyrien*, vol. 1 (Heidelberg: Carl Winter, 1920), fig. 201 = Leon

Another terracotta plaque shows a defecating person with a perfectly modelled pig (fig. 2).

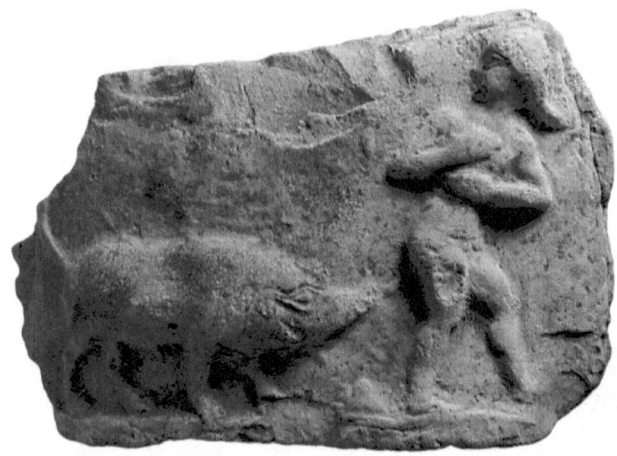

Fig. 2. Pig, catching the dung of a defecating person. Old Babylonian terracotta plaque, probably from Nippur, Eighteenth–Sixteenth century BCE. Courtesy of BIBLE+ORIENT Museum, Fribourg, Switzerland, VFig 2002.6.

According to Enkidu's curse in the Babylonian Gilgamesh epic, prostitutes had to live in the dirtiest places of the town.[40] Dogs and pigs who lived free in the roads of ancient Near Eastern towns connote the dirt of the streets, flies, mosquitos, and stench and therefore evoke disgust. In contrast, the lute connotes nice sounds, joy, feasts, and pleasure and therefore evokes delight and lust. The figure of the shitting *kurgarrû* (lower part of the image) playing music (upper part of the image)

Legrain, *Terracottas from Nippur*, PBS 16 (Philadelphia: University of Pennsylvania Press, 1930), n. 94 (Pennsylvania Museum, Philadelphia, Inv. 58–21986); on the "tablett hill," see Ruth Mayer-Opificius, *Das altbabylonische Terrakottarelief*, UAVA 2 (Berlin: de Gruyter, 1961), n. 580 (without figure; lost); and in the scribal quarter, see Donald Eugene McCown et al., *Temple of Enlil, Scribal Quarter, and Soundings: Excavations of the Joint Expedition to Nippur of the University Museum of Philadelphia and the Oriental Institute of the University of Chicago*, OIP 78 (Chicago: Oriental Institute of the University of Chicago, 1967), pl. 138, fig. 1. See also Baghdad, IM 9419 (according to a personal photo in the materials of Marie-Thérèse Barrelet).

[40] Andrew R. George, *The Babylonian Gilgamesh Epic* (Oxford: Oxford University Press, 2003), 639–40: "May the ground defile your fine-looking [garment!]/ May [the drunkard] smear [with durst your festive gown!] / ... / May [the junction] of the highway be where you sit! / [May the ruined houses be] where you sleep!" (7:109–117), etc.

represents human liminality between the sometimes disgusting materiality of human life and the longing for erotic and spiritual fulfillment of human desire. Music is evoked in this image as a strong apotropaic power. Even the barking dog, looking upwards, seems to be enchanted by the sounds of the lute. Not so the pig, sniffing and scuffing at the *kurgarrû*'s shit. Maybe the pig and dog represent two sides of animal behavior. If this is the case, the terracotta plaque not only confronts the material (defecating) and the spiritual (making music) world in the vertical direction of the scene but also "demonic" (pig) and "angelic" (dog) behavior in life, that is, in the horizontal direction of the scene. This interpretation of the behavior of the two animals fits well with the overall picture of the symbolism of the two animals in ancient Mesopotamia.[41]

As I have shown elsewhere,[42] the cowering musician, surrounded by wild animals, is the prototype of the male magician, who can banish the demonic world through his art. This figure takes shape in Ugaritic poetry as Aqhat, in Hebrew poetry as David and in Greek poetry as Orpheus. Not only the *kurgarrû*'s iconography but also his mythology shows striking parallels with the Orphic tradition. According to myth, the *kurgarrû* is created as a transgender being. Evidently the bridging of gender enables him to easily overcome the boundary between life and death. This is necessary for Ishtar's redemption from the underworld. As a punishment of his outrageous act, the *kurgarrû* is cursed by Ereshkigal, the Mistress of the Underworld, to live in the sewers, in the shadow of walls, and on thresholds, that is, in places where people defecated.[43] The myths of northern Greece tell us that Orpheus descends to the underworld for the liberation of Eurydice and returns safely after a failed mission. Frustrated by the result, he introduces boyish love in Thrace and thereby draws on the hatred of the Maenads, this being his punishment of trespassing the gender borders. In the case of David, the musician, his love to Jonathan is emphasized in 2 Sam 1:26, while any ability to trespass the way to Sheol is strictly omitted in the Hebrew Bible (but see 1 Sam 28).

We meet lute players again, surrounded by wild animals, centuries later on a Babylonian Kudurru, in a hymn to the city goddess of Arbela, and on the gate

---

[41] For the demonic character of the pig, see Thomas Staubli, "Warum man Hühner ass, aber keine Schweine: Biblische Speisetabus und ihre Folgen," in *"Im Schatten Deiner Flügel": Tiere in der Bibel und im Alten Orient*, ed. Othmar Keel and Thomas Staubli (Fribourg: Presses Universitaires, 2001), 47–50. For the wolf/dog as follower and layer of culture see Greger Larson et al., "Rethinking Dog Domestication by Integrating Genetics, Archeology, and Biogeography," *PNAS* 109 (2012): 8878–83.

[42] Thomas Staubli, "Magische Macht der Musik: Orpheus' orientalische Vorbilder," *Cardo* 16 (2018): 12–22.

[43] In other words, the places for transgender people in the ancient Babylonian society were urban, liminal, and stinky. The same is still the case in India; see Arundhaty Roy, *The Ministry of Utmost Happiness* (London: Hamish Hamilton, 2017).

reliefs of Sam'al. In each case, music is evoked as a magical power able to govern dangerous creatures. Interestingly, the motif of animal peace is an independent contribution of visual art that is not told explicitly in mythology. It is a pictorial illustration of the magical effect of music. On the myth's way westward, the lute, which is often the instrument of the armed god Reshef, was replaced by the lyre.

But the unvarnished motif of the shitting musician does not survive the Old Babylonian epoch. Its disgusting evocation was obviously too strong and led to the omission of the picture. The frightening side of the musician was henceforth represented by his armament. In fact, the *kurgarrû* tablet evokes smells and sounds. By combining the issue of shitting with music, it probably provoked a smile and thus was also a humoristic comment on human fugacity. This fits well the genre of terracotta tablets, which probably were a kind of apotropaica to be fixed on windows or house entrances.

3.2. Judean Sages and Prophets

Nevertheless, shit and shitting could be rhetorically evoked still in later periods, in order to provoke, to analyze, and to criticize, when the opportunity arose. For the Judean wisdom teacher, excretion, which leaves the body and disappears gradually, is a symbol of transience, a radical-materialistic *memento mori*. This argument is used as self-assurance for the pious in front of the egoist: the wicked and the godless are mortal like everybody. "They will perish forever like their own dung" (Job 20:7; cf. Sir 10:9).

A bitter note of protest inheres YHWH's command to the prophet Ezekiel to eat bread, prepared on "human dung" (גללי [צאת] האדם), in order to demonstrate to the public the anticipated misery of Jerusalem's remaining folk under Nebuchadnezzar's siege. Being a priest, Ezekiel avoided strictly contact with carcasses or any kind of rotten meat. At Ezekiel's plea God permits Ezekiel to replace the human dung by "cattle's dung" (צפועי הבקר), the product of herbivores and a traditional fuel in the Middle East (Ezek 4:9–15). The tenor of the prophet's symbolic acting is to stress the horror of Jerusalem's siege by evoking a feeling of disgust. On the literary level, the aspect of disgust is emphasized by the replacement of human dung by cattle's dung. The moral of the episode is that the reality was so shocking/disgusting that it was not possible for a Judean priest to represent it.[44]

Even more disgusting than the image of eating bread baked on human dung is the image of eating human feces. That is how the Assyrian Rabshakeh characterizes the beleaguered Jerusalemites: a people eating their own dung (צאת/חרא)

---

[44] Note, however, that the priestly code of ethics implied in this episode was modified by later rabbinic teaching. Excrements are regarded as more or less disgusting depending on circumstances and personal sensibilities (b. Yoma 30a).

and drinking their own urine (מים רגליו/שין) (2 Kgs 18:27), a horrific image well known from the Egyptian Book of the Dead (see above).

The sensation of disgust, triggered by excrements, also stands behind Zechariah's sarcastic prophetic polemics against Tyre, which ridicules the rich. In Zech 9:3 the city is said to have piled up silver like dust (עפר) and gold like shit (טיט). The accumulation of capital in the form of palaces, which should enhance prestige and honor, is unmasked as shameful, stinky, and therefore disgusting behavior. Similarly, Isaiah publicly criticizes the excessive feasting and drinking of priests and prophets. He describes their tables, completely covered with "filthy vomit" (קיא צאה; Isa 28:7–8). Binge drinking and vomiting by the upper class is iconographically represented in Late Bronze Age Egypt (fig. 3). In more general terms, but with the same feelings of disgust, Isaiah foretells that spirits of judgment and burning will wash the "filth" (צאת) of the daughters of Zion and the bloodstains of Jerusalem (Isa 4:4). The destruction of the house of Jeroboam is even compared to the burning of "dung" (גלל; 1 Kgs 14:10).

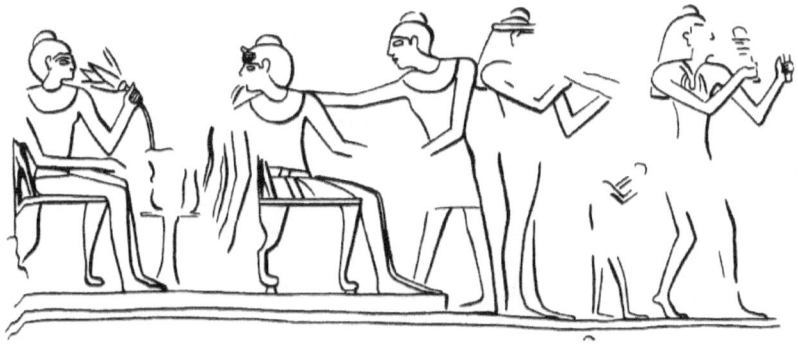

Fig. 3. An Egyptian of the elite vomits during a feast. A slave assists him. Fresco of a private tomb in Thebe around 1450 BCE. Drawing by Hildi Keel-Leu. Courtesy of Stiftung BIBEL+ORIENT, Fribourg, Switzerland.

3.3. Diogenes (and Till Eulenspiegel)

While the Judean sages highlight the symbolism of caducity, the need to defecate could also symbolize the equality not only of all humans but of all living beings. Thus, defecating in public was a philosophical manifest for the Cynic Diogenes of Sinope. Peter Sloterdijk interprets Diogenes's behavior as an aspect of pantomimic theory, which resists dividing our being between a higher human part and a lower animal part. As a consequence, the Cynic (dog-like) Diogenes overcomes his feelings of disgust whereas a (post)modern cynic would find everything disgusting.[45]

Given the universal disgust elicited by feces, its positive symbolism creates a sense of protest against social norms or established behaviors. For the Low-German anarchistic jester Till Eulenspiegel public shitting or objects made of feces became a common hoax by which to shock people or make them laugh at a cleric, the Jews of Frankfort, a shoemaker, a barber-surgeon, or a druggist. Evidently, the addressees of his hoaxes are mainly people who stress (moral) purity or cleanliness.[46]

4. Making Gods and Their Teachings Disgusting with Shit-Rhetoric

In the priestly Torah and cognate prophetic texts, the rhetoric of disgust plays a major role.[47] Disgust can be connected with land and people, sex, food and drink, unmoral acts, life and death, and to a high degree with the gods.[48]

---

[45] Peter Sloterdijk, *Kritik der zynischen Vernunft*, Edition Suhrkamp 1099 (Frankfurt: Suhrkamp, 1983), 289–90; English translation: Sloterdijk, *Critique of Cynical Reason*, trans. Michael Eldred, foreword Andreas Huyssen, Theory and History of Literature 40 (Minneapolis: University of Minnesota Press, 1987), 151.

[46] Wolfgang Lindow, ed., *Ein kurtzweilig Lesen von Dil Ulenspiegel: Nach dem Druck von 1515*, Universal-Bibliothek 1687 (Stuttgart: Reclam, 1978), see Historie 12, 36, 46, 52, 69, 90. An exceptional case is Historie 81, where Dil Ulenspiegel defecates in the kitchen of a very poor inn because he is unnerved by the children of the house making ca-ca behind the door.

[47] Thomas Kazen and Yitzhaq Feder examined the role of disgust for the Priestly system of pure and impure in the seminal view of Mary Douglas. Thomas Kazen, "The Role of Disgust in Priestly Purity Law: Insights from Conceptual Metaphor and Blending Theories," *Journal of Law, Religion and State* 3 (2014): 62–92; Kazen, "Disgust in Body, Mind, and Language: The Case of Impurity in the Hebrew Bible," in *Mixed Feelings and Vexed Passions: Exploring Emotions in Biblical Literature*, ed. F. Scott Spencer, RBS 90 (Atlanta: SBL Press, 2017), 97–116; Yitzhaq Feder, "Defilement and Moral Discourse in the Hebrew Bible: An Evolutionary Framework," *Journal of Cognitive Historiography* 3 (2016): 157–89; Feder, "Contamination Appraisals, Pollution Beliefs and the Role of Cultural Inheritance in Shaping Disease Avoidance Behavior," *Cognitive Science* (2016): 1561–85. Other articles focus on the role of disgust in identity formation, e.g., Carly L. Crouch, "What Makes a Thing Abominable? Observations on the Language of Boundaries and Identity Formation from a Social Scientific Perspective," *VT* 65 (2015): 516–41. For a critique of Mary Douglas's and others' theories of disgust, see already Edward B. Royzman and John Sabini, "Something It Takes to Be an Emotion: The Interesting Case of Disgust," *Journal for the Theory of Social Behaviour* 31 (2001): 29–59, esp. 40–41.

[48] For a more detailed analysis, see Thomas Staubli, "Disgusting Deeds and Disgusting Gods: Ethnic and Ethical Constructions of Disgust in the Hebrew Bible," *HeBAI* 6 (2017): 457–87.

With the strongest rhetoric available, the book of Deuteronomy tries to implement disgust for any non-Yahwistic cult: "Do not bring an abhorrent thing [i.e., a godly image] into your house, or you will be set apart for destruction like it. You must detest [שקץ] it with detestation and abhor [תעב] it with abhorrence, for it is set apart for destruction" (Deut 7:26). The terms תועבה and שקוץ are used from the times of Hosea until Hellenistic times to persecute non-Yahwistic worship (e.g., Isa 66:3; 1 Macc 1:54; 6:7). Furthermore, the legislators used fecal language to ensure the abhorrence of cult figures, which were made by the most skilled artists with the most precious materials and thus typically objects with a strong aesthetic attraction. The key term is גלולים (Deut 29:16; 1 Kgs 21:26; 2 Kgs 17:12; 21:21; 23:24). The root גלל refers to something round like the dung of goats and sheep. Therefore, the term probably connotes shit. Related to idols it means literally "shit-things."[49] It is certainly not by chance that Ezekiel favors the term גלולים for idols. He is especially sensitive to the interconnection of form, content, and emotions. The fecal association would evoke disgust. To stress the abomination of idolatry, Ezekiel also describes idolatry as whoring with lovers, whose nakedness is uncovered by those full of lust (Ezek 16:36). The priestly prophet's aim is to turn people away from their shit-things as they turn instinctively, driven by disgust, away from feces or from a person with shameless behavior (Ezek 14:6). The veneration of shit-things is for him an act that defiles (Ezek 36:18) and needs to be cleansed (Ezek 36:25).

Ezekiel's sensitivity for moral disgust, which is elicited in the obedience to gods other than YHWH, is echoed in the legislation of the Holiness Code: "I will destroy your high places and cut down your incense altars; I will heap your carcasses on the carcasses of your shit-things. I will abhor you" (Lev 26:30). At the very end of a series of punishments, YHWH shall destroy the very source of Israel's misdeeds, the shit-things. They will be destroyed together with their worshippers. The image of the carcasses of the Israelites heaped on the carcasses of the idols not only underlines dramatically the connection of idolatry and injustice according to the Holiness Code; it also evokes rhetorically a feeling of disgust in the reader or hearer of this sentence.

---

[49] The Zürcher Bibel translates "Mistgötzen," the NRSV "idol." In Palmyrenian language *gllh* corresponds to Greek στήλη λιθίνη, "stone stele." Ezekiel 20:7–8 urges the people to throw away the גלולי מצרים. Maybe he was rather referring to scarabs, the most widespread type of amulets in the Levant. These miniature idols were associated with dung also on a biological level, because the beetle cuts perfectly round balls out of heaps of dung. See Christian Herrmann, *Ägyptische Amulette aus Palästina/Israel: Mit einem Ausblick auf ihre Rezeption durch das Alte Testament*, OBO 138 (Fribourg: Presses Universitaires; Göttingen: Vandenhoeck & Ruprecht, 1994), 83–87.

While rhetorical efforts to evoke disgust in order to win support for a social or political aim is known also from the Greek polis,[50] the manner of making other gods disgusting by strong rhetorical means seems to be an ancient Israelite peculiarity. It was a very effective way to regulate the moral behavior of the people in a systematic way. The idols must be detested for ideological reasons, for they were considered to be the source of immoral offerings and an immoral way of life. According to the prophets, they represent a wrong ethical code. Ezekiel states explicitly that the mind of the idolaters follows the mind of their idols (Ezek 11:21). Jeremiah holds that Baal commanded abominable rules like the burning of children, which YHWH did not command, decree, or enter his mind (Jer 19:5). In the Holiness Code's view, the natives of the country followed "abominable rules" (חקות התועבת; Lev 18:30), rules that were decreed by their gods (see fig. 4). In contrast to the Deuteronomist, who holds that the Israelites have the duty to expel the natives (Deut 7), for the Holiness Code the behavior of the natives does not directly justify their expulsion by the Israelites. The Holiness Code formulates the view that they are vomited out by the "land" (ארץ; Lev 18:28).

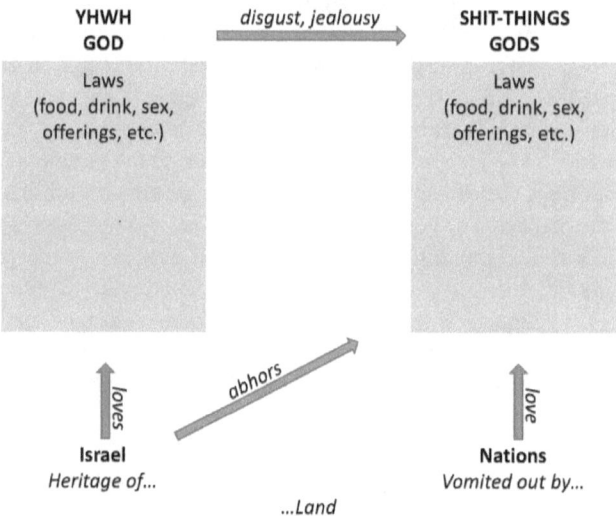

Fig. 4. The Holiness Code's view of the relationship between Israel and the nations, YHWH and the gods.

---

[50] Thomas Cirillo, "Transferable Disgust in Demosthenes 54: Against Conon," *Syllecta classica* 20 (2009): 1–30; for a wide range of examples of the resonance of the emotion of disgust in Greek society, see now Donald Lateiner and Dimos Spatharas, eds., *The Ancient Emotion of Disgust* (Oxford: Oxford University Press, 2017).

The land is conceptualized like a person with senses and emotions. According to this view the practices of the inhabitants of the land evoke a spontaneous feeling of disgust in mother earth/the land, and the inhabitants are vomited out. Paradoxically, the plausibility of this concept seems to be based on ancient Canaanite mythology in which the land is personified as a living being, a goddess, who gives birth to plants after being fertilized by the weather god.[51]

5. Conclusion

It is clear that fecal matter causes disgust in the ancient Near East. Basically, the emotion of fecal disgust provoked two very different behaviors: First and primarily, in daily life people tried to eliminate excrements by defecating in a secluded place or in flowing waters or by digging a hole for the excrements. Magic could help eliminate the contact with feces. Second, the effect of disgust triggered by excrements was also used on a moral level to provoke (*kurgarrû*, prophets, cynics, etc.) and to deter (Ezekiel, Holiness Code, etc.).

The different treatments of fecal disgust illustrates perfectly the ambivalence of the emotion "disgust." On the one hand, disgust seems to arise spontaneously as a natural defense against certain dangers. On the other hand, the examples in sections 3 and 4 make it clear that disgust is a socially constructed emotion; that is, feelings of disgust that can be recalled in a collective must first be built up in this collective with great rhetorical strain.

The efforts made in ancient Israel to render invisible human feces (section 1) and the efforts made in Egypt to magically prevent scatophagy postmortem (section 2) indirectly indicate the strong emotional stimuli and feelings caused by feces. Contrariwise, the purpose of fecal language used by prophets and priests (sections 3 and 4) may have been intended to make present something otherwise absent. The prophets and priests mobilized senses and emotions via strong imagery in order to achieve a certain moral behavior as efficiently as possible.

Bibliography

Allen, Thomas George. *The Book of the Dead or Going Forth by Day: Ideas of the Ancient Egyptians Concerning the Hereafter as Expressed in Their Own Terms*. SAOC 37. Chicago: The University of Chicago Press, 1974.

---

[51] Othmar Keel and Silvia Schroer, *Eva—Mutter alles Lebendigen: Frauen und Göttinnenidole aus dem Alten Orient*, 3rd ed. (Fribourg: Presses Universitaires, 2010), 21, 112–29, 164–71; the fertility rites took place in the week of the new year around the autumnal equinox, see Thomas Staubli, "Bull Leaping and Other Images and Rites of the Southern Levant in the Sign of Scorpius," *UF* 41 (2009): 611–30.

Angyal, András. "Digust and Related Aversions." *Journal of Abnormal and Social Psychology* 36 (1941): 393–412.
Archi, Alfonso et al. *The Prosopography of Ebla: Lettera G* 47 (2011): http://www.sagas.unifi.it/upload/sub/eblaweb/dbase_prosopografia/g.pdf
Barrelet, Marie-Thérèse. *Figurines et reliefs en terre cuite de la Mésopotamie antique.* Bibliothèque archéologique et historique 85. Paris: Geuthner, 1968.
Baumgarten, Albert I. "The Temple Scroll, Toilet Practices, and the Essenes." *Jewish History* 10 (1996): 9–20.
Blocher, Felix. "Gaukler im Alten Orient." Pages 79–111 in *Außenseiter und Randgruppen: Beiträge zu einer Sozialgeschichte des Alten Orients.* Edited by Volkert Haas. Xenia 32. Konstanz: Universitätsverlag, 1992
Cirillo, Thomas. "Transferable Disgust in Demosthenes 54: Against Conon." *Syllecta classica* 20 (2009): 1–30.
Crouch, Carly L. "What Makes a Thing Abominable? Observations on the Language of Boundaries and Identity Formation from a Social Scientific Perspective." *VT* 65 (2015): 516–41.
Curtis, Valerie, and Adam Biran. "Dirt, Disgust, and Disease: Is Hygiene in Our Genes?" *Perspectives in Biology and Medicine* 44 (2001): 17–31.
Darwin, Charles. *The Expression of the Emotions in Man and Animals.* Chicago: University of Chicago Press, 1965.
Ebeid, Nabil I. *Egyptian Medicine in the Days of the Pharaohs.* Cairo: The General Egyptian Book Organization 1999.
Edzard, Dietz Otto. "Zur Ritualtafel der sog. 'Love Lyrics.'" Pages 57–69 in *Language, Literature, and History, Philological and Historical Studies Presented to Erica Reiner.* Edited by Francesca Rochberg-Halton. AOS 67. New Haven: American Oriental Society, 1987.
Elwood, Lisa S., and Bunmi O. Olatunji. "A Cross-Cultural Perspective on Disgust." Pages 99–122 in *Disgust and Its Disorders: Theory, Assessment, and Treatment.* Edited by Bunmi O. Olatunji and Dean McKay. Washington DC: American Psychological Association, 2009.
Fallon, April E., Paul Rozin, and Patricia Pliner. "The Child's Conception of Food: The Development of Food Rejections with Special Reference to Disgust and Contamination Sensitivity." *Child Development* 55 (1984): 566–75.
Feder, Yitzhaq. "Contamination Appraisals, Pollution Beliefs and the Role of Cultural Inheritance in Shaping Disease Avoidance Behavior." *Cognitive Science* (2016): 1561–85.
———. "Defilement and Moral Discourse in the Hebrew Bible: An Evolutionary Framework." *Journal of Cognitive Historiography* 3 (2016): 157–89.
Fessler, Daniel M. T., Alexander P. Arguello, Jeannette M. Mekdara, and Ramon Macias. "Disgust Sensitivity and Meat Consumption: A Test of an Emotivist Account of Moral Vegetarianism." *Appetite* 41 (2003): 31–41.
Frahm, Eckart. "Prophetie." *RlA* 11 (2006): 7–11.
Frandsen, Paul John. "BWT: Divine Kingship and Grammar." Pages 151–58 in *Linguistik, Philologie, Religion.* Vol. 3 of *Akten des vierten internationalen Ägyptologenkongresses, München 1985.* Edited by Sylvia Schoske. Hamburg: Buske, 1989.

———. "Durkheim's Dichotomy Sacred: Profane and the Egyptian Category *bwt.*" Pages 149–74 in vol. 1 of *Millions of Jubilees: Studies in Honor of David P. Silverman*. Edited by Zahi Hawass and Jennifer Houser Wegner. Cairo: Conseil suprême des antiquités de l'Égypte, 2010.

———. "Faeces of the Creator or the Temptations of the Dead." Pages 25–62 in *Ancient Egyptian Demonology: Studies in the Boundaries between the Demonic and the Divine in Egyptian Magic*. Edited by P. Kousoulis. Leuven: Peters, 2011.

———. "On the Avoidance of Certain Forms of Loud Voices and Access to the Sacred." Pages 975–1000 in part 2 of *Egyptian Religion: The Last Thousand Years; Studies Dedicated to the Memory of Jan Quaegebeur*. Edited by Willy Clarysse, Antoon Schoors, and Harco Willems. Leuven: Peeters, 1998.

———. "On Fear of Death and the Three *bwts* Connected with Hathor." Pages 131–48 in *Gold of Praise: Studies on Ancient Egypt in Honor of Edward F. Wente*. Edited by Emily Teeter and John A. Larson. Chicago: Oriental Institute of the University of Chicago, 1999.

Groneberg, Brigitte. "Die sumerisch-akkadische Inanna/Ištar: Hermaphroditos?" *WO* 17 (1986): 25–46.

Hannig, Rainer. *Großes Handwörterbuch Ägyptisch-Deutsch (2800–950 v. Chr.): Die Sprache der Pharaonen*. 5th ed. Mainz: von Zabern, 2009.

George, Andrew R. *The Babylonian Gilgamesh Epic*. Oxford: Oxford University Press, 2003.

Haidt, Jonathan. "The Moral Emotions." Pages 852–70 in *Handbook of Affective Sciences*. Edited by Richard J. Davidson, Klaus R. Scherer, and H. Hill Goldsmith. Oxford: Oxford University Press, 2003.

Haidt, Jonathan, Paul Rozin, Clark Mccauley, and Sumio Imada. "Body, Psyche, and Culture: The Relationship between Disgust and Morality." *Psychology and Developing Societies* 9 (1997): 107–31.

Hasenfratz, Hans-Peter. *Die Toten Lebenden: Eine religionsphänomenologische Studie zum sozialen Tod in archaischen Gesellschaften; Zugleich ein kritischer Beitrag zur sogenannten Strafopfertheorie*. BZRGG 24. Leiden: Brill, 1982.

Haul, Michael. *Stele und Legende: Untersuchungen zu den keilschriftlichen Erzählwerken über die Könige von Akkade*. Göttinger Beiträge zum Alten Orient 4. Göttingen: Universitätsverlag, 2009.

Herrmann, Christian. *Ägyptische Amulette aus Palästina/Israel: Mit einem Ausblick auf ihre Rezeption durch das Alte Testament*. OBO 138. Fribourg: Presses Universitaires; Göttingen: Vandenhoeck & Ruprecht, 1994.

Hornung, Erik. *Altägyptische Höllenvorstellungen*. ASAW 59.3. Berlin: Akademieverlag, 1968.

Joachim, Heinrich. *Papyros Ebers: Das älteste Buch über Heilkunde*. Berlin: de Gruyter, 1890.

Josephus, Flavius. *The Works of Flavius Josephus*. Translated by William Whiston. Auburn: John E. Beardsley, 1895.

Kadish, Gerald E. "The Scatophagous Egyptian." *JSSEA* 9 (1979): 203–17.

Kazen, Thomas. "Disgust in Body, Mind, and Language: The Case of Impurity in the Hebrew Bible." Pages 97–116 in *Mixed Feelings and Vexed Passions: Exploring*

Emotions in Biblical Literature. Edited by F. Scott Spencer. RBS 90. Atlanta: SBL Press, 2017.

———. "The Role of Disgust in Priestly Purity Law: Insights from Conceptual Metaphor and Blending Theories." *Journal of Law, Religion and State* 3 (2014): 62–92.

Keel, Othmar, and Silvia Schroer. *Eva—Mutter alles Lebendigen: Frauen und Göttinnenidole aus dem Alten Orient*. 3rd ed. Fribourg: Presses Universitaires, 2010.

Knohl, Israel. *Sanctuary of Silence: The Priestly Torah and the Holiness School*. Minneapolis: Fortress, 1995.

Lambert, Wilfried G. "Prostitution." Page 127–57 in *Außenseiter und Randgruppen: Beiträge zu einer Sozialgeschichte des Alten Orients*. Edited by Volkert Haas. Xenia 32. Konstanz: Universitätsverlag, 1992.

Larson, Greger et al. "Rethinking Dog Domestication by Integrating Genetics, Archeology, and Biogeography." *PNAS* 109 (2012): 8878–83.

Lateiner, Donald, and Dimos Spatharas, eds. *The Ancient Emotion of Disgust*. Oxford: Oxford University Press, 2017.

Legrain, Leon. *Terracottas from Nippur*. PBS 16. Philadelphia: University of Pennsylvania Press, 1930.

Lindow, Wolfgang, ed. *Ein kurtzweilig Lesen von Dil Ulenspiegel: Nach dem Druck von 1515*. Universal-Bibliothek 1687. Stuttgart: Reclam, 1978.

MacGinn, Colin. *The Meaning of Disgust*. Oxford: Oxford University Press, 2011.

Maul, Stefan M. "*Kurgarrû* und *assinnu* und ihr Stand in der babylonischen Gesellschaft." Pages 159–72 in *Außenseiter und Randgruppen: Beiträge zu einer Sozialgeschichte des Alten Orients*. Edited by Volkert Haas. Xenia 32. Konstanz: Universitätsverlag, 1992.

Mayer-Opificius, Ruth. *Das altbabylonische Terrakottarelief*. UAVA 2. Berlin: de Gruyter, 1961.

McCown, Donald Eugene, et al. *Temple of Enlil, Scribal Quarter, and Soundings: Excavations of the Joint Expedition to Nippur of the University Museum of Philadelphia and the Oriental Institute of the University of Chicago*. OIP 78. Chicago: Oriental Institute of the University of Chicago, 1967.

Meissner, Bruno. *Babylonien und Assyrien*. Vol. 1. Heidelberg: Carl Winter, 1920.

Miller, William I. *The Anatomy of Disgust*. Cambridge: Harvard University Press, 1997.

Mineka, Susan, and Michael Cook. "Mechanisms Involved in the Observational Conditioning of Fear." *Journal of Experimental Psychology General* 122 (1993): 23–38.

Nussbaum, Martha C. *Hiding from Humanity: Disgust, Shame, and the Law*. Princeton: Princeton University Press, 2004.

Parayre, Dominique. "Les suidés dans le monde syro-mésopotamien aux époques historiques." *Topoi Suppl* 2 (2000): 141–206.

Pizarro, David, Yoel Inbar, and Chelsea Helion. "On Disgust and Moral Judgment." *Emotion Review* 3 (2011): 267–68.

Roy, Arundhaty. *The Ministry of Utmost Happiness*. London: Hamish Hamilton, 2017.

Royzman, Edward B., and John Sabini. "Something It Takes to Be an Emotion: The Interesting Case of Disgust." *Journal for the Theory of Social Behaviour* 31 (2001): 29–59.

Rozin, Paul, and April E. Fallon. "A Perspective on Disgust." *Psychological Review* 94 (1987): 23–41.

Rozin, Paul, Jonathan Haidt, and Clark R. McCauley. "Disgust." Pages 637–53 in *Handbook of Emotions*. Edited by M. Lewis and J. Haviland. 2nd ed. New York: Guilford, 2000.

Rozin, Paul, Linda Millman, and Carol Nemeroff. "Operation of the Laws of Sympathetic Magic in Disgust and Other Domains." *Journal of Personality and Social Psychology* 50 (1986): 703–712.

Sallaberger, Walther, and Miguel Civil. *Der babylonische Töpfer und seine Gefäße: Nach Urkunden altsumerischer bis altbabylonischer Zeit sowie lexikalischen und literarischen Zeugnissen*, Mesopotamian History and Environment 2/3. Gent: University of Gent, 1996.

Shupak, Nili. "The Abomination of Egypt: New Light on an Old Problem" [Hebrew]. Pages 271–94 in *Marbeh Hokmah: Studies in the Bible and the Ancient Near East in Loving Memory of Victor Avigdor Huowitz*. Edited by Shamir Yona et al. Beer-Sheva: Gen-Gurion University of the Negev Press, 2015.

Sloterdijk, Peter. *Critique of Cynical Reason*. Translated by Michael Eldred. Foreword by Andreas Huyssen. Theory and History of Literature 40. Minneapolis: University of Minnesota Press, 1987.

———. *Kritik der zynischen Vernunft*. Edition Suhrkamp 1099. Frankfurt: Suhrkamp, 1983.

Staubli, Thomas. "Bull Leaping and Other Images and Rites of the Southern Levant in the Sign of Scorpius." *UF* 41 (2009): 611–30.

———. "Disgusting Deeds and Disgusting Gods: Ethnic and Ethical Constructions of Disgust in the Hebrew Bible." *HeBAI* 6 (2017): 457–87.

———. "Von Ausscheidungen und Ekel." Pages 264–69 in *Menschenbilder der Bibel*. Edited by Thomas Staubli and Silvia Schroer. Ostfildern: Patmos Verlag, 2014.

———. "Warum man Hühner ass, aber keine Schweine: Biblische Speisetabus und ihre Folgen." Pages 46–57 in *"Im Schatten Deiner Flügel": Tiere in der Bibel und im Alten Orient*. Edited by Othmar Keel and Thomas Staubli. Fribourg: Presses Universitaires, 2001.

Takács, Gábor. *Etymological Dictionary of Egyptian*. Vol. 2. Leiden: Brill, 2009.

Tigay, Jeffrey H. *Deuteronomy*. Philadelphia: Jewish Publication Society of America, 1996.

Topmann, Doris. *Die "Abscheu"-Sprüche der altägyptischen Sargtexte: Untersuchungen zu Textemen und Dialogstrukturen*, Göttinger Orientforschungen 4/39. Wiesbaden: Harrassowitz, 2002.

Vermès, Géza. *The Dead Sea Scrolls in English*. 3rd ed. Harmondsworth: Penguin Books, 1990.

von Lieven, Alexandra. "'Where There Is Dirt There Is System': Zur Ambiguität der Bewertung von körperlichen Ausscheidungen in der ägyptischen Kultur." *Studien zur Altägyptischen Kultur* 40 (2011): 287–300.

Zandee, Jan. *Death as an Enemy according to Ancient Egyptian Conceptions*. SHR 5. Leiden: Brill, 1960.

SENSES LOST IN PARADISE?
ON THE INTERRELATEDNESS OF SENSORY AND ETHICAL
PERCEPTIONS IN GENESIS 2–3 AND BEYOND

Dorothea Erbele-Küster

With "Senses Lost in Paradise" I allude to the epic poem "Paradise Lost," written by John Milton in 1667.[1] In this piece, the author retells and expands the creation story of Gen 2–3; he wrestles with the fate of the first humans who—after eating the fruit of insight into good and bad—no longer live in paradise. Milton, presupposing as I do a link between aesthetics and ethics, inquires: "Will it not be found ... that what is beautiful is ... true; and what is at once both beautiful and true is, of consequence, agreeable and good?"[2]

A common trait of the exhaustive modern interpretation history of the paradise story in Gen 2–3 is a disregard for the role of aesthetics and in particular the senses.[3] It seems that after gripping the fruit of knowledge, as induced by the senses, the trust in the use of the senses for acquiring knowledge of good and bad is lost. As a result, interpretation often focuses on the ambiguous outcome and long-term consequences of the first humans' actions (i.e., expulsion of the garden). Even those interpreters who believe that the acquisition of knowledge was

---

My thanks go out to the organizers of the conference Annette Schellenberg and Thomas Krüger. The article is the outcome of continuous discussions on the occasion of lecturing and teaching on the topic. I am especially grateful to Tamar Frank, Ellen Kerber, Nikolett Móricz, Steven M. Philp, Greg Schmidt Goering and an anonymous reader for their careful reading and comments on earlier versions.

[1] John Milton, *Paradise Lost: A Poem Written in Ten Books* (London: Parker, 1667).
[2] Milton, *Paradise Lost*, 2:268–69.
[3] The exceptions prove the rule: Gerhard von Rad comments on the emergence of the different senses (in a positive way), naming hearing, smell, sight, and taste. Gerhard von Rad, *Das erste Buch Mose*, 10th ed., ATD 2/4 (Göttingen: Vandenhoeck & Ruprecht, 1976), 73. Phyllis Trible stresses the oral sense. According to her this leads to the shift of humans to "moral responsibility." Phyllis Trible, *God and the Rhetoric of Sexuality*, OBT 2 (Philadelphia: Fortress 1978), 86.

inevitable leave out the role that the senses play in the dramaturgy of the story. I invert the common reading: tasting the attractive fruits in the creation myth is not the origin of sin but the origin of the senses and hence the origin of the capability of humans to grasp the good (and eventually the bad).[4] In order to make this argument, I shall examine the Hebrew concept of "good" (טוב) as an aesthetical and ethical concept in Gen 2–3. Indeed a paradox seems to be that knowledge is gained through disobedience.[5] I shall focus on the role of the sensory perception as a means to acquiring ethical perception in this narrative and other wisdom literature in the Hebrew Bible, mainly the book of Proverbs.[6]

The book of Proverbs demonstrates that there are two different ways of using the senses: acquiring wisdom and warning against folly.[7] I shall argue—by reading Gen 3 through the lens of Proverbs—that sensory perception of the good is indispensable for human discernment. In Gen 3, for the first time in the narrated story of humanity in the Hebrew Bible, the first woman, makes uses of her senses. Therefore, this story seems to answer the questions: "How are the senses of the first human beings portrayed? If there is a fall from grace, does this come about through the misuse of any particular sense?"[8] Genesis 2–3 develops, through narrative, how the senses become involved in gripping the knowledge of good and evil.

Before starting, I must clarify two key terms: *ethics* and *aesthetics*. Aesthetics refers to the Greek word αἴσθησις, meaning perception or sense. Hence aesthetical

---

[4] For the history of interpretation, see Frederick R. Tennant, *The Sources of the Doctrines of the Fall and Original Sin* (New York: Schocken, 1968); Elizabeth A. Clark, "Heresy, Asceticism, Adam, and Eve: Interpretations of Genesis 1–3 in the Later Latin Fathers," in *Genesis 1–3 in the History of Exegesis: Intrigue in the Garden*, ed. Gregory Allen Robbins (Lewiston, NY: Mellen, 1988), 99–133.

[5] On the notion of paradox in the story, see Deanne Westbrook, "Paradise and Paradox," in *Mappings of the Biblical Terrain: The Bible as Text*, ed. Vincent L. Toller (Lewisburg: Bucknell University Press, 1990), 121–43. Westbrook identifies in Gen 2–3 a current literary strategy that does not try to resolve antithetical components.

[6] I subsume the creation narrative in Gen 2–3 under the vast label of wisdom literature as the text is about introducing relevant categories and themes within wisdom literature such as "good and evil" and human finitude. For the discussion on the denotation of wisdom literature as genre, see Mark R. Sneed, ed., *Was There a Wisdom Tradition? New Prospects in Israelite Wisdom Studies*, AIL 23 (Atlanta: SBL Press, 2015).

[7] Greg Schmidt Goering, "Attentive Ears and Forward-Looking Eyes: Disciplining the Senses and Forming the Self in the Book of Proverbs," *JJS* 66 (2015): 242–64.

[8] David Howes and Constance Classen, "Conclusion: Sounding Sensory Profiles," in *The Varieties of Sensory Experience: A Sourcebook in the Anthropology of the Senses*, ed. David Howes (Toronto: University of Toronto Press 1991), 280. See chapter 1 above in the present volume.

experience overlaps with sensory experience.⁹ The second term, ethics, refers to the concern for the good. Ethics, as an analytical endeavor, rises from lived practice.

Ethics as discourse on good and evil, as I use the term, is neither restricted to modern philosophical treatises nor to the legal directives found in the Hebrew Bible.¹⁰ Along with others in the field,¹¹ I assume that one can read texts from the Hebrew Bible philosophically. This is true because the texts themselves address philosophical questions either explicitly or implicitly. Even if philosophical approaches to the Hebrew Bible are not common, it has been argued that the corpus can be considered a part of Western philosophy in antiquity. Moreover, I assume that ethical directives are found throughout the Hebrew Bible. Traditionally, within Hebrew Bible studies ethical questions have been discussed primarily in connection with legal texts, since ethics tend to be equated with normative or legal requirements. As a consequence, there is resistance to considering literary genres beyond legal texts as they seemingly possess no explicit normative claim. However, other genres, like narratives and poetical-lyrical sayings, also teach ethical lessons through their aesthetics, as we shall see. It is therefore appropriate to include proverbial sayings and a creation narrative in my examination of Hebrew Bible ethics here.

Finally, an underlying presupposition of my argument is that our worldview is shaped by language.¹² The investigation of semantic fields will therefore serve

---

⁹ Although they overlap, these two modes of perception stem from different scholarly fields: where aesthetics is used in the arts, sensory perception belongs to the field of cognitive sciences and cultural anthropology. See Jason Michael Peck, "Ethics," in *German Aesthetics: Fundamental Concepts from Baumgarten to Adorno*, ed. J. D. Mininger and Jason Michael Peck, New Directions in German Studies 16 (New York: Bloomsbury, 2016), 77: "Aesthetics referring to the Greek αἰστονομαι ("I perceive, I sense") beyond the study of poetics and arts in general, would be the science of sensory perception." See also Berys N. Gaut, "Ethics and Aesthetics," in *The Routledge Companion to Aesthetics*, ed. Berys N. Gaut and Dominic McIver Lopes (London: Routledge, 2001), 341–52.

¹⁰ See Henri Frankfort et al., *The Intellectual Adventure of Ancient Man: An Essay on Speculative Thought in the Ancient Near East* (Chicago: University of Chicago Press, 1946), 10–11. The volume has been edited in midst the collapse of the modern western civilization while speaking of the logic of mythopoetic thought.

¹¹ See Eckart Otto, "Die Geburt des moralischen Bewusstseins: Die Ethik der Hebräischen Bibel," in *Bibel und Christentum im Orient: Studien zur Einführung der Reihe "Orientalia Biblica et Christiana,"* ed. Eckart Otto and Siegbert Uhlig, OBC 1 (Glückstadt: Augustin, 1991), 63–87; John Barton, *Ethics in Ancient Israel* (Oxford: Oxford University Press, 2014), 2–4.

¹² See Meir Malul, *Knowledge, Control and Sex: Studies in Biblical Thought, Culture and Worldview* (Tel Aviv: Archaeological Centre, 2002), 67–69 (esp. remarks on cognitive anthropology).

as the basis for classifying sensory experiences and their roles concerning the reflection on the Hebrew term for "good." My linguistic analysis will take into consideration the specific cultural notion of the senses in the Hebrew Bible, as well as presuppose that sensory experiences transmit embodied knowledge since the sensory organs play a major role in acquiring insight. I shall combine this philological and cultural anthropological reading with a philosophical approach.[13] The aim is to highlight the contribution of sensory experiences to the process of judgment, an enactment of ethics. This will lead to an appraisal of sensory experience (aesthetics) for ethical learning.

THE SENSORY PERCEPTION OF KNOWLEDGE OF GOOD AND EVIL IN GENESIS 2–3

The paradox that (the perception of) what is good and beautiful turns out to be fatal is the starting point for my investigation of the role of the senses in ethical decision making according to Gen 2–3. Or in the words of Eve, as offered by Milton: "Naming thee the tree of knowledge, knowledge both of good and evil; forbids us then to taste."[14] Long time the history of interpretation has focused on how to understand the phrasing "knowledge (of) good and evil." One can identify mainly four interpretations which are interwoven:[15] (1) It is understood as a merism composed of a binary pair meaning "knowledge of everything" (omniscience, which is restricted to God and should hence be forbidden). (2) It denotes coming to age and maturity (cf. Deut 1:39) within a psycho-mythical setting.[16] (3) It refers to sexual knowledge; after the ingestion of the fruit, the humans realize that they

---

[13] The latter seems quite common up to the middle of the last century. Herold Stern pleads that "a philological analysis of such key ethical terms as 'good' and 'evil' cannot be separated from a philosophical discussion." One has to understand the concepts of a particular culture. Having stated this, he gives no further methodological hints how this should be done. Herold Stern, "The Knowledge of Good and Evil," *VT* 8 (1958): 405.

[14] Milton, *Paradise* Lost, 9:751–53.

[15] Out of the post-enlightenment historical-critical interpretation history, I quote just a few. A landmark is Julius Wellhausen's interpretation: The expression of knowledge of good and bad in Gen 2–3 is about if things are useful, beneficial, or harmful for human beings. It is not about their metaphysical value; rather, it stands for the civilization of humankind. Julius Wellhausen, *Prolegomena zur Geschichte Israels*, 5th ed. (Berlin: Reimer, 1899), 305–7. Karl Budde in his lengthy discussion of Wellhausen's position, comes to the conclusion that is about "sittliche Erkenntnis." Karl Budde, *Die Biblische Urgeschichte (Gen 1–12,5)* (Giessen: Ricker, 1883), 65–70.

[16] Samuel R. Driver identifies two interwoven meanings of the knowledge of good and bad: as passing from innocence in childhood to knowledge and as acquisition of the moral order. Samuel R. Driver, *The Book of Genesis*, 10th ed. (London: Methuen, 1916), 46, 56.

are naked and feel ashamed.[17] (4) Finally, as I will argue, it stands for the capability of ethical reflection and the possibility to make choices (cf. with number 1).[18] Following the narrative drama, the philosophical question arises: why should this tree of knowledge of good and bad, which was good and attractive to the senses according to the narrator (Gen 2:9), be forbidden to taste? Indeed, it is self-contradictory that usufruct is forbidden.

The scene is set in Gen 2, where we read about the garden and its beautiful trees. All of the trees, we are told, may serve as food (v. 7) except for the tree of knowledge of good and evil, which God forbids (vv. 16–17). It is important to note that the woman had not yet been created when God's prohibition was uttered. This juxtaposition—between the pleasurable trees and the forbidden knowledge—is a portentous prolepsis to the conflict in the following chapter, where a new actor, the snake, enters the narrative. Here, in Gen 3, the serpent and the woman discuss the forbidden tree, and the dialogue quickly leads to the turning point of the narrative, eating the fruit. The outcome of the dialogue between the woman and the serpent reads as follows:

> The woman saw that the tree was good for eating, and a delight for the eyes, and that the tree was desirable as a source of insight. And she took of its fruit and ate; she gave also some to her man who was with her, and he ate. (Gen 3:6)

---

[17] See Robert Gordis, with a decisive rejection of the moral and cognitive interpretation. At the same time, strangely enough, within this interpretation in sexual terms he includes moral categories. Robert Gordis, "The Knowledge of Good and Evil in the Old Testament and the Dead Sea Scrolls," in *Poets, Prophets and Sages: Essays in Biblical Interpretation*, ed. Robert Gordis (Bloomington: Indiana University Press, 1971), 198–216. Bo Reicke adheres this view. He insists that the sexual knowledge belongs to the broader field of the so-called arts of civilization. Bo Reicke, "The Knowledge Hidden in the Tree of Paradise," *JSS* 1 (1956): 193–201. Malul expands on this: "Thus, sexual knowledge in the case of Adam … meant for all practical reasons being transformed, as well transferred, into the bounds of civilization, or the specific social group in question, and being accorded the status of a full member with all the privileges (and obligations) that it entails" (*Knowledge, Control and Sex*, 297). According to Michaela Bauks acquiring wisdom has sexual overtones: "Die Semantik von Gen 2–3 (שכל, נחמד, תאוה, ערום hif., ידע, נגע, טוב-רע) zeige eine Ambivalenz an, die zwischen weisheitlichen Anleihen und libidinösen Deutungen changierend Sexualität als Parabel für die Vernunft deutet." Michaela Bauks "Erkenntnis und Leben in Gen 2–3: Zum Wandel eines ursprünglich weisheitlichen geprägten Lebensbegriffs," *ZAW* 127 (2015): 20–42.

[18] See Rainer Albertz, "'Ihr werdet sein wie Gott': Gen 3,1–7 auf dem Hintergrund des alttestamentlichen und des sumerisch-babylonischen Menschenbildes," *WO* 24 (1993): 89–111.

Different senses are addressed: sight ("she saw," "the eyes"), taste ("good for eating"), and perhaps even smell (implied by the notion of good for tasting). Finally, the story is about touching, as the woman seizes the fruit.[19] The text primarily uses verbal expressions for the sensory perceptions. One sensory organ is explicitly named: the eyes, which is linked to the act of seeing (in Hebrew organs represent the sensory actions they invoke). In other words, multiple sensory experiences are involved in grasping the fruit of knowledge.

There is also a conflation of good (טוב) as attractive for the senses and good (טוב) as morally adequate. The word טוב is used by the narrative voice to describe the gold of the land (Gen 2:12) and by God to declare that is not good for the first human be on its own (Gen 2:18). Finally, it is used twice to describe the tree of knowledge, with dual meaning (Gen 2:9). The narrator describes that "every tree [is] desirable to the sight and good for food ... and the tree of the knowledge of good and evil" (Gen 2:9; cf. 2:17; 3:5, 22).[20] The first refers to the aesthetic dimension implying an overall positive notion: the tree is said to be good to eat. The second notion introduces an ambiguity as it is juxtaposed to evil. It is perplexing that out of something good (for eating) can flow evil, or at least the knowledge of it.

The storyline becomes even more complex because the ingestion of its fruit is forbidden. Last but not least, as the narrative moves forward, we discover that the knowledge of good and bad has no beneficial results; in fact, at first glance it is destructive. This entangled setup results in attributing טוב an ambiguous overtone. On the one hand, טוב defines the forbidden tree in ethical and epistemological terms; it is the tree of knowledge of good and evil. On the other hand, as the preposition ל indicates, טוב means that something is adequate for a particular purpose—in this case: eating. The same tree that brings knowledge of good and evil is good for eating, in a context of several sensory experiences. This multifaceted aesthetical and ethical use of טוב makes it a crucial term for the story.[21] It fits in with the other puns of the narrative, like the wordplay that links the term for the first human being (אדם) to the material from which he is made, the earth (האדמה), or like the notion that knowing (ידע) refers to different acts of insight (ethical, sexual, aesthetical).

---

[19] Interestingly the woman herself referred to touching earlier when she alluded to the prohibition of God. According to her, God did even forbid to touch the fruit (see Gen 3:3). See Nicole L. Tilford, *Sensing World, Sensing Wisdom: The Cognitive Foundation of Biblical Metaphors* (Atlanta: SBL Press, 2017), 98. Tilford stresses the permanence of touch.

[20] A crucial point for the interpretation of the tree of knowledge of good and bad is its juxtaposition to the tree of life (see below).

[21] See for a similar argument, Wellhausen, *Prolegomena*, 305–7. According to Wellhausen, there is an overlap of sensory and utilitarian aspects in the use of in Gen 2–3. He maintains that the expression has only an ethical stretch insofar the consequences of a value or an act are beneficial or harmful.

The aesthetic aspect of טוב is often articulated through the notion of "seeing" (see Gen 1; 24:16; 26:7; 1 Sam 16:2; 2 Sam 11:2; Esth 1:2–3).[22] This makes beauty, according to Ingeborg Höver-Johag, something that resides in the eye of the beholder.[23] Note again the use of the word aesthetics here. An act of perception unites different aspects of the observed object: assessing its physical, sensual, and utilitarian values. The perception of beauty and goodness is also an act of analytical evaluation. This becomes obvious when one considers the parallel use of verbs such as to know (Gen 3:7), the opening of the eyes (Gen 3:7) and insight (Gen 3:6). Humans have been able to see since their creation, yet—after eating of the fruit—their eyes are said to be opened.[24]

Furthermore, the sensation of the fruit is qualified as pleasant. Although the woman evaluates the tree by sight, the tree also appeals to her through the stimulation of other senses: pleasure and taste. She sees that the fruit is good for eating. Hence there is a link between the sense of sight and taste. Its attractiveness is stressed by the use of נחמד ("desirable") next to טוב ("good") (Gen 3:6).[25] It is also "a delight [תאוה] to the eyes" (Gen 3:6); תאוה is a sapiential term, which has both negative (Prov 21:25, 26) and positive (Prov 10:24; 11:23; 13:12, 19; 19:22) overtones in Proverbs. It is also used in Ps 10:17 to speak of the destitute's longing (תאוה) for liberation.

The tree is desirable to the woman because of the promise it makes: to be a source of insight. The meaning of the *hiphil* verb שכל is "to be insightful and, as a result, successful" in accordance with the so-called action-consequence nexus, that is, the idea that wicked deeds will bring disastrous consequences and good deeds will bring good consequences (see Prov 1:3; 10:5, 19).[26] שכל is a common verb in wisdom literature and belongs to the semantic field of טוב ("good").[27] The primary meaning of the verb שכל is to look, implying that looking brings about understanding. The sense of sight seems to be implied. The verb שכל expresses cognition and its result and often occurs alongside verbs of sensory perception.[28]

---

[22] Matthias Augustin speaks of "dynamisch-funktional." Matthias Augustin, "Schönheit," *NBL* 3:497.

[23] Ingeborg Höver-Johag, "טוב," *ThWAT* 3:315–39.

[24] See Malul, *Knowledge, Control and Sex*, 103–6, 147, 168: "To see that indicates an evaluation of the situation and not just sight or consciousness, especially with the complement כי־טוב ראה."

[25] Cf. Prov 21:20 and Ps 19:11 חמד.

[26] Klaus Koch, "Gibt es ein Vergeltungsdogma im Alten Testament?," *ZTK* 52 (1955): 1–42.

[27] Cf. Prov 1:3; 10:5, 19; 14:35; 15:24; 16:20, 23; 17:2, 8; 19:14; 21:11, 12, 16; Job 22:2; 33:20; 34:27, 35; Sir 17:6–7.

[28] See Paul Humbert, *Etudes sur le Récit du Paradis et de la chute dans la Genèse*, Mémoires de l'Université de Neuchâtel 14 (Neuchâtel: Secrétariat de l'Université, 1940), 94–97; and Malul, *Knowledge, Control and Sex*, 103–6, 128–29.

As a result of the stimulus of the different senses, the woman picks the fruit. The prehension of the fruit in turn leads to comprehension. The woman and the man next to her acquire knowledge through eating.[29] Taste and ingestion turn into moral understanding; hence, perception turns into action. In this first part, I have outlined how the senses have been involved in the perception, prehension, and acquisition of insight into good and bad. The garden story is about the invention, failure, and success of the senses. From our analyses of the use of the senses in this story—namely, sight, taste (smell may be included), touch, and speech—we shall move to a broader discussion of the semantic field and classification of the senses.

THE CLASSIFICATION OF THE SENSES IN CONTEXTS OF ETHICAL TEACHINGS

In our analysis of Gen 2–3, two salient features of the senses have been identified. First, sensory perception is characterized as pleasure. Second, next to sight, taste plays a prominent role in ethical insight. As we shall see in this section, these are common characteristics of the senses according to wisdom literature. I shall expand our investigation of the role of the senses for ethical discernment to teachings in Proverbs. Earlier research has been focused on ranking the senses. However, our analysis has identified that the senses are commonly used as tools for discernment (see below).

Pleasure, the Senses, and Ethics

The book of Proverbs can be classified as pedagogical literature drawing on embodied experiences and the notion of pleasure. Its cogent sayings stimulate the senses in order to induce certain behaviors. Or to put it in another way: "Sensory pleasure (and displeasure) is closely linked ... to moral judgement."[30] Hence it is a book that treats issues concerning the senses in educational practices.[31]

---

[29] See Frank Crüsemann, "Essen als Akt der Verinnerlichung von Normen und Fähigkeiten," in *Essen und Trinken in der Bibel: Ein literarisches Festmahl für Rainer Kessler zum 65. Geburtstag*, ed. Michaela Geiger, Christl M. Maier, Uta Schmidt, and Rainer Kessler (Gütersloh: Gütersloher Verlagshaus, 2009), 85–100. See also Dorothea Erbele-Küster, "Eat this Scroll (Ezekiel 3): Reading as Eating with Special Reference to 'Niddah' (Menstruation)," *Canon and Culture 3* (2009): 5–22.

[30] Yael Avrahami, *The Senses of Scripture: Sensory Perception in the Hebrew Bible*, LHBOTS 545 (New York: T&T Clark, 2012), 167.

[31] According to the cultural anthropologists Howes and Classen, "Conclusion," 269–70, one can identify through the importance of certain senses in childrearing processes and in educational practices the cultural understanding of the senses.

In her recent monograph *Poetic Ethics in Proverbs*, Anne Stewart builds on this idea. She identifies four discrete models of ethical teaching: a model of rebuke, a model of motivation, a model of desire, and a model of imagination.[32] Regarding the model of desire, she distinguishes between the desire of the wicked and the fool, on one hand (Prov 13:25; 21:10), and, on the other hand, the desire of the wise (13:5; 21:15). Her argument is that wisdom is gained through sensory appeal. I shall develop this relation between pleasure, the senses, and ethics in the sage's longing for the good.

Wisdom is often depicted as an edible plant and thus associated with a sweet taste. Proverbs 13:12 equates desire with the tree of life: "desire fulfilled is a tree of life." One may read this as a sophisticated allusion to the tree of life that is mentioned in the garden story of Gen 2–3 next to the tree of knowledge of good and bad. However, Prov 13 may likewise be read as an independent literary layer that does not presuppose Gen 2–3.[33] In either case, it is clear from other instances in Proverbs that the book combines the tree of life with the acquisition of wisdom (e.g., Prov 11:30). Personified Wisdom is "a tree of life to them that lay hold upon her, and happy is every one that holds her fast" (Prov 3:18). Furthermore, the sensory experience of touch is referred to by making the point that the sensation of grasping and holding leads to the prehension of happiness and wisdom.

In these and other passages from Proverbs, the role of the senses in the process of acquiring wisdom is assessed positively. Whereas in Gen 3 the desire for the tree of life turns out to be fatal, in Proverbs, the craving converts itself into the source of life. In a similar way Prov 24:13–14 appeals to the sense of taste to foster one's desire toward wisdom:

> Eat honey, my son, for it is good, sweet dripping honey on your palate.
> Know this: (such is) wisdom for your throat [נפש].
> If you find it there will be things beyond you and your expectation will not be cut off.

Here, two sensory organs are explicitly mentioned: the palate (חך), as the seat of the taste, and the throat (נפש), as the organ that governs the intake of breath and

---

[32] Anne Stewart, *Poetic Ethics in Proverbs: Wisdom Literature and the Shaping of the Moral Self* (Cambridge: Cambridge University Press, 2016).

[33] Eckart Otto, "Die Paradieserzählung Genesis 2–3: Eine nachpriesterliche Lehrerzählung in ihrem religionshistorischen Kontext," in *"Jedes Ding hat seine Zeit ...": Studien zur israelitischen und altorientalischen Weisheit für Diethelm Michel zum 65. Geburtstag*, ed. Anja Angela Diesel, Reinhard G. Lehmann, Eckart Otto, and Andreas Wagner, BZAW 241 (Berlin: de Gruyter, 1996), 174: "Das gilt auch für das Motiv des Lebensbaumes, das in den Proverbien mehrfach belegt ist (s. i. f.), dort aber Gen 2–3 nicht voraussetzt. Erst nachkanonisch in Test. Levi 18,10f; 4 Esra 8,52; 4 Makk 16,18; Apc 2,7; 22,1f.14.19 wird diese Verbindung hergestellt."

food, which can stand for longing and the person as a whole.[34] Actually, the text simply refers to the sensory organs, taking them as a signifier for the sensory perception. Through this the embodied notion of the sensory perception is stressed.[35] As the organs taste the sweetness and attractiveness of honey, they taste wisdom and long for it. Wisdom is toothsome like fluid honey. "The first line employs a literal directive for the student to savor the sweet substance, the taste of which is embellished in the second half of the line."[36] Interpretations like this one suggest that honey serves as a metaphor for how wisdom is to be appropriated or how abundant and affecting wisdom is.[37] Through the parallel use of the organs, the sweet taste of honey is like the pleasure of wisdom and vice versa. The ingested food becomes part of the person. It nourishes and creates the moral self as words do.[38]

Taste of Ethics

As stated earlier there is no umbrella or epistemological term for the senses in Hebrew. Still, one can identify some general traits. There seems to be a close relation between taste, judgment, and the senses in several texts. As the Latin *sapere* can mean both "to taste" and "to know," in Hebrew the verb "to taste" may

---

[34] For the embodied concept of the term נפש, see Dorothea Erbele-Küster, "Gender in Gesenius Revisited," in *Biblische Exegese und hebräische Lexikographie: Das "Hebräisch-deutsche Handwörterbuch" von Wilhelm Gesenius als Spiegel und Quelle alttestamentlicher Forschung, 200 Jahre nach seiner ersten Auflage*, ed. Stefan Schorch, and Ernst-Joachim Waschke, BZAW 427 (Berlin: de Gruyter, 2013), 41–55; and Bernd Janowski, "Die lebendige *næpæš*: Das Alte Testament und die Frage nach der 'Seele,'" in *Der nahe und der ferne Gott*, Beiträge zur Theologie des Alten Testaments 5 (Neukirchen-Vluyn: Neukirchner, 2014), 73–116.

[35] For the embodied conception of the senses in the Hebrew Bible in general and in particular for this text, see Greg Schmidt Goering, "Honey and Wormwood: Taste and the Embodiment of Wisdom in the Book of Proverbs," *HBAI* 5 (2016): 23–41.

[36] Stewart, *Poetic Ethics in Proverbs*, 148: "The saying [in Prov 24] operates with sensory perception. Identifying wisdom's desirability by its taste, and the opening description of nature's honey makes the saying more pressing and tangible."

[37] Yael Avrahami, "The Study of Sensory Perceptions in the Hebrew Bible: Notes on Method," *HBAI* 5 (2016): 4, speaks of "sensory metaphors" or "figurative use" and Tilford, *Sensing World, Sensing Wisdom*, 187 of a "complex metaphor."

[38] See Schmidt Goering, "Honey and Wormwood," 33.

encompass the act of perception in general.³⁹ Although the root טעם ("taste, perceive") is not used in Gen 3, the more common verb אכל ("to eat") plays a prominent role.⁴⁰

The sense of taste often occurs with female figures (Proverbs; Gen 2–3; and 1 Sam 25). Proverbs 11:22 speaks of a woman whose good taste (i.e., sense) has departed her. The woman who is appraised for her wisdom in trade "tastes that her merchandise is good" (Prov 31:18).⁴¹ In his article on taste, Aaron Schart comments on this association and argues that a woman's special knowledge of taste comes through the preparation of food.⁴² Often interpreters understand the Hebrew lexeme טעם ("taste") in women as a sense of food (esp. 1 Sam 25). They limit taste in these instances to a physiological process, excluding "common sense" as the meaning of taste. This narrow reading assumes a dualistic view of the embodied sense of taste versus a cognitive common sense. This leads to the view that women are associated with the body, whereas men are equated with reason. Indeed, the Hebrew notion of the senses is embodied, but this holds true for reason (heart) as well. Tasting is discriminating. Therefore, the modern binary notion of body and reason/mind or sensation and cognition are blurred. "Taste works as marker of wisdom, because, like wisdom, taste bridges bodily and cognitive functions."⁴³ Perception for the sake of knowledge is embodied. Furthermore, the lexeme for taste stands in these instances for discriminating abilities, referring to the sense of wisdom in the woman.⁴⁴

In summary, our analysis of taste in different strands of wisdom literature has shown that this particular sense is an act of cognitive evaluation. Hence sensory perception involves ethical judgment. Physical appreciation, taste, and ingestion lead to understanding. In the garden story, the tree and its fruit coincide with the fruit of wisdom. Something which is טוב ("good") is worth striving for.⁴⁵ Sensory perception (aesthetics) and ethical perception coincide in this term. Good taste seems to be a virtue belonging to the knowledgeable and is praised in characters who possess it.

---

³⁹ See Malul, *Knowledge, Control and Sex*, 105, 130–33 on the role of taste in the epistemic process.

⁴⁰ See Avrahami, *Senses of Scripture*, 93: "It is noteworthy that neither a sharp semantic distinction exists between the common verb to eat and the rare verb to taste, nor the tasting process and eating."

⁴¹ The only other time the root is used in Prov 26:16.

⁴² See Aaron Schart, "Geschmack," WiBiLex (2009): https://www.bibel wissenschaft.de/stichwort/66598/.

⁴³ Schmidt Goering, "Honey and Wormwood," 27.

⁴⁴ See Schmidt Goering, "Honey and Wormwood," 25.

⁴⁵ See Höver-Johag, "טוב," 318.

Classification of Senses as Ethical Tools

In order to describe the epistemological concept of the senses and eventually compare it with concepts from other cultures, a major focus in earlier studies has been to rank and classify the senses.[46] In this section I shall take up the question of how to classify the senses and assess the implication of the senses for the ethical discernment and hence the interconnectedness between the aesthetical and ethical.

The controversy regarding which mode of perception is granted dominion plays a crucial role in evaluating the bearing of the senses in the garden story of Gen 2–3. In the history of interpretation, two assumptions are common: first, listening is prioritized over sight; second, the senses of taste and touch are regarded as the primary mode of interaction for infants, in contrast to the higher senses of listening or hearing (note that both are regarded as superior to the other senses).[47] These assumptions have resulted in the aforementioned distrust of the senses and their disregard when it comes to discernment. This holds true even beyond the interpretation history of Gen 2–3.

Yael Avrahami argues for the priority of sight in the Hebrew Bible, as it is a term for witness and first-hand learning.[48] Yet, this is a minority position. In addition one should note that the aural perception (listening) is often linked with the heart, the sensory organ for understanding.[49] In her listing of expressions used in the learning and teaching process of wisdom literature, Nili Shupak omits verbs referring to the sensual experiences of sight and taste.[50] Shupak starts the list with the aural sense, the verb שמע ("to listen"), underlining that at the base of learning lies obedience. One of the influential defenders of this prioritization is Hans Walter Wolff. He claims that hearing generally has supremacy over sight in the

---

[46] This is also the case for David Howes and Constance Classen, *Ways of Sensing: Understanding the Senses in Society* (London: Routledge, 2014), as they move from "sensory orders" to "ways of sensing," the title of their recent book.

[47] This goes along with the interpretation of Gen 2–3 as a socialization myth. It is about becoming adult.

[48] See Avrahami, *Senses of Scripture*, 232-276: chapter 5. The Centrality of Sight.

[49] According to Avrahami, sensory imagery portrays emotional experiences (*Senses of Scripture*, 163). In the Hebrew Bible physical, emotional, and intellectual senses are intertwined.

[50] Nili Shupak, "Learning Methods in Ancient Israel," *VT* 53 (2003): 416-26. Towards the end of her article she notes metaphorical expressions linked to the learning process referring to Prov 24:13–14 and stating that wisdom is compared to honey.

Hebrew Bible.[51] Since hearing is linked to speech (e.g., Prov 15:32; 18:21), it is a characteristic of the reasonable nature of human beings.[52]

Sight and taste, however, are the most prominent senses of Gen 3, and they are allotted the greatest vocabulary. As the story is about humankind's first use of the senses, this may be taken as an argument that sight has priority over other modes of perception, especially hearing. Further, at first glance, the story seems to contain no mention of the aural sense (hearing). Yet, although the woman had not yet been created at the moment of God's utterance, the woman rephrases the speech of God, which presupposes that she has listened to God's command. This may be why interpreters argue that the story is about disobedience, not listening to the command of God. The conclusion one may draw from this for a hierarchy of the senses would be that when sight and taste take priority over listening one is led to misconduct and failure. Yet, each sense is *sine qua non*, and—as explained above—the sense of sight is intrinsically linked with the sense of taste in our story.

While unraveling the role of the senses, there seems to be an inclination to subsume the senses under a third category: understanding. "Of particular importance in this regard is to determine which sense is most associated with knowledge and understanding."[53] I have argued that eating in Gen 3 and taste in general is that sense in the Hebrew Bible. Yet, on an epistemological level I ask myself if this is the proper way to describe the role of the senses. According to this classification, understanding would become a super-sense or even be located beyond the senses. However, in wisdom literature understanding is a sense; more precisely, the ways of sensing are interrelated with the ways of knowing. Testing is, truly, knowing.

Trust in Senses Regained?[54]

We moved from senses lost to trust in senses regained. A crucial argument has been that sensory perception is indispensable for humankind's initial acquaintance with good and evil. As discussed above, according to the final stretch of the story in Gen 2–3, privileging the senses of sight and taste over the sense of hearing leads to ambivalent knowledge and to expulsion from the garden.

In light of what our study has shown about how sensory experience functions in terms of learning to discern ethically, I have compared Gen 2–3 and Proverbs.

---

[51] See Hans Walter Wolff, *Anthropology of the Old Testament*, trans. Margaret Kohl (London: SCM, 1974), 74–75.

[52] Malul argues in favor of a combination of a culture of the eye and a culture of the ear as central for the epistemic process (*Knowledge, Control and Sex*, 144–48, esp. 147).

[53] See David Howes and Constance Classen, "Conclusion," 264.

[54] See John Milton, *Paradise Regain'd: A Poem in IV Books, to Which Is Added Samson Agonistes* (Starkey: London, 1671).

The latter fosters ethical education by aesthetic means and the former is a philosophical reflection on good and bad in a narrative disguise.

In documenting the first involvement of the senses in the acquisition of ethical insight into good and evil, Gen 3 confronts us with both the necessity *and* the ambivalence of the senses. My intention has been to decode the role of the senses regarding ethical discernment. In the history of interpretation, the consumption of the fruit in the creation myth (that is, the desire for it) was equated with forbidden lust, thus, dismissing the role of sense perception in our ethical behavior. However, when one pays attention to the senses in the story, it becomes clear that acquiring comprehension is portrayed as attractive and as an analytical act. In the context of the myth, to reach for the fruit constitutes a violation of a commandment. On the narrative level, nevertheless, this is not seen as irrefutably negative. In fact, it is necessary in order to enable human beings to distinguish between good and evil and, therefore, act in an ethical manner. Genesis 3 builds on the assumption that what is "good" is also "good to eat," playing with the notion of desire. The narrative is about the ambivalence of human decision-making and the role of sense perception in this process.[55] Sensory perception is necessary, albeit ambiguous. Our analysis has led to an appraisal of the senses and their contribution to ethical decision-making. Genesis 3 outlines the benefits and pitfalls of using the senses for prehension of insight. In the narrative, the tempting taste of the good is the good itself: to taste implies to assess. The proverbial sayings induce us (how) to use the senses.

BIBLIOGRAPHY

Albertz, Rainer. "'Ihr werdet sein wie Gott': Gen 3,1–7 auf dem Hintergrund des alttestamentlichen und des sumerisch-babylonischen Menschenbildes." *WO* 24 (1993): 89–111.
Augustin, Matthias. "Schönheit." *NBL* 3:497–98.
Avrahami, Yael. *The Senses of Scripture: Sensory Perception in the Hebrew Bible*. LHBOTS 545. New York: T&T Clark, 2012.
———. "The Study of Sensory Perceptions in the Hebrew Bible: Notes on Method." *HBAI* 5 (2016): 3–22.
Barton, John. *Ethics in Ancient Israel*. Oxford: Oxford University Press, 2014.

---

[55] Annette Schellenberg speaks of "Ambivalenz der menschlichen Erkenntnisfähigkeit." Annette Schellenberg, *Erkenntnis als Problem: Qohelet und die alttestamentliche Diskussion um das menschliche Erkennen*, OBO 188 (Freiburg, CH: Universitätsverlag; Göttingen: Vandenhoeck & Ruprecht, 2002), 240–47. See also Hermann Spieckermann, "Ambivalenzen: Ermöglichte und Verwirklichte Schöpfung in Gen 2f," in *Verbindungslinien: Festschrift für Werner H. Schmidt zum 65. Geburtstag*, ed. Axel Graupner, Holger Delkurt, Alexander B Ernst, and Lutz Aupperle (Neukirchen-Vluyn: Neukirchener Verlag, 2000), 363–76.

Bauks, Michaela. "Erkenntnis und Leben in Gen 2–3: Zum Wandel eines ursprünglich weisheitlichen geprägten Lebensbegriffs." *ZAW* 127 (2015): 20–42.
Budde, Karl. *Die Biblische Urgeschichte (Gen 1–12,5)*. Giessen: Ricker, 1883.
Clark, Elizabeth A. "Heresy, Asceticism, Adam, and Eve: Interpretations of Genesis 1–3 in the Later Latin Fathers." Pages 99–133 in *Genesis 1–3 in the History of Exegesis: Intrigue in the Garden*. Edited by Gregory Allen Robbins. Lewiston, NY: Mellen, 1988.
Crüsemann, Frank. "Essen als Akt der Verinnerlichung von Normen und Fähigkeiten." Pages 85–100 in *Essen und Trinken in der Bibel: Ein literarisches Festmahl für Rainer Kessler zum 65. Geburtstag*. Edited by Michaela Geiger, Christl M. Maier, Uta Schmidt, and Rainer Kessler. Gütersloh: Gütersloher Verlagshaus, 2009.
Driver, Samuel R. *The Book of Genesis*. 10th ed. London: Methuen, 1916.
Erbele-Küster, Dorothea. "Eat this Scroll (Ezekiel 3): Reading as Eating with Special Reference to 'Niddah' (Menstruation)." *Canon and Culture* 3 (2009): 5–22.
———. "Gender in Gesenius Revisited." Pages 41–55 in *Biblische Exegese und hebräische Lexikographie: Das "Hebräisch-deutsche Handwörterbuch" von Wilhelm Gesenius als Spiegel und Quelle alttestamentlicher Forschung, 200 Jahre nach seiner ersten Auflage*. Edited Stefan Schorch, and Ernst-Joachim Waschke. BZAW 427. Berlin: de Gruyter, 2013.
Frankfort, Henri, H. A. Frankfort, John A. Wilson, Thorkild Jacobsen, and William A. Irwin. *The Intellectual Adventure of Ancient Man: An Essay on Speculative Thought in the Ancient Near East*. Chicago: University of Chicago Press, 1946.
Gaut, Berys N. "Ethics and Aesthetics." Pages 341–52 in *The Routledge Companion to Aesthetics*. Edited by Berys N. Gaut and Dominic McIver Lopes. London: Routledge, 2001.
Gordis, Robert. "The Knowledge of Good and Evil in the Old Testament and the Dead Sea Scrolls." Pages 198–21 in *Poets, Prophets and Sages: Essays in Biblical Interpretation*. Edited by Robert Gordis. Bloomington: Indiana University Press, 1971.
Höver-Johag, Ingeborg. "טוב." *ThWAT* 3:315–39.
Howes, David, and Constance Classen. "Conclusion: Sounding Sensory Profiles." Pages 257–88 in *The Varieties of Sensory Experience: A Sourcebook in the Anthropology of the Senses*. Edited by David Howes. Toronto: University of Toronto Press 1991.
———. *Ways of Sensing: Understanding the Senses in Society*. London: Routledge, 2014.
Humbert, Paul. *Etudes sur le Récit du Paradis et de la chute dans la Genèse*. Mémoires de l'Université de Neuchâtel 14. Neuchâtel: Secrétariat de l'Université, 1940.
Janowski, Bernd. "Die lebendige *næpæš*: Das Alte Testament und die Frage nach der 'Seele.'" Pages 73–116 in *Der nahe und der ferne Gott*. Beiträge zur Theologie des Alten Testaments 5. Neukirchen-Vluyn: Neukirchner, 2014.
Koch, Klaus. "Gibt es ein Vergeltungsdogma im Alten Testament?" *ZTK* 52 (1955): 1–42.
Malul, Meir. *Knowledge, Control and Sex: Studies in Biblical Thought, Culture and Worldview*. Tel Aviv: Archaeological Centre, 2002.
Milton, John. *Paradise Lost: A Poem Written in Ten Books*. London: Parker, 1667.
———. *Paradise Regain'd: A Poem in IV Books, to Which Is Added Samson Agonistes*. Starkey: London, 1671.
Otto, Eckart. "Die Geburt des moralischen Bewusstseins: Die Ethik der Hebräischen Bibel." Pages 63–87 in *Bibel und Christentum im Orient: Studien zur Einführung der*

Reihe *"Orientalia Biblica et Christiana."* Edited by Eckart Otto and Siegbert Uhlig. obc 1. Glückstadt: Augustin, 1991.

———. "Die Paradieserzählung Genesis 2–3: Eine nachpriesterliche Lehrerzählung in ihrem religionshistorischen Kontext." Pages 167–92 in *"Jedes Ding hat seine Zeit ... ": Studien zur israelitischen und altorientalischen Weisheit für Diethelm Michel zum 65. Geburtstag*. Edited by Anja A. Diesel, Reinhard G. Lehmann, Eckart Otto, and Andreas Wagner. BZAW 241. Berlin: de Gruyter, 1996.

Peck, Jason Michael. "Ethics." Pages 76–84 in *German Aesthetics: Fundamental Concepts from Baumgarten to Adorno*. Edited by J. D. Mininger and Jason Michael Peck. New Directions in German Studies 16. New York: Bloomsbury, 2016.

Rad, Gerhard von. *Das erste Buch Mose*. 10th ed. ATD 2/4. Göttingen: Vandenhoeck & Ruprecht, 1976.

Reicke, Bo. "The Knowledge Hidden in the Tree of Paradise." *JSS* 1 (1956): 193–201.

Schart, Aaron. "Geschmack." WiBiLex (2009): https://www.bibel wissenschaft.de/stichwort/66598/

Schellenberg, Annette. *Erkenntnis als Problem: Qohelet und die alttestamentliche Diskussion um das menschliche Erkennen*. OBO 188. Freiburg, CH: Universitätsverlag; Göttingen: Vandenhoeck & Ruprecht, 2002.

Schmidt Goering, Greg. "Attentive Ears and Forward-Looking Eyes: Disciplining the Senses and Forming the Self in the Book of Proverbs." *JJS* 66 (2015): 242–64.

———. "Honey and Wormwood: Taste and the Embodiment of Wisdom in the Book of Proverbs." *HBAI* 5 (2016): 23–41.

Shupak, Nili. "Learning Methods in Ancient Israel." *VT* 53 (2003): 416–26.

Sneed, Mark R., ed. *Was There a Wisdom Tradition? New Prospects in Israelite Wisdom Studies*. AIL 23. Atlanta: SBL Press, 2015.

Spieckermann, Hermann. "Ambivalenzen: Ermöglichte und Verwirklichte Schöpfung in Gen 2f." Pages 363–76 in *Verbindungslinien: Festschrift für Werner H. Schmidt zum 65. Geburtstag*. Edited by Axel Graupner, Holger Delkurt, Alexander B Ernst, and Lutz Aupperle. Neukirchen-Vluyn: Neukirchener Verlag, 2000.

Stern, Herold. "The Knowledge of Good and Evil." *VT* 8 (1958): 405–18.

Stewart, Anne. *Poetic Ethics in Proverbs: Wisdom Literature and the Shaping of the Moral Self*. Cambridge: Cambridge University Press, 2016.

Tennant, Frederick R. *The Sources of the Doctrines of the Fall and Original Sin*. New York: Schocken, 1968.

Tilford, Nicole L. *Sensing World, Sensing Wisdom: The Cognitive Foundation of Biblical Metaphors*. Atlanta: SBL Press, 2017

Trible, Phyllis. *God and the Rhetoric of Sexuality*. OBT 2. Philadelphia: Fortress 1978.

Wellhausen, Julius. *Prolegomena zur Geschichte Israels*. 5th ed. Berlin: Reimer, 1899.

Westbrook, Deanne. "Paradise and Paradox." Pages 121–43 in *Mappings of the Biblical Terrain: The Bible as Text*. Edited by Vincent L. Toller. Lewisburg: Bucknell University Press, 1990.

Wolff, Hans Walter. *Anthropology of the Old Testament*. Translated by Margaret Kohl. London: SCM, 1974.

HOME BUT NOT HEALED:
HOW THE SENSORY PROFILES OF PROPHETIC UTOPIAN VISIONS INFLUENCE PRESENTATIONS OF DISABILITY

Kirsty L. Jones

1. INTRODUCTION

Prophetic utopian visions are exciting but dangerous things. When authors construct their ideal future, they expose what they perceive is wrong with the present.[1] When issues like disability are involved, the dangers are obvious.[2] Two Old Testament utopian texts, Isa 35:5–8 and Jer 31:7–9, are so similar that a degree of dependency is likely, yet they present sensory disabilities in a very different manner.

In this chapter, I argue that these differences are heavily influenced by the sensory profiles of Isaiah and Jeremiah. I use sensory analysis alongside methodology associated with inner-biblical exegesis to highlight the similarities and differences between the texts and the significance of these.

A version of this paper was produced in partial fulfilment of the MPhil at the University of Cambridge. I wish to thank my advisor, Nathan MacDonald, for his generous and stimulating support.

[1] Ehud Ben Zvi, "Utopias, Multiple Utopias, and Why Utopias at All? The Social Roles of Utopian Visions in Prophetic Books within Their Historical Context," in *Utopia and Dystopia in Prophetic Literature*, ed. Ehud Ben Zvi, Publications of the Finnish Exegetical Society 92 (Göttingen: Vandenhoeck & Ruprecht, 2006), 55–85; Stephan James Schweitzer, "Utopia and Utopian Literary Theory: Some Preliminary Observations," in Ben Zvi, *Utopia and Dystopia*, 23.

[2] Kim's study of disability and cure in North Korea is a striking example of how disabilities are eradicated from desired futures, and the implications of this on the present. See Eunjung Kim, *Curative Violence: Rehabilitating Disability, Gender, and Sexuality in Modern Korea* (Durham: Duke University Press, 2017).

Applying the established methodological principles of inner-biblical exegesis to these texts shows that a relationship between them is fairly certain.[3] They have a high proportion of lexical and thematic parallels (underlined below):

⁷ כי־כה אמר יהוה	⁵ אז תפקחנה עיני <u>עורים</u>
<u>רנו</u> ליעקב שמחה	ואזני חרשים תפתחנה:
וצהלו בראש הגוים	⁶ אז ידלג כאיל <u>פסח</u>
השמיעו הללו ואמרו	<u>ותרן</u> לשון אלם
הושע יהוה את־עמך	כי־נבקעו במדבר <u>מים</u>
את שארית ישראל:	<u>ונחלים</u> בערבה:
⁸ הנני מביא אותם מארץ צפון	⁷ והיה השרב לאגם
וקבצתים מירכתי־ארץ	וצמאון למבועי מים
בם <u>עור ופסח</u>[4]	בנוה תנים רבצה
הרה וילדת יחדו	חציר לקנה וגמא:
קהל גדול ישובו הנה:	⁸ <u>והיה־שם מסלול ודרך</u>
⁹ בבכי יבאו	<u>ודרך</u> הקדש יקרא לה
ובתחנונים אובילם[5]	<u>לא</u>־יעברנו טמא
<u>אוליכם אל־נחלי מים</u>	והוא־למו
<u>בדרך</u> ישר <u>לא</u> יכשלו בה	<u>הלך דרך</u> ואוילים <u>לא</u> יתעו:

---

[3] See, e.g., David M. Carr, "Method in Determination of Direction of Dependence: An Empirical Test of Criteria Applied to Exodus 34,11–26 and Its Parallels," in *Gottes Volk am Sinai: Untersuchungen zu Ex 32–34 und Dtn 9–10*, ed. Matthias Köckert and Erhard Blum, VWGTh 18 (Gütersloh: Gütersloher Verlag, 2001); Michael Fishbane, *Biblical Interpretation in Ancient Israel* (Oxford: Clarendon, 1985), 1; Nathan MacDonald, *Priestly Rule: Polemic and Biblical Interpretation in Ezekiel 44*, BZAW 467 (Berlin: de Gruyter, 2015); William A. Tooman, *Gog of Magog: Reuse of Scripture and Compositional Technique in Ezek 38–39*, FAT 2/52 (Tübingen: Mohr Siebeck, 2011).

[4] OG: καὶ συνάξω αὐτοὺς ἀπ' ἐσχάτου τῆς γῆς ἐν ἑορτῇ φασεκ· καὶ τεκνοποιήσῃ ὄχλον πολύν, καὶ ἀποστρέψουσιν ὧδε. In comparing the MT and OG of Isa 53:10, Schipper suggests that a desire to translate away disability is present in the OG. Jeremy Schipper, *Disability and Isaiah's Suffering Servant*, Biblical Reconfigurations (Oxford: Oxford University Press, 2011), 60–82. Further investigation of this proposed tendency might investigate Jer 31:8 [OG 38:8]. See also Douglas Rawlinson Jones, *Jeremiah*, NCB (London: Marshall Pickering, 1992), 388; Emanuel Tov, "Did the Septuagint Translators Always Understand Their Hebrew Text?," in *De Septuaginta: Essays in Honor of John W. Wevers on His Sixty-Fifth Birthday*, ed. Albert Pietersma and Claude Cox (Mississauga, ON: Benben, 1984), 61–62.

[5] OG: ἐν κλαυθμῷ ἐξῆλθον καὶ ἐν παρακλήσει ἀνάξω (Jer 38:9). Often, OG has ἐξέρχομαι when MT has יצא; the OG Jeremiah attests ἐξέρχομαι 39 times, 37 of these in verses where the MT has יצא. The exceptions are here and 51:32 (Gk. 28:32). MT "and with pleas of mercy" (ובתחנונים) differs by one consonant from the Hebrew equivalent (ובתנחונים) to the OG reading "and with consolations/comfort" (ἐν παρακλήσει). MT aligns with Jer 3:21, OG with Jer 16:7. See, e.g., Barbara A. Bozak, *Life Anew: A Literary-Theological Study of Jer. 30–31*, AnBib 122 (Rome: Pontifical Biblical Institute, 1991), 84; Carl Heinrich Cornill, *Das Buch Jeremia (Classic Reprint)* (London: Forgotten Books, 2015), 335.

כי־הייתי לישראל לאב
ואפרים בכרי הוא: ס

⁷ For thus says YHWH:
"Sing aloud with gladness for Jacob,
and raise shouts for the chief of the nations;
Proclaim, give praise, and say,
'O YHWH, save your people,
the remnant of Israel.'"
⁸ Behold, I will bring them from the North country,
and gather them from the ends of the earth,
among them the blind man and the lame man,[6]
the pregnant woman and she who is in labor, together.
A great company, they shall return here.
⁹ With weeping they shall come,
and with pleas for mercy I will lead them back,
I will cause them to walk by streams of water,
by a straight way in which they shall not stumble.
For I am a father to Israel,
and Ephraim is my firstborn.
(Jer 31:7–9)

⁵ Then the eyes of the blind will be opened,
and the ears of the deaf unstopped.
⁶ Then the lame man will leap like a deer,
and the tongue of the mute man sing.
For in the wilderness water will gush forth,
and streams in the desert.
⁷ The burning sand will become a pool,
the thirsty ground bubbling springs.
In the place of jackals, their resting place,
there will be grass, reeds and papyrus.[7]
⁸ And in that place there will be a highway,[8]
it will be called the holy way;
the unclean will not pass on it.
It will be for those who walk on the way,
wicked fools will not stagger about on it. (Isa 35:5–8)

---

[6] The "man" is not necessarily male; however, translating as "man" preserves singular substantive adjectives and a personal nuance arguably lacking with "person."

[7] Or, "grass will be(come) reeds and rushes." Some amend this clause and read חצר (habitation) in place of חציר. See Otto Kaiser, *Isaiah 1–39*, trans. R. A. Wilson, OTL (Philadelphia: Westminster, 1974), 361; Peter D. Miscall, *Isaiah 34–35: A Nightmare/A Dream*, JSOTSup 281 (Sheffield: Sheffield Academic, 1999), 103 no. 114; John N. Oswalt, *The Book of Isaiah: Chapters 1–39*, NICOT (Grand Rapids: Eerdmans, 1986), 619.

[8] Or, "a highway-way." ודרך is omitted in 1QIsa and Syr; MT is sometimes regarded as corrupt, with the duplication of ודרך explained as dittography. MT preserves a parallel through repeating ודרך, difficult to convey when מסלול is translated highway. Both being a highway and being holy describe the way. OG describes the road through two collocations (ἐκεῖ ἔσται ὁδὸς καθαρὰ καὶ ὁδὸς ἁγία κληθήσεται). See David A. Dorsey, *Roads and Highways of Ancient Israel*, ASOR Library of Biblical and Near Eastern Archaeology (Baltimore: John Hopkins University Press, 1991), 223.

When the shared lexemes and themes are traced in the broader contexts of Isaiah and Jeremiah, a strong case can be made that Jeremiah used Isaianic material. The way theme is an obvious example. It is difficult to imagine the book of Isaiah without reference to the way,[9] and the motif of a straight/level way (through the root ישר) is found scattered throughout the book of Isaiah (see, e.g., Isa 26:7; 40:3; 45:2, 13). However, Jeremiah only uses it in chapter 31.

Like the theme of the way, lexemes and the theme of disability are foreign to Jeremiah. The theme of disability occurs so frequently in Isaiah, however, that themes of blindness and deafness have been incorporated into theories about the book of Isaiah's development.[10] Isaiah uses precise terms for the disabilities blind, deaf, and mute (עור, חרש, אלם) more than any Old Testament book and frequently uses them within the obduracy motif. Jeremiah refers to faulty sight and hearing as spiritual impairment but never uses the terms blind and deaf or attests specific terms for disabilities outside of Jer 31:7–9.[11] This suggests that the use of the lexemes עור and פסח (lame), like the way theme, are Isaianic imports taken into Jer 31:7–9. I argue that these disabilities are reinterpreted in Jeremiah, where they are used to develop a distinctive line on sensory disability in accordance with Jeremiah's sensory profile.

Why would Jeremiah reuse an existing text? For many reasons. Isaiah's vision is very idealistic, but Jeremiah's is more realistic. Isaiah's emphasizes radical discontinuity, Jeremiah's continuity. Jeremiah seems more attuned to the needs of a hurting people than Isaiah's extravagant proclamation does.[12] Prophetic

---

[9] Hans M. Barstad, *A Way in the Wilderness: The "Second Exodus" in the Message of Second Isaiah*, JSS Monograph Series 12 (Manchester: University of Manchester, 1989), 44 (for overview); Bernard Duhm, *Das Buch Jesaja*, HAT 3.1 (Göttingen: Vandenhoeck & Ruprecht, 1922), 462; Ernst Haag, "Der Weg zum Baum des Lebens: Ein Paradiesmotiv in Buch Jesaja," in *Künder des Wortes: Beiträge zur Theologie der Propheten; Festschrift Josef Schreiner zum 60. Geburstag*, ed. Lothar Ruppert, Peter Weimar, and Erich Zenger (Würzburg: Echter, 1982), 40; Bo H. Lim, *The "Way of the Lord" in the Book of Isaiah*, LHBOTS 522 (London: T&T Clark, 2010), 60; Øystein Lund, *Way Metaphors and Way Topics in Isaiah 40–55*, FAT 28 (Tübingen: Mohr Siebeck, 2007), 2–3; Gary V. Smith, *Isaiah 1–39*, NAC 15A (Nashville: Broadman & Holman, 2007), 580.

[10] Ronald Ernest Clements, "Patterns in the Prophetic Canon: Healing the Blind and the Lame," in *Canon, Theology, and Old Testament Interpretation: Essays in Honor of Brevard S Childs*, ed. Gene M. Tucker, David L. Petersen, Robert R. Wilson, and Brevard S. Childs (Philadelphia: Fortress, 1988), 189–200.

[11] This is analogous to contemporary Western use of disability language in a figurative manner. *Lame* is rarely used as a specific term for impaired ambulance, but it is used figuratively: "that is a lame argument" whereas a specific term is avoided: "that is a paraplegic argument."

[12] Kathleen O'Connor, "Jeremiah's Two Visions of the Future," in Ben Zvi, *Utopia and Dystopia*, 86–104 (90).

utopian visions not only address cognitive dissonance,[13] they create it. Dissonance may occur when visions are not realized (immediately or eventually) in the way envisaged[14] or when the "best imaginable"[15] is not an imaginable best. The contexts of proclamation and reception may also be discordant; as things change so must words; on these grounds it is natural that textual reuse would occur. Visions are interpreted and reformulated so that hope can sound clearly.

After providing an overview of the sensory profiles of Isaiah and Jeremiah and their use of the senses in their obduracy motifs, I consider sight/blindness, hearing/deafness, kinaesthesia/lameness, and briefly touch upon speech/mutism. I conclude by discussing the impact of this discussion for the exegesis of the two visions.

2. Sensory Profiles

Exegetes rarely consider how the senses are used in Isaiah and Jeremiah when they label the disabilities of Isa 35 and Jer 31 as metaphorical (spiritual) or literal (physical/somatic).[16] Even when investigating the relationship between these texts, few works on the relationship between Isa 35 and Jer 31 venture to explain why sensory impairment might be presented differently in these texts. R. E. Clements suggests that Jer 31 may have been composed before Isa 35, "during a period when the healing of the lame was not yet understood as a sign of Israel's eschatological renewal."[17] Benjamin D. Sommer makes the move from literal to metaphorical part of the amplification of Jer 31:7–9 in Isa 35:4–10.[18] An exclusively metaphorical or literal nuance is described, and both scholars represent an understanding that "events, acts and people" to which a text refers "have a literal reference when they first appear but come to have an increasingly metaphorical significance as they reappear."[19]

---

[13] Ben Zvi, "Utopias," 82.

[14] See Robert P. Carroll, *When Prophecy Failed: Reactions and Responses to Failure in the Old Testament Prophetic Traditions* (London: SCM, 1979).

[15] Ben Zvi, "Utopias," 56.

[16] E.g., Ronald Ernest Clements, *Isaiah 1–39*, New Century Bible Commentary (Grand Rapids: Eerdmans, 1994), 276; Jerome, *Commentary on Jeremiah*, trans. Michael Graves, Ancient Christian Texts (Downers Grove, IL: InterVarsity Press, 2011), 191; Kaiser, *Isaiah 1–39*, 328; Oswalt, *Book of Isaiah*, 624; John D. W. Watts, *Isaiah 34–66*, WBC 25 (Waco, TX: Nelson, 1987), 15.

[17] Clements, *Isaiah 1–39*, 28.

[18] Benjamin D. Sommer, *A Prophet Reads Scripture: Allusion in Isaiah 40–66*, Contraversions (Stanford, CA: Stanford University Press, 1998), 46.

[19] John Goldingay, *Models for Interpretation of Scripture* (Grand Rapids: Eerdmans, 1995), 63–64.

These perspectives make a simplistic distinction between literal and metaphorical and envisage a linear progression between the two. In this chapter, I will refer to figurative and somatic emphases, but I recognize that it is a false dichotomy to place figurative over-against somatic, especially since sensory metaphors have clear roots in somatic processes. Clements and Sommer also fail to consider the different sensoria of two different authors. Because the Old Testament is the product of multiple authors and redactors, working in various places and times, it is impossible to maintain that there is an Old Testament sensorium.[20] Individual books have their own sensoria, because individual authors and groups do, just as they do in contemporary societies.

Recognizing the distinctions between the sensoria represented in the Old Testament and the West, and the differences between the sensoria of Old Testament texts, may help biblical scholars. I advance that the sensory profiles (or sensory rhetorics) of the works naturally influence their different views on sensory disability. Investigating these differences within a reused text helps the exegesis of the visions and the role of sensory disability within them.

Isaiah 35 and Jer 31 treat sensory disabilities very differently, but this is often overlooked. In Isaiah, people are healed to come home. The lame and mute join in the movement and music of the returning people. The blind and deaf have their faculties restored. In Jeremiah, people come home but are not healed. The way of return changes for them, not they for the return.

I argue that this key difference is due in part to the different sensory rhetorics of Isaiah and Jeremiah. These differences are striking from the openings of the two books. The book of Isaiah claims to be the vision (חזון) of Isaiah saw (חזה); Isaiah sees words and oracles (2:1; 13:1). The book of Jeremiah claims to be the words (דבר) of Jeremiah to whom YHWH's word (דבר) came (see, e.g., Jer 1:1–13). Throughout the canonical contexts of Isa 35 and Jer 31, differences in how the senses are used are striking, as this brief overview demonstrates.

2.1. Isaiah

With somatic experience as the basis of many of Isaiah's metaphors, Isaiah is not so much written on the body[21] but through the language of the body. Isaiah does

---

[20] See Yael Avrahami, *The Senses of Scripture: Sensory Perception in the Hebrew Bible*, LHBOTS 545 (New York: T&T Clark, 2012), 113: "the sensorium as reflected in the Hebrew Bible." I suggest that the term *sensorium* should be considered a heuristic lens through which to view senses in various contexts, not an indicative tool to wield upon analysis, especially textual analysis.

[21] See Robert P. Carroll, "Blindsight and the Vision Thing: Blindness and Insight in the Book of Isaiah," in *Writing and Reading the Scroll of Isaiah*, ed. Craig C. Broyles and Craig A. Evans, vol. 1, VTSup 70.1 (Leiden: Brill, 1997), 82.

not always differentiate between the role of the senses in the same way as other Old Testament books and uses different senses to describe perception and apperception, cognitive and somatic responses and results, and qualitative evaluations of people, things, and events.

Isaiah often uses sensory language, especially language about vision and audition, in a nonsomatic way. Seeing and hearing, eyes and ears, blindness and deafness are often used to describe nonsensory process and failures, failures which are evident in the book's obduracy motif.

Isaiah uses simile (59:10), and often metaphor, to link visual perception, cognition, and action (or lack thereof):

His watchmen are <u>blind</u>, all of them do not know,	צפו [צפיו] <u>עורים</u> כלם לא ידעו
all of them are <u>mute</u> dogs,	כלם כלבים <u>אלמים</u>
they cannot bark.	לא יוכלו לנבח
Sleeping, lying down,	הזים שכבים
loving to slumber. (Isa 56:10)	אהבי לנום:

Whilst being mute or silent (אלם) means that one cannot bark (נבח), being blind (עור) means that one cannot know (ידע).

A key passage for understanding the obduracy motif in Isaiah links cognition to vision and audition:

⁹ And he said, "go and say this to the people:	⁹ ויאמר לך ואמרת לעם הזה
'<u>hear indeed</u>, but do not understand;	<u>שמעו שמוע</u> ואל־תבינו
<u>see indeed</u>, but do not know.'	<u>וראו ראו</u> ואל־תדעו:
¹⁰ Make fat the hearts of this people,	¹⁰ השמן לב־העם הזה
and their <u>ears</u> heavy, and their <u>eyes</u> blind;	<u>ואזניו</u> הכבד <u>ועיניו</u> השע
lest they <u>see with their eyes, hear with their ears</u>,	פן־<u>יראה בעיניו ובאזניו ישמע</u>
and know in their hearts, and turn, and be healed." (Isa 6:9–10; see also 44:18)	ולבבו יבין ושב ורפא לו:

Read alongside Isa 43:8, where having eyes and ears does not prevent blindness and deafness, the metaphor of impaired sensory perception as impaired cognitive and spiritual apperception is clear.

Isaiah also connects deafness to the obduracy motif, highlighting that having an open ear leads to obedience:

And the <u>ears</u> of the deaf <u>unstopped</u>.[22] (Isa 35:5b)	ואזני חרשים <u>תפתחנה</u>:

---

[22] OG "will hear" (ἀκούω).

> The Lord YHWH has <u>unstopped</u>[23] my <u>ear</u>, אדני יהוה <u>פתח־לי אזן</u>
> and I was not rebellious, ואנכי לא מריתי
> I did not turn back (Isa 50:5) אחור לא נסוגתי:

And linking the closed ear to a lack of knowledge, and transgression:

> You have never heard, גם לא־שמעת
> you have never known, גם לא ידעת
> from of old <u>your ear has not been opened</u>. גם מאז <u>לא־פתחה</u>
> For I knew you would surely act treacherously, <u>אזנך</u>
> and from the womb you were called a transgressor. (Isa 48:8) כי ידעתי בגוד תבגוד
> ופשע מבטן קרא לך:

Isaiah's past and present is conceptualized and communicated through this distinctive obduracy motif and the extensive use of visual and audial tropes; YHWH's acts can be heard and seen, but people do not see or hear, looking to (trusting) other powers and being wise in their own eyes (5:22). By dulling and sharpening perceptive and cognitive faculties, YHWH's sovereignty in creating and removing disability is stressed, and the precedent is set for the restoration of ability in the future.

The blindness and deafness, which characterized the people's predicament, is removed from the future; the eyes and ears of the blind people and deaf people are not so much physically opened as spiritually. Spiritual blindness and deafness are endemic problems in Isaiah's present. This makes it likely that they will be removed in his utopia.[24]

2.2. Jeremiah

Kinaesthesia is overwhelming connected to obedience and disobedience, right and wrong actions; not only walking, but running, coming and going, sitting, standing and turning or returning:

> How can you say, "I am not unclean, איך תאמרי לא נטמאתי
> I have not <u>gone after</u> the Baals"? אחרי הבעלים לא <u>הלכתי</u>
> Look at your <u>way</u> in the valley, ראי <u>דרכך</u> בגיא
> know what you have done; דעי מה עשית
> a swift young camel, <u>bolting in her ways</u>. בכרה קלה <u>משרכת</u>
> (Jer 2:23) <u>דרכיה</u>:

---

[23] OG "opened" (ἀνοίγω), as in Isa 48:8.
[24] See Jeremy Schipper, "Why Does Imagery of Disability Include Healing in Isaiah?," *JSOT* 39 (2015): 319–33.

> | Therefore, their way will be to them | לכן יהיה <u>דרכם</u> להם |
> | like slippery <u>paths</u> in the darkness, | <u>כחלקלקות</u> באפלה |
> | <u>they will be driven away, and will fall</u> in them. (Jer 23:12a–b) | <u>ידחו ונפלו</u> בה |

A whole range of kinaesthetic activity is used to establish and describe boundary markers; where and how people move shows who they are:[25]

> | ¹⁷ I did not <u>sit</u> in the company of the revelers, | ¹⁷ לא־<u>ישבתי</u> בסוד־משחקים |
> | and I did not exult. | ואעלז |
> | Because of your hand upon me, <u>I sat</u> alone, | מפני ידך בדד <u>ישבתי</u> |
> | for you had filled me with indignation ... | כי־זעם מלאתני: ס״ |
> | ¹⁹ Therefore thus says YHWH: | ¹⁹ לכן כה־אמר יהוה |
> | "if you <u>return</u>, <u>I will restore</u> you, | אם־<u>תשוב ואשיבך</u> |
> | before me <u>you will stand</u>. | לפני <u>תעמד</u> |
> | If what is pure <u>goes out from you</u>, not what is worthless, | ואם־<u>תוציא</u> יקר מזולל |
> | | כפי תהיה |
> | you will be as my mouth, | <u>ישבו</u> המה אליך |
> | they will <u>turn</u> to you, | ואתה לא־<u>תשוב</u> אליהם: |
> | but you will not <u>turn</u> to them." |
> | (Jer 15:17, 19a) |

Orality is frequently used to refer to discernment or manifestation of a person's nature:

> | Everyone deceives his neighbor, | ואיש ברעהו יהתלו |
> | and <u>no one speaks</u> the truth; | ואמת <u>לא ידברו</u> |
> | they have taught their <u>tongue to speak</u> lies; | למדו <u>לשונם דבר</u>־שקר |
> | they weary themselves committing iniquity. | העוה נלאו: |
> | (Jer 9:4 [Eng. 5]) |

It is also closely linked to providing or relaying revelation. Reception and response to this revelation are often conveyed through oral tropes:

> | Hear the word | שמעו את־<u>הדבר</u> |
> | that YHWH <u>speaks</u> to you, | אשר <u>דבר</u> יהוה עליכם |
> | O house of Israel. (Jer 10:1) | בית ישראל: |

In Jeremiah, there is a link between seeing and not seeing with reference to cognition, but the relationship between visual perception and perceiving YHWH's

---

[25] It would be interesting to bring discussion of kinaesthesia into studies of spatiality in the Old Testament, asking not only where people and things are, but their manner of being in and getting to places.

ways is weaker than in Isaiah. The reverse is true for hearing and not hearing, and walking and not walking.

Alongside kinaesthesia, the highly audiocentric book of Jeremiah often uses audition with nonsomatic nuances:

<u>Hear</u> this,	שמעו־נא זאת
foolish and mindless people,	עם סכל ואין לב
<u>eyes they have- but they do not see,</u>	עינים להם ולא יראו
<u>ears they have- but they do not hear.</u> (Jer 5:21)	אזנים להם ולא ישמעו:

Audition and kinaesthesia, I argue, crown Jeremiah's sensorium, particularly when perception of and response to divine revelation are described.[26] Because audition is so important in Jeremiah, and lack of audial perception is the obvious antonym to this, aural tropes are used in the obduracy motif, and Jeremiah describes a people with uncircumcised ears, who do not, or cannot, listen and obey. Kinaesthetic action is also used to connote response to revelation, or lack thereof; the risk of being unsound and walking in the wrong way features in Jeremiah's critique of the present. Because Jeremiah's sensorium emphasizes audial and kinaesthetic activity in a different way to Isaiah, it is natural that the obduracy motif is presented differently in each book. Jeremiah does not have a problem with blindness. It is the elective deafness of the people and their wayward movement that causes their predicament. Considering the disabilities and senses in these two works will further illustrate this difference.

3. Blindness and Sight

Like the way (דרך) in Isaiah and Jeremiah, the term blind (עור) has different nuances in different contexts. Isaiah is the most likely source context for both lexeme and theme: the book of Isaiah contains a high proportion of the Old Testament attestations of עור (11 of 26 occurrences) as well as almost all of the nonsomatic uses of the term. Jeremiah attests the adjective עור once (31:8), and the related

---

[26] The audiocentricity of Jeremiah is similar to that of Deuteronomy and the DtrH. See Rachel Raphael, *Biblical Corpora: Representations of Disability in Hebrew Biblical Literature*, LHBOTS 445 (London: T&T Clark, 2008), 30–31. The Deuteronomistic corpus prioritizes aural over visual revelation, with obedience and disobedience frequently delineated when people who hear or do not hear are referred to. Sensory disability is never, however, described with the term חרש. For the Deuteronomist, both people and idols are sensorally disabled, in contrast to the sensorally able YHWH. See Saul M. Olyan, "The Ascription of Physical Disability as a Stigmatizing Strategy in Biblical Iconic Polemics," *JHS* 9 (2009): art. 14; Raphael, *Biblical Corpora*, 42–43, 46; and Gerhard von Rad, *Deuteronomy*, OTL (Philadelphia: Westminster, 1966), 124.

verb (which is absent in Isaiah) is used to describe the physical blinding of Zedekiah (Jer 39:7; 52:11).

Visual language is not only used in Isaiah's call; it also develops the prophetic persona.[27] Because Isaiah has eyes which have seen YHWH (6:4–7), but the people have blind eyes, the prophet can call them to see in their blindness and can chastise their inability to perceive.[28] פקח is conjugated with עין eighteen times in the Old Testament, three times in Isaiah (Isa 35:5; 37:17; 42:7), and ears once (Isa 42:20). This opening can be somatic/sensory, leading to visual perception (Gen 21:19; 2 Kgs 6:17), or metaphorical, leading to cognitive apperception (Gen 3:5, 7). The opening of eyes in Isa 35:5 looks back to the pronouncement of Isa 6 and forward to the mission of the servant:[29]

To open the eyes that are blind,[30]	לפקח עינים עורות
to bring out from the dungeons the prisoners,	להוציא ממסגר אסיר
from the prison the ones who sit in darkness.	מבית כלא ישבי חשך:
(Isa 42:7)	

Isaiah's references to figurative eyes and sight are extensive. Jeremiah, however, uses eye(s) figuratively far less than Isaiah, often associating them with emotional expression (e.g., 9:1, 18; 13:17; 14:17; 31:16), as well as visual perception and cognitive evaluation. Though the inability of eyes to see is discussed in Jer 5:21, the adjective blind עור is never used, and the verb עור only refers to physical blindness. This suggests that the use of עור in Jer 31:7–9 also refers to physical blindness.

עור is given a nonsomatic/spiritual nuance in Isaiah, where it is used to evaluate past and present obduracy, communicate failure, and imagine a future without it. In Jeremiah, these associations are lost and adapted, partially the result

---

[27] See Aitken for discussion of four ways that the motif of hearing and seeing occur in Isaiah and their respective purposes. Kenneth T. Aitken, "Hearing and Seeing: Metamorphoses of a Motif in Isaiah 1–39," in *Among the Prophets: Language, Image and Structure in the Prophetic Writings*, ed. Philip R. Davies and David J. A. Clines, JSOTSup 144 (Sheffield: JSOT Press, 1993), 12–41.

[28] Carroll, "Blindsight," 83. The prophet's call to see occurs, e.g., in Isa 40:16; 42:18; 49:18; 51:1, 2, 6; 60:4; 63:15 where the imperative of ראה is used. Isaiah is also able to speak to the people because he has clean lips, whilst they do not (6:4–7), and able to speak well (38:9), whilst others speak falsely (32:7; 59:3; see also 9:15). Isaiah uses oral tropes far less frequently, however, than visual ones.

[29] See Clements, "Patterns"; Hugh Godfrey Maturin Williamson, *The Book Called Isaiah: Deutero-Isaiah's Role in Composition and Redaction* (Oxford: Clarendon, 1994), 46–51.

[30] The only attestation of the adjective in the feminine plural.

of Jeremiah's sensoria; blindness has primarily, but not exclusively, somatic overtones. The role of vision and the eyes in Isaiah's rhetoric and the thematic development of revelation, obduracy, and renewal makes it probable that the language of blindness to sight in the utopian vision of chapter 35 refers to spiritual blindness and sight. Because Jeremiah uses the same language in a different way, does not present blindness as an endemic problem of the future, and is composing an ultimately more realistic vision of the future in chapter 31, it is likely that the blindness in this chapter is literally/somatically sensory blindness.

4. DEAFNESS AND HEARING

Just as the Old Testament frequently pairs sight and hearing and eyes and ears, it regularly pairs blind and deaf (חרש).[31] Different books pair vision and audition to a different extent; Isaiah only ever uses deaf with blind, and seven of the twenty uses of ear(s) (אז) in this text are with eye(s) (עין). In the more audiocentric book of Jeremiah, ear(s) are used more often, but they are only paired with eye(s) once (5:21). Isaiah and Jeremiah both refer to ears to describe audial reception and spiritual attention to about the same extent.

Isaiah often uses this pairing in the obduracy motif. The people do not only fail to see what YHWH has done and what they are doing; they also fail to hear YHWH's words and right instruction. The people are deaf, and Isaiah contains over half of the Old Testament attestations of this relatively rare adjective (29:18; 35:5; 42:18, 19; 43:8). Elsewhere in the Old Testament, deafness, divinely ordained or humanly determined, physical or elective, commonly relates to the communicative inability to perceive (and apperceive) human communication and divine revelation and to respond appropriately. In Isa 35:5–8, I argue, the pair blind and deaf refers to a spiritual inability to receive and respond to revelation. Spiritual disability, not sensory disability, has characterized the past and present predicament of the people and will be removed in the future.

In this utopia, the time of impaired sight ends and so too does the time of impaired hearing. Isaiah associates opening (פתח), of captives, heavens, rivers, and ears, with an approaching age of salvation, and attests 22 of the verb's 136 occurrences. Ear(s) never occur with the verb פתח outside of Isaiah,[32] a book which highlights that having an open ear leads to obedience. On these grounds, it is logical to suggest that the sight and deafness, which are restored in Isaiah's vision of the future, are spiritual impairments.

Audial tropes are prevalent in Jeremiah and used to describe the obduracy of the people, as well as to discuss revelation and response. However, Jeremiah never

---

[31] See Avrahami, *Senses of Scripture*, 69; Hans-Joachim Kraus, *Biblisch-theologische Aufsätze* (Neukirchener Verlag: Neukirchener Vluyn, 1972), 84–101.

[32] Used in 2 Chr 6:40; 7:15; Neh 1:6 of eyes (in parallel with ears being קשב).

uses the word "deaf" (חרש); Jeremiah refers to ears, which are not inclined (נטה).[33] In Jeremiah, defective hearing occurs frequently alongside reference to wayward kinaesthesia, which work together to connect obduracy (attitude) and disobedience (action):

But they did not listen,	ולא שמעו
and did not incline their ear,	ולא־הטו את־אזנם
but they walked in their counsels,	וילכו במעצות
in the stubbornness of their wicked hearts,	בשררות לבם הרע
and they went backward and not forward.	ויהיו לאחור ולא
(Jer 7:24)	לפנים:

In Jeremiah's utopia, constructed in Jer 31, it is therefore notable that the pairing of kinaesthesia and vision, not deafness, is found. If Jeremiah spoke of the inclusion of people who were deaf, without them being healed, it would be more likely, given his sensory profile, to suggest that he describes a figurative impairment.

5. Lameness and Walking

Disability is removed from Isaiah's utopia, but not Jeremiah's. In Isa 35:6 it is not necessarily clear what is removed; if Isaiah proclaims the healing of nonsomatic blindness and deafness, are lameness and mutism also to be understood thus? The lame man and mute man of Isa 35:6 receive far less scholarly attention than the blind and deaf of Isa 35:5, and vagueness pervades some comments on the nature of their healing.[34] Vagueness may arise from a desire to label the healing event as either "metaphorical" or "physical"[35] but, I suggest, also stems from not understanding Isaiah's sensory profile.

I advance that the grouping of disabilities in Isa 35:5–6 does not render, or make "apparent,"[36] the healing of all four as "not at all metaphorical, but the healing of actual physical infirmities."[37] Differences between the disabilities of verses 5 and 6 go beyond the use of plural substantive adjectives for blind and deaf but singular for lame and mute. Sensory analysis of Isaiah and Jeremiah has shown that in neither book are kinaesthesia and orality used in the same way as vision and audition. Metaphorical nuances for the terms used for lame (פסח) and mute

---

[33] Jer 7:24, 26; 11:8; 17:23; 25:4; 34:14; 35:15; 44:5.

[34] See in particular, Smith, *Isaiah 1–39*, 580; Watts, *Isaiah 34–66*, 540–41.

[35] Claire R. Matthews, *Defending Zion: Edom's Desolation and Jacob's Restoration (Isaiah 34–35) in Context*, BZAW 236 (Berlin: de Gruyter, 1995), 132. Cf. also David Stacey, *Isaiah*, Epworth Commentaries (London: Epworth, 1993), 212.

[36] Joseph Blenkinsopp, *Isaiah 1–39*, AB 19 (New York: Doubleday, 2000), 457.

[37] Matthews, *Defending Zion*, 132. See also Clements, "Patterns," 198; Lim, *"Way of the Lord,"* 140, for one understanding of all four disabilities.

(אלם) are dormant in Isaiah and Jeremiah, and I argue that they are also dormant in Isa 35 and Jer 31. Removal of lameness and mutism in Isaiah is a physical healing; in Jeremiah physically lame people travel on the way. Spiritual connotations may be present, but they are not accentuated.

Of the fourteen attestations of lame (פסח) in the Old Testament, two are in Isaiah and one in Jeremiah. Almost exclusively somatic nuances are present throughout the corpus. Half of the attestations of lame (פסח) are with blind (עור), and Saul Olyan suggests that this, and the frequent pairing of feet and the head (רגל and ראש), connotes a merism of impairment.[38] However, the head is linked to various sensory faculties; kinaesthesia is often paired with hearing and speech, not only sight.[39]

In Isaiah, the pairing of lameness and mutism (פסח/אלם) are not otherwise found in Isaiah, and they are certainly not used to build a motif in the same way that blindness and deafness are. Kinaesthesia is sometimes used in Isaiah to describe obedience and disobedience, but hardly to the same extent as in Jeremiah.

If somatic ambulatory ability, rather than obedience or faithfulness, is connoted by the healing of the lame man, I advance that the clustering of kinaesthetic verbs in Isa 35:8–9 emphasizes that the healing of the lame man facilitates his inclusion amongst the people travelling to Zion.[40] Isaiah, however, goes beyond facilitation and exaggerates the effect of the lame man's transformation. When Isaiah proclaims this healing, a simile is used, and exceptional ability is promised; he does not walk but leaps (דלג) like a deer (איל). Rare in the Old Testament, leaping (דלג) primarily refers to outstanding ambulatory ability, sometimes resulting from transformation.[41] The two unusual words used in this simile are paralleled in the richly multi- and intersensory text of Songs:

Then shall the lame man <u>leap like a deer</u>. (Isa 35:6a)	אז ידלג כאיל פסח
[8] The voice of my Beloved! Behold, he comes, <u>leaping</u> over the mountains, bounding over the hills.	⁸ קול דודי הנה־זה בא <u>מדלג</u> על־ההרים מקפץ על־הגבעות:

---

[38] Saul M. Olyan, "'Anyone Blind or Lame Shall Not Enter the House': On the Interpretation of Second Samuel 5:8b," *CBQ* 60 (1998): 226 n. 12.

[39] For kinaesthesia + hearing, see, e.g., Deut 26:17; Prov 5:7; 8:32; Jer 7:23–24; 9:13; 11:8; 13:10; 16:12; 24:6; 32:23; 44:23. For kinaesthesia + speech, see, e.g., Prov 26:7; Isa 33:15; Jer 1:6; 2:20; 35:15.

[40] Scalise erroneously writes that in Isaiah, healing occurs when the people reach Zion. Gerald L. Keown, Pamela J. Scalise, and Thomas G. Smothers, *Jeremiah 26–52*, WBC 27 (Nashville: Nelson, 1995), 115.

[41] 2 Sam 22:30; Ps 18:30 [29]; Songs 2:8; Zeph 1:9; Sir 36:31.

> ⁹ My beloved is like a gazelle,
> or a young <u>deer</u>. (Songs 2:8–9a)

> ⁹ דומה דודי לצבי
> או לעפר <u>האילים</u>

Beauty, lack of defect (Songs 4:7), and ability are equated.⁴² In Isa 54:1, exceptional future ability in place of disability is again described, and transformation and rejoicing (רנן) are linked as in Isa 35:5–8:

> "<u>Sing</u>, O barren one who did not bear,
> break forth into <u>singing</u>, and cry out, one who has
>   not been in labor.
> For greater are the children of the desolate one,
> than the children of the one who is married," says
>   YHWH. (Isa 54:1)

> <u>רני</u> עקרה לא ילדה
> פצחי <u>רנה</u> וצהלי לא־חלה
> כי־רבים בני־שוממה
> מבני בעולה אמר יהוה:

Isaiah's other attestation of פסח, however, does not describe a transformation from disability to ability but describes ability alongside disability, highlighting the diversity of utopias even within one (canonical) prophetic work:

> Then prey and spoil in abundance will be divided;
> <u>the lame</u> will plunder the prey.
> (Isa 33:23, cf. Ps 68:12)

> אז חלק עד־שלל מרבה
> <u>פסחים</u> בזזו בז:

In Jeremiah, the pair blind and lame (not deaf and lame) may have been used to reflect the usual pairing in the Old Testament. However, because Jeremiah frequently pairs audition and kinaesthesia and attaches figurative nuances, I suggest that the pairing strives to avoid figurative interpretation of the blind and lame in Jer 31:7–9. Pairing of kinaesthesia and sight, feet and eyes, I suggest, does not (*contra* Avrahami) render these senses "semantically equivalent."⁴³ Associative links are present (as in perception and action of eyes and feet), but the associative link is not semantic equivalence because perception, apperception and response are distinguished through different sensory actions.

In Jeremiah, as I have posited, kinaesthesia is understood and used differently with stronger figurative overtones than vision does. This might suggest that the lameness referred to in Jer 31 is, then, also figurative. However, if this was the case, I would expect similar language of the inability to walk to in the rest of the book. Instead, Jer 31 uses the very specific lexeme, פסח, and a pairing of lameness and blindness. In this chapter, like in Isa 33:23, I argue that disability remains and

---

⁴² Saul M. Olyan, "Disability in the Prophetic Utopian Vision," in *Disability in the Hebrew Bible: Interpreting Mental and Physical Differences* (Cambridge: Cambridge University Press, 2008), 87.

⁴³ Avrahami, *Senses of Scripture*, 82 n. 71.

shows YHWH's willingness and ability to work transformation alongside (not through or by removing) variations in the human physical condition.

6. Mutism and Speaking

Isaiah contains two of the six occurrences of the adjective mute (אלם)[44] in the Old Testament (cf. 59:10) and one of the related verb (53:7). Though Jeremiah uses oral verbs more frequently than Isaiah, it never uses the root אלם. In the Old Testament, an explicit link between the somatic and cognitive processes of orality is present, as oral communication sometimes reflects "the actual process of thought,"[45] not only the communication of thought. Mutism is, therefore, related to cognitive and communicative disability.[46]

In this respect, it is like blindness, but unlike blindness it is rarely connected to exclusion and impurity. Isaiah uses the root to link disabled communication with the inability to perform an allotted task (Isa 56:10), but when the servant is described as mute (through the verb in Isa 53:10), silence is linked to the fulfilment of a task. Although, in Isaiah as elsewhere in the Old Testament, people who cannot speak often cannot act and participate, they are not presented as spiritually or morally deficient.

Looking to the context of Isa 35, and to other utopian visions in Isaiah, the emphases on singing, shouting and proclaiming are clear. In Isa 35:6, the tongue sings (רנן), a verb only used with לשון here and in Ps 51:16 (Eng. 14). When the mute man's tongue is healed in Isaiah, silence turns to shouting, and the transformed tongue rejoices with the transformed wilderness:

And the tongue of the mute man <u>sing</u>. (Isa 35:6b)	ותרן לשון אלם

| [1] The wilderness and the dry land will be glad; the desert will rejoice and blossom as the crocus; [2] abundantly it will blossom, and it will rejoice, with joy and <u>singing</u>. The glory of Lebanon will be given to it, the majesty of Carmel and Sharon. They shall see the glory of YHWH, the majesty of our God. (Isa 35:1–2) | [1] יששום מדבר וציה ותגל ערבה ותפרח כחבצלת: [2] פרח תפרח ותגל אף גילת ורנן כבוד הלבנון נתן־לה הדר הכרמל והשרון המה יראו כבוד־יהוה הדר אלהינו: ס |

---

[44] See Exod 4:11; 56:10; Pss 31:19; 38:14; 39:3, 10; Prov 31:8; Ezek 3:26; 24:27; 33:22; Hab 2:18; Dan 10:15.

[45] Avrahami, *Senses of Scripture*, 84.

[46] See also the use of blind and deaf of the servant (Isa 42:19) and others.

Healing enables participation. This brief sensory analysis suggests that transformation of the lame man and mute tongue is not proclaimed because lameness and mutism are endemic problems of the past and present. Instead, this healing displays radical transformation in tangible, touchable bodies, bodies which can now participate in the return to Zion. In Isaiah, every clean and transformed body, every clear and responsive heart can come home.

7. Conclusion

Jeremiah never uses specific terms for disability and often pairs kinaesthetic inability with aural, not visual inability. Because of this, I suggest that the adaptation of Isa 35:5–8 in Jer 31:7–9 is one which seeks to avoid exclusively figurative understandings lameness, as well as blindness. Comparing the presentation of these disabilities in Isaiah and Jeremiah, I have discussed the striking variance between these texts; in Isaiah, people must be healed to come home, but in Jeremiah they come home without being healed.

Isaiah makes nonsomatic blindness and deafness a central failure of the people and an endemic problem with the past and present. As one who has seen, Isaiah is qualified to exhort the people to see, criticize blindness, and promise its future removal. The role of vision, the pairing of vision and audition, and the use of language relating to these senses in a nonsomatic way all support the evaluation that Isa 35:5 refers to nonsomatic disability and healing. Reversal of perceived deficiency is not the reversal of physical blindness and deafness, but spiritual blindness and deafness.

I have established that a different sensory rhetoric underpins Jeremiah and that the book's sensorium pairs audition and kinaesthesia more than audition and vision. The obduracy motif is developed through language of hearing and walking, or not hearing and not walking; Jeremiah uses these tropes to critique and evaluate the past and present. Because terms for sensory disability are unattested outside of Jer 31:7–9, and because the root עור is not used in Jeremiah with a nonsomatic nuance, I maintain that the text emphasizes somatic blindness. In Jeremiah, visual inability is less problematic than the inability to hear or walk. Blindness is not healed in the future because it is not an inherent wrong to be removed, but is included to show that homecoming is not dependent on healing.

Studying the sensory profiles of these two visions, in the context of Isaiah and Jeremiah at large, provided suggestions of how and why two related visions have such striking differences. The differences between the presentation of disability in these texts, I have advanced, arises from a different use of sensory tropes, especially to present the past and present failings of the people. Transformation in Isaiah reflects this, as healing enables spiritual perception and somatic participation. In Jeremiah, transformation is changed to facilitation, with participation possible for those whose disabilities remain. Homecoming and healing and the presence of disabilities in utopias come into a sharper focus when sensory profiles are considered and enable exegesis to attend to significant variations with fresh perspectives.

BIBLIOGRAPHY

Aitken, Kenneth T. "Hearing and Seeing: Metamorphoses of a Motif in Isaiah 1–39." Pages 12–41 in *Among the Prophets: Language, Image and Structure in the Prophetic Writings*. Edited by Philip R. Davies and David J. A. Clines. JSOTSup 144. Sheffield: JSOT Press, 1993.

Avrahami, Yael. *The Senses of Scripture: Sensory Perception in the Hebrew Bible*. LHBOTS 545. New York: T&T Clark, 2012.

Barstad, Hans M. *A Way in the Wilderness: The "Second Exodus" in the Message of Second Isaiah*. JSS Monograph Series 12. Manchester: University of Manchester, 1989.

Ben Zvi, Ehud. "Utopias, Multiple Utopias, and Why Utopias at All? The Social Roles of Utopian Visions in Prophetic Books within Their Historical Context." Pages 55–85 in *Utopia and Dystopia in Prophetic Literature*. Edited by Ehud Ben Zvi. Publications of the Finnish Exegetical Society 92. Göttingen: Vandenhoeck & Ruprecht, 2006.

Blenkinsopp, Joseph. *Isaiah 1–39*. AB 19. New York: Doubleday, 2000.

Bozak, Barbara A. *Life Anew: A Literary-Theological Study of Jer. 30–31*. AnBib 122. Rome: Pontifical Biblical Institute, 1991.

Carroll, Robert P. "Blindsight and the Vision Thing: Blindness and Insight in the Book of Isaiah." Pages 79–93 in *Writing and Reading the Scroll of Isaiah*. Edited by Craig C. Broyles and Craig A. Evans. Vol. 1. VTSup 70.1. Leiden: Brill, 1997.

———. *When Prophecy Failed: Reactions and Responses to Failure in the Old Testament Prophetic Traditions*. London: SCM, 1979.

Carr, David M. "Method in Determination of Direction of Dependence: An Empirical Test of Criteria Applied to Exodus 34,11–26 and Its Parallels." Pages 107–40 in *Gottes Volk am Sinai: Untersuchungen zu Ex 32–34 und Dtn 9–10*. Edited by Matthias Köckert and Erhard Blum. VWGTh 18. Gütersloh: Gütersloher Verlag, 2001.

Clements, Ronald Ernest. *Isaiah 1–39*. New Century Bible Commentary. Grand Rapids: Eerdmans, 1994.

———. "Patterns in the Prophetic Canon: Healing the Blind and the Lame." Pages 189–200 in *Canon, Theology, and Old Testament Interpretation: Essays in Honor of Brevard S Childs*. Edited by Gene M. Tucker, David L. Petersen, Robert R. Wilson, and Brevard S. Childs. Philadelphia: Fortress, 1988.

Cornill, Carl Heinrich. *Das Buch Jeremia (Classic Reprint)*. London: Forgotten Books, 2015.

Dorsey, David A. *Roads and Highways of Ancient Israel*. ASOR Library of Biblical and Near Eastern Archaeology. Baltimore: John Hopkins University Press, 1991.

Duhm, Bernard. *Das Buch Jesaja*. HAT 3.1. Göttingen: Vandenhoeck & Ruprecht, 1922.

Fishbane, Michael. *Biblical Interpretation in Ancient Israel*. Oxford: Clarendon, 1985.

Goldingay, John. *Models for Interpretation of Scripture*. Grand Rapids: Eerdmans, 1995.

Haag, Ernst. "Der Weg zum Baum des Lebens: Ein Paradiesmotiv in Buch Jesaja." Pages 35–52 in *Künder des Wortes: Beiträge zur Theologie der Propheten; Festschrift Josef*

Schreiner zum 60. Geburstag. Edited by Lothar Ruppert, Peter Weimar, and Erich Zenger. Würzburg: Echter, 1982.
Jerome. *Commentary on Jeremiah*. Translated by Michael Graves. Ancient Christian Texts. Downers Grove, IL: InterVarsity Press, 2011.
Jones, Douglas Rawlinson. *Jeremiah*. NCB. London: Marshall Pickering, 1992.
Kaiser, Otto. *Isaiah 1–39*. Translated by R. A. Wilson. OTL. Philadelphia: Westminster, 1974.
Keown, Gerald L., Pamela J. Scalise, and Thomas G. Smothers. *Jeremiah 26–52*. WBC 27. Nashville: Nelson, 1995.
Kim, Eunjung. *Curative Violence: Rehabilitating Disability, Gender, and Sexuality in Modern Korea*. Durham: Duke University Press, 2017.
Kraus, Hans-Joachim. *Biblisch-theologische Aufsätze*. Neukirchener Verlag: Neukirchener Vluyn, 1972.
Lim, Bo H. *The "Way of the Lord" in the Book of Isaiah*. LHBOTS 522. London: T&T Clark, 2010.
Lund, Øystein. *Way Metaphors and Way Topics in Isaiah 40–55*. FAT 28. Tübingen: Mohr Siebeck, 2007.
MacDonald, Nathan. *Priestly Rule: Polemic and Biblical Interpretation in Ezekiel 44*. BZAW 467. Berlin: de Gruyter, 2015.
Matthews, Claire R. *Defending Zion: Edom's Desolation and Jacob's Restoration (Isaiah 34–35) in Context*. BZAW 236. Berlin: de Gruyter, 1995.
Miscall, Peter D. *Isaiah 34–35: A Nightmare/A Dream*. JSOTSup 281. Sheffield: Sheffield Academic, 1999.
O'Connor, Kathleen. "Jeremiah's Two Visions of the Future." Pages 86–104 in *Utopia and Dystopia in Prophetic Literature*. Edited by Ehud Ben Zvi. Publications of the Finnish Exegetical Society 92. Göttingen: Vandenhoeck & Ruprecht, 2006.
Olyan, Saul M. "'Anyone Blind or Lame Shall Not Enter the House': On the Interpretation of Second Samuel 5:8b." *CBQ* 60 (1998): 218–27.
———. "The Ascription of Physical Disability as a Stigmatizing Strategy in Biblical Iconic Polemics." *JHS* 9 (2009): art. 14.
———. "Disability in the Prophetic Utopian Vision." Pages 78–92 in *Disability in the Hebrew Bible: Interpreting Mental and Physical Differences*. Cambridge: Cambridge University Press, 2008.
Oswalt, John N. *The Book of Isaiah: Chapters 1–39*. NICOT. Grand Rapids: Eerdmans, 1986.
Rad, Gerhard von. *Deuteronomy*. OTL. Philadelphia: Westminster, 1966.
Raphael, Rachel. *Biblical Corpora: Representations of Disability in Hebrew Biblical Literature*. LHBOTS 445. London: T&T Clark, 2008.
Schipper, Jeremy. *Disability and Isaiah's Suffering Servant*. Biblical Reconfigurations. Oxford: Oxford University Press, 2011.
———. "Why Does Imagery of Disability Include Healing in Isaiah?" *JSOT* 39 (2015): 319–33.
Schweitzer, Stephan James. "Utopia and Utopian Literary Theory: Some Preliminary Observations." Pages 13–26 in *Utopia and Dystopia in Prophetic Literature*. Edited by Ehud Ben Zvi. Publications of the Finnish Exegetical Society 92. Göttingen: Vandenhoeck & Ruprecht, 2006.

Smith, Gary V. *Isaiah 1–39*. NAC 15A. Nashville: Broadman & Holman, 2007.
Sommer, Benjamin D. *A Prophet Reads Scripture: Allusion in Isaiah 40–66*. Contraversions. Stanford, CA: Stanford University Press, 1998.
Stacey, David. *Isaiah*. Epworth Commentaries. London: Epworth, 1993.
Tooman, William A. *Gog of Magog: Reuse of Scripture and Compositional Technique in Ezek 38–39*. FAT 2/52. Tübingen: Mohr Siebeck, 2011.
Tov, Emanuel. "Did the Septuagint Translators Always Understand Their Hebrew Text?" Page 53–70 in *De Septuaginta: Essays in Honor of John W. Wevers on His Sixty-Fifth Birthday*. Edited by Albert Pietersma and Claude Cox. Mississauga, ON: Benben, 1984.
Watts, John D. W. *Isaiah 34–66*. WBC 25. Waco, TX: Nelson, 1987.
Williamson, Hugh Godfrey Maturin. *The Book Called Isaiah: Deutero-Isaiah's Role in Composition and Redaction*. Oxford: Clarendon, 1994.

THE ROLE OF SENSES IN LAMENTATIONS 4

Marianne Grohmann

"Which senses are emphasized or repressed, and by what means and to which ends?"[1]—This question, formulated by David Howes and Constance Classen as a general tool for analyzing the senses in any culture, is relevant for the Hebrew Bible as well. The overall image is that seeing and hearing are predominant in the texts of the Hebrew Bible, reflecting a certain hierarchy of senses. There have been many discussions about the prevalence of hearing or seeing in the Hebrew Bible. While Thorleif Boman's thesis "that for the Hebrew the most important of his senses for the experience of truth was his hearing" has been influential, the consensus today is that both of these senses—seeing and hearing—are equally important in the texts of the Hebrew Bible.[2] In the context of knowledge, understanding, and learning, we often find combinations of sight and hearing.[3]

Yet, new research about the senses in the ancient Near East has called for an investigation of the other three senses as well, that is, touch, smell, and taste, which have been traditionally overlooked.[4] In addition to that, some researchers include kinaesthesia and speech, thereby developing a septasensory model of senses.[5] These discussions indicate that "other cultures do not necessarily divide

---

[1] David Howes and Constance Classen, "Conclusion: Sounding Sensory Profiles," in *The Varieties of Sensory Experience: A Sourcebook in the Anthropology of the Senses*, ed. David Howes (Toronto: University of Toronto Press, 1991), 259. See chapter 1 above in the present volume.

[2] Thorleif Boman, *Hebrew Thought Compared with Greek* (New York: Norton, 1970), 206. For an example of the consensus today, see Christian Frevel, "Altes Testament," in *Menschsein*, ed. Christian Frevel and Oda Wischmeyer, NEB.T 11 (Würzburg: Echter, 2003), 38–41. For recent discussion against Boman's thesis, see, e.g., Yael Avrahami, *The Senses of Scripture: Sensory Perception in the Hebrew Bible*, LHBOTS 545 (New York: T&T Clark, 2012), 28–31. See also David Howes and Jan Dietrich in this volume.

[3] See Avrahami, *Senses of Scripture*, 69–74.

[4] See Mark M. Smith, *Sensing the Past: Seeing, Hearing, Smelling, Tasting, and Touching in History* (Berkeley: University of California Press, 2007), 18.

[5] Avrahami, *Senses of Scripture*, 75–93, 109–12. See also Greg Schmidt Goering and Thomas Krüger in this volume.

the sensorium as we do."⁶ Now, we do not find any systematization or classification of senses in the Hebrew Bible. Its sensory profile can only be deduced from texts and language. Therefore, some of the questions formulated by Howes and Classen are very helpful for investigating the language of senses in the Hebrew Bible:

- What words exist for the different senses?
- Which sensory perceptions have the greatest vocabulary allotted them (sounds, colors, odors)?
- How are the senses used in metaphors and expressions?⁷

The senses are linked with the body: "in the Hebrew Bible, the senses are embodied experiences, whereby each sense is semantically associated with a particular organ that operates it."⁸ So we ask: which body parts are linked with the senses?

According to the pluralistic and holistic concept of human being in the ancient Near East, the senses in the Hebrew Bible express more than perception; they represent some kind of *"personales und soziales Beziehungshandeln"*: there is a connection between personal contact, social relationship, emotions, and the senses.⁹ The senses facilitate communication between humans and between humans and God.

For pragmatic reasons, the following article concentrates on one example text, Lam 4, and focuses on the verses that describe activities of the five classical senses or activate them in a certain way.

Lamentations 4, an anonymous poetic text in the form of an alphabetic acrostic in twenty-two strophes, refers directly to the destruction of Jerusalem and the deportation of part of its inhabitants into exile in 587 BCE. The song elaborates the suffering of the people from siege and starvation. The contrast between the glorious past and the present suffering is viewed from the perspective of former elites and representatives of the city.¹⁰ Some commentators argue that this text was written immediately after the destruction of Jerusalem, because it describes

---

⁶ Howes and Classen, "Conclusion," 257.

⁷ Howes and Classen, "Conclusion," 262.

⁸ Avrahami, *Senses of Scripture*, 2.

⁹ Frevel, "Altes Testament," 40; see also Ulrike Steinert, *Aspekte des Menschseins im Alten Mesopotamien: Eine Studie zu Person und Identität im 2. und 1. Jt. v. Chr.*, CM 44 (Leiden: Brill, 2012), 121.

¹⁰ See Christian Frevel, *Die Klagelieder*, NSKAT 20.1 (Stuttgart: Katholisches Bibelwerk, 2017), 40.

the happenings in a shocking way.[11] Others argue that the vivid descriptions reflect conscious literary and stylistic decisions from a later but still exilic time.[12] After all, the last two verses, Lam 4:21–22, indicate a possible change of fate. Lamentations 4 combines elements of ancient Mesopotamian city laments, the genre of keen/laments after death—for example, the introductory cry איכה (vv. 1, 2), the contrast between former glory and present misery—and biblical language from the book of Psalms and prophetic literature.[13]

Hearing

According to the literary genre of Mesopotamian city laments,[14] Lam 4 contains an interchange between different voices: a narrator (vv. 1–16), the "we" of the inhabitants of the city or their representatives (vv. 17–20), and maybe a messenger or prophet at the end (vv. 21–22). Although we have no evidence of actual performances of Lamentations, the change of voices renders Lam 4—as well as the other songs in Lamentations—a dramatic character.[15] "This ability to shift points of view gives the city laments depth, an ability to express a variety of views and feelings without seeming contradictory."[16]

The significant cry איכה, an exclamation of despair and lament, opens the song and is repeated at the beginning of verse 2. Depending on the translation, איכה either is audible as onomatopoetic sigh, cry, or shouting ("alas")[17] or it lacks acoustic quality ("how"; cf. Deut 1:12, Song 1:7, NRSV, JPS).

In verses 14 and 15 we find "the nations" (גוים) "shouting" (קרא) and "talking" (אמר) about the people of Jerusalem, but altogether the sense of hearing plays a rather small role in this song. The ear or special qualities of sounds are not mentioned. The text does not say anything explicit about hearing or listening. This can

---

[11] See Ulrich Berges, *Klagelieder*, HThKAT (Freiburg: Herder, 2002), 236–39. See also Klaus Koenen, *Klagelieder (Threni)*, BKAT 20 (Neukirchen-Vluyn: Neukirchener Verlag, 2015), 317.

[12] See Frevel, *Die Klagelieder*, 39, 275.

[13] See Frederick W. Dobbs-Allsopp, *Weep, O Daughter of Zion: A Study of the City-Lament Genre in the Hebrew Bible*, BibOr 44 (Rome: Pontifical Biblical Institute, 1993). See also Marc Wischnowsky, *Tochter Zion: Aufnahme und Überwindung der Stadtklage in den Prophetenschriften des Alten Testaments*, WMANT 89 (Neukirchen-Vluyn: Neukirchener Verlag, 2001).

[14] See, e.g., Nili Samet, *The Lamentation over the Destruction of Ur*, MC 18 (Winona Lake, IN: Eisenbrauns, 2014).

[15] See Frevel, *Die Klagelieder*, 25.

[16] Dobbs-Allsopp, *Weep, O Daughter of Zion*, 32.

[17] Adele Berlin, *Lamentations: A Commentary*, OTL (Louisville: Westminster John Knox, 2002), 98.

be interpreted as a purposeful negation of the sense of hearing, the voicelessness of death after the destruction of Jerusalem. It might go too far, but maybe the concept of the "Sanctuary of Silence"—the absence of sounds and noise in many priestly texts describing the cult—stands in the background of this lack of acoustic signals.[18]

This lack of acoustic signals is characteristic for Lam 4, but not for all five songs in the book of Lamentations: Lam 2, probably the oldest of the songs, has many different sounds: for example, "mourning and lamentation" (תאניה ואניה, v. 5); the "clamor, voice, noise" (קול) of the enemies (v. 7); the "hissing" (שרק) both of neighbors (v. 15) and enemies (v. 16); even the "shout, scream" of the heart (צעק לבם, v. 18). These manifold acoustic signals make Lam 2 "the loudest song."[19] Yet, even in this song with many sounds and signals addressing the sense of hearing, we find the negation and inversion of the sense of hearing: "the silencing" or "sitting down in silence" (דמם) of the elders (v. 10).

VISION

After the exclamation איכה, the song addresses the eye in verse 1–2:

1a	How the gold has grown dim,	איכה יועם זהב
	how the pure gold is changed!	ישנא הכתם הטוב
1b	The sacred stones lie scattered	תשתפכנה אבני־קדש
	at the head of every street.	בראש כל־חוצות
2a	The precious children of Zion,	בני ציון היקרים
	worth their weight in fine gold—	המסלאים בפז
2b	how they are reckoned as earthen pots,	איכה נחשבו לנבלי־חרש
	the work of a potter's hands![20]	מעשה ידי יוצר

Verse 1a almost works as a heading of the song: the contrast between former brightness and present darkness, another typical element both of Mesopotamian laments and the biblical laments,[21] is described with the contrast of colors in verses 1, 2, 5, 7, and 8. The colors of the past are: "gold" or "fine gold" (זהב, כתם טוב, and

---

[18] See Israel Knohl, *The Sanctuary of Silence: The Priestly Torah and the Holiness School* (Winona Lake, IN: Eisenbrauns, 2007). See also Annette Schellenberg, "'Ein beschwichtigender Geruch für JHWH': Zur Rolle der Sinne im Kult," in *Anthropologie(n) des Alten Testaments*, ed. Jürgen van Oorschoot and Andreas Wagner, VWGTh 42 (Berlin: Evangelische Verlagsanstalt, 2015), 139.

[19] Frevel, *Die Klagelieder*, 146.

[20] The English translation follows NRSV, if not indicated otherwise.

[21] See Dobbs-Allsopp, *Weep, O Daughter of Zion*, 39. See also Koenen, *Klagelieder*, 315.

פז); "scarlet" or "carmine" (תולע)[22]; "white" (like snow, like milk)[23]; "redder than corals" (אדם מפנינים); and the color of "sapphire" (ספיר), blue, often identified with Lapis lazuli.[24] These colors representing former glory, wealth, and an ideal of beauty (Song 5:10–16) are not visible in the present situation of the song. They are mentioned to stimulate the "inner eye," the imagination. The colors—both the bright colors of the past and the darkness of the present situation—are attributed to the בני ציון היקרים ("the precious children of Zion," v. 2) and the נזירים ("princes, consecrated, Nazirites," v. 7),[25] parallel terms for the noble citizens of Jerusalem.

The contrast of colors, addressing the eye, is continued in verses 7–8a:

7a	Her princes were purer than snow, whiter than milk;	זכו נזיריה משלג צחו מחלב
7b	their bodies were more ruddy than coral, their hair like sapphire.	אדמו עצם מפנינים ספיר גזרתם
8a	Now their visage is blacker than soot; they are not recognized[26] in the streets.	חשך משחור תארם לא נכרו בחוצות

The quality usually ascribed to these colors has "changed" (שנא; v. 1) to their opposite: the gold has become dark (עמם, v. 1). The colors of the present situation of despair are black and dark: אשפתות ("ash heaps") in verse 5 hint at the grey color of dust or the brown color of dung. The princes' תאר ("form, look, appearance") has become "darker than black" (v. 8) or "blacker than soot" (NRSV). Common terms of visual perception—תאר, derived from ראה ("seeing") and נכר ("recognize")—do not work anymore. The princes of the city have become so dark that they are not recognizable any more. The terms תאר and נכר ("recognize") belong to the world field of vision. The verse is an example of the fact that seeing

---

[22] תולע, occurring mainly in postexilic texts, is a worm or scale insect, living on the carmine tree or bush, producing red, scarlet colorant—see Koenen, *Klagelieder*, 327; Frevel, *Die Klagelieder*, 282–83; Wolfgang Zwickel, "Färben in der Antike," in *Edelsteine in der Bibel*, ed. Wolfgang Zwickel (Mainz: Philipp von Zabern, 2002), 43–44.

[23] The color white is expressed with the verbs זכך ("to be bright, pure," not in the sense of ritual purity, but in the sense of brightness) in a comparison with snow and צחח ("to dazzle") in comparison with milk. While the verbs hint at brightness in a general way, the color white is expressed via the comparisons.

[24] See Koenen, *Klagelieder*, 331–34. See also the Lamentation over the Destruction of Ur: "My precious metals and lapis lazuli have been scattered about; 'My possessions!' I shall cry" (Samet, *Lamentation*, 69).

[25] The context makes it plausible to understand *Nazirites* in a wide sense of "consecrated, selected" people (see Koenen, *Klagelieder*, 330).

[26] Another possible translation of this *niphal* form is: "they are not recognizable" (see Berlin, *Lamentations*, 99).

is more than plain sight; it has many other connotations, for example, "recognizing." Contrasting former glory to present misery is typical for the lamentation of the dead or keen.[27]

An escalation of darkness is the blindness in verse 14a:

> 14a Blindly they wandered through the streets,   נעו עורים בחוצות
> so defiled with blood   נגאלו בדם

Those who should see, do not see anymore. It is open in the text who is the blind subject: either the priests and prophets mentioned in verse 13,[28] the people in general,[29] a combination of both,[30] or the righteous people (צדיקים) mentioned in verse 13b.[31]

נעו עורים maybe "refers to the groping, stumbling progress ... of someone who has (just) become blind" (cf. Zeph 1:17).[32] However, physical blindness is not a logical consequence of hunger and starvation. Thus, more plausible is an understanding of blindness in a metaphoric sense, which is very common in prophetic literature: "The visionaries have become blind (cf. Isa 56:10) and there is no new divine utterance to illumine the darkness in which they find themselves (// Ps 36:10 and 119:105). This is the situation which we now see reflected in the physical condition of the prophets: spiritually broken, all their strength has been sapped from their bodies. Thus blind, they falter through the city streets."[33] The dichotomy between sight and blindness in metaphoric meaning is part of a conceptual system of contrasts: life—death; light—darkness; wisdom—foolishness; choice—rejection; good—evil.[34]

In opposition to the red colors of the past—children who were brought up in scarlet fabrics (v. 5b), bodies redder than coral (v. 7b)—the present color—beside black, grey, and brown—is the redness of blood.

The climax of not seeing lies at the end of the first part of the song, in verse 16:

---

[27] See Hedwig Jahnow, *Das hebräische Leichenlied im Rahmen der Völkerdichtung*, BZAW 36 (Giessen: Töpelmann, 1923), 99.

[28] See Johan Renkema, *Lamentations*, HCOT (Leuven: Peeters, 1998), 530.

[29] See Lena-Sofia Tiemeyer, "The Question of Indirect Touch: Lam 4,14; Ezek 44,19 and Hag 2,12–13," *Bib* 87 (2006): 67–68.

[30] Berlin, *Lamentations*, 104: "The priests and prophets are a metonym for the people ('a kingdom of priests,' Exod 19:6), who are rejected and scattered by God."

[31] See Hans-Joachim Kraus, *Klagelieder (Threni)*, 3rd ed., BKAT 20 (Neukirchen-Vluyn: Neukirchener Verlag, 1968), 80.

[32] Renkema, *Lamentations*, 530.

[33] Renkema, *Lamentations*, 532.

[34] See Avrahami, *Senses of Scripture*, 276.

16a	The LORD himself has scattered them, he will regard them no more;	פני יהוה חלקם לא יוסיף להביטם
16b	no honor was shown to the priests, no favor to the elders.	פני כהנים לא נשאו זקנים [וזקנים] לא חננו

In a literal reading it is not "the LORD himself" but פני יהוה ("YHWH's face"), in parallelism to "the face of the priests," indicating YHWH's presence as God-king in the temple and as a body part responsible for care and attention;[35] it is the פני יהוה that "divided, scattered" them. The combination of the verb חלק with YHWH's face is quite unusual. The second part of the first parallelism in verse 16a describes the end of God's look: "he does not see them any more, he will regard them no more."

Verse 16 makes clear that seeing is more than perception: God's attention, care and help are connected with his look—נבט ("to look, regard" in the sense of attention, honor, favor, and care)—a motive throughout the book of Lamentations and in the Hebrew Bible in general. Another word for attention is נשא פנים ("to lift up the face")—like in the blessing (Num 6:26): "the face of the priests"; to lift up someone's face in Hebrew means: "to treat someone as eminent" or "to honor someone."[36] Seeing is more than a physical process; it includes active attention and dynamic presence.[37] It is not clear who is the subject of verse 16b: it can be a general, impersonal description of the missing attention—in parallelism with mercy—to priests and elders.

The caring look of both God and humans is absent here. The whole poem can be interpreted as a cry for God's help, care, and attention, but "God does not look at the people or answer them (v. 16)."[38] We find parallels of the deity hiding its organs of perception—ear, eye, and heart—in Sumerian Emesal prayers (first millennium BCE): the deity does not regard its own city because it is so engaged in the act of devastation: "Your eyes [i-bi_2-zu] do not rest in order to look favorably [u_6-di-de_3] (at your city)!"[39]

While the first part of the song ends with God's absent caring look, the second part opens with the eyes of the people in verse 17. The eyes, sensual organs usually responsible for sight, do not work the way they should. Colors affect the

---

[35] Friedhelm Hartenstein, *Das Angesicht "JHWHs": Studien zu einem höfischen und kultischen Bedeutungshintergrund in den Psalmen und in Exodus 32–34*, FAT 55 (Tübingen: Mohr Siebeck, 2008), 284. See also Koenen, *Klagelieder*, 349.

[36] Renkema, *Lamentations*, 543.

[37] Thomas Staubli and Silvia Schroer, *Menschenbilder der Bibel* (Ostfildern: Patmos Verlag, 2014), 199.

[38] Berlin, *Lamentations*, 104.

[39] Uri Gabbay, *Pacifying the Hearts of the Gods: Sumerian Emesal Prayers of the First Millennium BC*, Heidelberger Emesal-Studien 1 (Wiesbaden: Harrassowitz, 2014), 31.

eye; the eye is activated in the process of reading but mentioned only one time, in verse 17a:

17a	Our eyes failed, ever watching vainly for help;[40]	עודינה [עודינו] תכלינה עינינו אל־עזרתנו הבל
17b	we were watching eagerly for a nation that could not save.	בצפיתנו צפינו אל־גוי לא יושע

כלה means "to fail, finish, become weak,"[41] in combination with the eyes: "to become blind." In addition to that, the phrase has the connotation "to swelter" (*"verschmachten, sich nach etwas verzehren"*) (Ps 119:82, 123), "to long for something, to wait anxiously"[42] (cf. Lam 2:11): the eyes stand for the longing look. The weakness of the eyes is in the same line as the blindness in verse 14.

Another root for "watching, looking out" in this verse is the verb צפה, in combination with the noun צפיה, a *hapax legomenon* that can mean "peering on a certain object" here, maybe from a watch post or tower[43]—a look which does not see the expected here.

Altogether, Lam 4, like the whole book of Lamentations, stresses the aspect of seeing, looking, and perceiving (Lam 1:7–12, 18, 20; 2:16, 20; 3:1, 36, 50, 59–60, 63; 4:16; 5:1). It is an appeal to the reader to participate in the suffering and pain of the city. We find an inversion of the sense of vision in Lam 4; it does not work as is expected. The sense of sight is linked with God's caring attention, which is missing in the situation after the destruction of Jerusalem.

The fact that aspects of sight occur at the end of the first part of the song (v. 16) and at the beginning of the second part (v. 17) has a parallel in Lam 1, a text that might have been composed at a similar time. Also in Lam 1 seeing works as an attention marker in an appeal to God (vv. 9, 11, 12, 20) and in framing verses of the song. Like in Lam 4 it finishes the first part of the song (v. 11) and is taken up again at the beginning of the second part (v. 12).

In the discussion about the prevalence of hearing versus seeing, Lam 4 has more aspects of sight than of acoustic signals.

---

[40] The Hebrew text is a nominal clause, without a verb for seeing, literally: "to our help—in vain"; see Berlin, *Lamentations*, 100: "(looking) for our help, for naught."

[41] "All the while our eyes wore out" (see Berlin, *Lamentations*, 100, 102).

[42] Koenen, *Klagelieder*, 351–52; Franz Josef Helfmeyer, "כלא," *TDOT* 7:163–64.

[43] Koenen, *Klagelieder*, 352. Berlin provides the most literal translation: "we watched and watched" (*Lamentations*, 100).

Tasting

Lamentations 4 describes the sense of tasting in the context of famine and starvation, which are consequences of the destruction and breakdown of Jerusalem (שבר; v. 10b). In this text, we cannot only understand טעם as the sense of tasting,[44] but the sense of taste does appear in the context of the elementary needs for food and drink (cf. Lam 1:11; 2:12). Hunger and thirst are illustrated with intensive images in verses 3–5 and 9–11. Body parts mentioned in the context of eating are the "breast" (שד) in connection with nursing; the "tongue" (לשון) sticking on the palate (חך, "gum, the roof of the mouth"), a description of thirst; and the "hands" (ידים) becoming cruel. In addition to that, food (bread, produces of the field) and drink are missing: the present situation is one of hunger and thirst. Like other songs in Lamentations (e.g., Lam 1:11), this text describes the lack of basic supply as a consequence of the siege.[45]

In Lam 4:3–4 the children and very young people are described as being affected in particular by starvation, violence, and death:

3a	Even the jackals offer the breast and nurse their young,	גם־תנין [תנים] חלצו שד היניקו גוריהן
3b	but my people has become cruel, like the ostriches in the wilderness.	בת־עמי לאכזר כי ענים [כיענים] במדבר
4a	The tongue of the infant sticks to the roof of its mouth for thirst;	דבק לשון יונק אל־חכו בצמא
4b	the children beg for food, but no one gives them anything.	עוללים שאלו לחם פרש אין להם

While verse 3 is formulated from the perspective of the parents, verse 4 describes thirst and hunger from the viewpoint of the small children. The animals mentioned in verse 3, jackals and ostriches,[46] are associated with wilderness (Isa 13:21; Jer 50:39; Mic 1:8). Both animals share negative connotations and are associated with loneliness (Job 30:29): "inhabiting ruins and uttering eerie cries that sound like keening."[47] The difference in their care for the young animals is unique in this imagery. While ינק (v. 3b) is the common verb for breastfeeding, חלץ ("to bare, uncover"; v. 3a) as well as the differentiation between the two animals in their brood care is rather unusual. Target of the animal metaphor is the "cruelty" (אכזר) of "the daughter of my people" (בת־עמי).[48] "The Judean mothers are contrasted

---

[44] See Pierre van Hecke in this volume.
[45] Berlin, *Lamentations*, 102.
[46] In the *qere*: כַּיְעֵנִים.
[47] Berlin, *Lamentations*, 106.
[48] The Septuagint reads the plural form here.

with jackals, who, although thought of as despicable animals, at least suckle their offspring, and they are compared to ostriches, who were believed to abandon their eggs (Job 39:13–17)."[49]

Verse 4 describes the thirst and hunger of babies and small children in a drastic way: the term דבק is a verb of contact, thus belonging to the sense of touch. The phrase of the "tongue sticking to the roof of the mouth" can either mean thirst (Ps 22:16) or the inability to speak or cry (Ezek 3:26; Job 29:10; Ps 137:6): "The infants are so weak from starvation that they no longer cry when hungry."[50] This description corresponds with the silence, the missing acoustic signals in Lam 4. The small children beg, ask for "bread" (לחם), but no one gives it to them.[51]

Verse 5 shows a strong contrast and addresses many senses: taste, sight, touch, and even smell.

| 5a | Those who feasted on[52] delicacies perish in the streets; | האכלים למעדנים נשמו בחוצות |
| 5b | those who were brought up[53] in purple cling to ash heaps. | האמנים עלי תולע חבקו אשפתות |

Elementary needs are addressed here, no tasting in the sense of different tastes. The only noun describing a special quality of food belongs to the past: the "delicacies" (מעדנים) in verse 5, those who ate or "were used to eat"[54] מעדנים. The noun, derived from the root עדן ("enjoy"), occurs in Gen 49:20 in the blessing of Jacob for Gad as "delicacies, delights of a king," in parallelism to "fat bread." In Prov 27:17, it has the meaning "delight, pleasure." The "eating" (אכל) of "delicacies" stands in a contradictory parallelism to the contemporary situation of "perishing" (שמם, "becoming deserted, devastated") in the streets. The former eating of delicacies is contrasted with the "eating, consuming" (אכל) fire in Lam 4:11.

These descriptions of dire need, hunger, and problems with food supply are in contradiction with texts such as Jer 39–40, which are intended to convey hope

---

[49] Berlin, *Lamentations*, 106; Frevel, *Die Klagelieder*, 279–81; Koenen, *Klagelieder*, 325.
[50] Berlin, *Lamentations*, 106.
[51] NRSV understands the bread *pars pro toto* for food. The "breaking" (פרס) of bread can be a possible acoustic association to this verse.
[52] Literally: "those who ate delicacies."
[53] אמן evokes associations of nourishing as well: "being brought up, nourished by a wet nurse."
[54] Koenen, *Klagelieder*, 327.

for a new beginning. One explanation may be that immediately after the destruction of Jerusalem, supplies in the city were obviously scarcer than in rural areas and during subsequent periods.[55]

While eating delicacies is contrasted to perishing in the streets in Lam 4:5 as a description of state, it is formulated as a curse in other places, for example, in the Curse of Agade: "May your aristocrats, who eat fine food, lie down in hunger" (CA 249).[56]

"The cause of the degradation is the famine of the siege, and its effects are described in a realistic sequence in which starvation weakens the population: first the children, who are starving (vv. 3–4); then the adults, whose health deteriorates precipitously (vv. 5–9); then the ultimate trope for starvation: cannibalism (v. 10)."[57] However, a list of all population groups mentioned in the book of Lamentations shows that it was not only the weakest that suffered. It reveals a diverse picture of the urban population including some or even all strata and groups of society.[58] "The picture is … a drastic reversal of fortunes, socially and physically, caused by the ravages of wartime famine."[59]

In verse 9, hunger is contrasted to "the products, fruits of the field" (תנובת שדי) (Deut 32:13; Judg 9:11; Isa 27:6; Ezek 36:30), derived from the root נוב ("to grow, develop"):

9a	Happier were those pierced by the sword than those pierced by hunger,	טובים היו חללי־חרב מחללי רעב
9b	whose life drains away,[60] deprived of the produce of the field.	שהם יזובו מדקרים מתנובת שדי

The מ before תנובת שדי expresses separation: "Without the produce of the field"—"Thus they are pierced by the lack of food."[61]

---

[55] See Rainer Kessler, *Sozialgeschichte des Alten Israel: Eine Einführung* (Darmstadt: Wissenschaftliche Buchgesellschaft, 2006), 131. See also Oded Lipschits, *The Fall and Rise of Jerusalem: Judah under Babylonian Rule* (Winona Lake, IN: Eisenbrauns, 2005), 190.

[56] Jerrold S. Cooper, *The Curse of Agade*, The John Hopkins Near Eastern Studies (Baltimore: Johns Hopkins University Press, 1983), 240.

[57] Berlin, *Lamentations*, 103.

[58] See Berlin, *Lamentations*, 13–15.

[59] Berlin, *Lamentations*, 103.

[60] Literally: "they flow out, pierced."

[61] Berlin, *Lamentations*, 108. See LSUr 389: "Those of the city who were not given over to weapons, died of hunger," cited according to Dobbs-Allsopp, *Weep, O Daughter of Zion*, 72.

In verse 10 the situation of hunger gains a climax in "maternal cannibalism":[62]

10a	The hands of compassionate women have boiled their own children;	ידי נשים רחמניות בשלו ילדיהן
10b	they became their food[63] in the destruction of my people.[64]	היו לברות למו בשבר בת־עמי

While Lam 2:20 formulates the situation that mothers might even eat their children as a question and sets it in an appeal to God to see, to look, Lam 4:10 describes a situation of mothers even "boiling" their children: "The picture of women devouring their children is a particularly gruesome form of cannibalism signifying extreme famine; it is a reversal of the natural order in which women feed their children."[65] The motif of cannibalism is found in descriptions of famine in the Hebrew Bible (Lev 26:29; Deut 28:53–57; 2 Kgs 6:26–30; Jer 19:9; Ezek 5:10) and in Assyrian sources, for example, in Esarhaddon's Succession Treaty: "just as [thi]s ewe has been cut open and the flesh of [her] young has been placed in her mouth, may they make you eat in your hunger the flesh of your brothers, your sons and your daughters."[66]

"This motif may be an exaggeration that does not correspond to reality, but the image that it conjures up is extremely effective."[67] In Lam 4:10 it gets a specific variant in the oxymoron that the women are described as "compassionate," and they are not only eating, but their hands that should break bread for the children (v. 4b) are "boiling" their offspring.

This is the only place in the Hebrew Bible where "boiling" has "hands" as subject, not persons: "By using ידי, the poets render the mechanistic character of the women's actions: their hands are at work but they themselves are not really present."[68]

According to verse 10b, the children become ברות, a special meal of mourning, grief, and solace after the death of somebody (2 Sam 12:17; 13:7; 7:10; Ps 69:22):

---

[62] See Hendrik Ludolph Bosman, "The Function of (Maternal) Cannibalism in the Book of Lamentations (2:20 and 4:10)," *Scriptura* 110 (2012): 152–65.

[63] The form לִבְרוֹת *lebārôt* is quite unclear. Some, e.g., Koenen, *Klagelieder*, 301, 305, change the vowels to לְבָרוּת *lebārût*, following the Septuagint and other ancient translations, and translate "zu einem Notessen."

[64] Literally: "the daughter of my people."

[65] Berlin, *Lamentations*, 75.

[66] Simo Parpola and Kazuko Watanabe, *Neo-Assyrian Treaties and Loyalty Oaths*, SAA 2 (Helsinki: Helsinki University Press, 1988), 28–58 (Esarhaddon's Succession Treaty): §69, lines 547–550.

[67] Berlin, *Lamentations*, 76.

[68] Renkema, *Lamentations*, 519.

the only food remaining is ברות, the dead children being both the reason for mourning and the meal of solace. The literary motif of teknophagy is known in ancient Near Eastern texts but not in laments: it serves as an illustration of the dramatic situation of destruction, cruelty, and starvation. It cannot be deduced from these parallels that it reflects some kind of historic reality.[69]

SMELL

The nose, God's nose, is mentioned two times in the text, verses 11 and 20.

11a	The LORD gave full vent to his wrath; he poured out his hot anger,[70]	כלה יהוה את־חמתו שפך חרון אפו
11b	and kindled a fire in Zion that consumed its foundations.	ויצת־אש בציון ותאכל יסודתיה

If we follow the line of active and passive aspects in the senses,[71] this talking about the nose—as synonym of breath—would be the active side. This has nothing to do with smelling as a passive process of perception. The emotion attributed the nose is anger and wrath.[72] This angry blowing of the nose is combined, in parallelism, with the "eating, consuming" (אכל) fire (Deut 4:24; Isa 30:30; Ezek 15:7).[73] The fire can be both real fire, which accompanies the destruction of the city, and a metaphor for divine emotions.[74] The "eating" of the fire is metaphoric. The fire addresses many senses: touching, temperature, seeing, tasting, and smelling.

Smelling as a passive process of perception might be a connotation in verse 5: אשפתות ("dust, ash, dung heaps") generate associations of dust, death, garbage, and bad smell. It addresses the eye: grey, black, maybe brown colors—and the nose: bad smell. Garbage is the place of poor people (1 Sam 2:8; Ps 113:7).[75] Disgust is linked with bad smell, which is very common in the ancient Near East.[76]

Again verse 20 addresses more than one sense:

---

[69] Koenen, *Klagelieder*, 175–80.
[70] Literally: "he poured out the burning anger of his nose."
[71] See Pierre van Hecke in this volume.
[72] See Avrahami, *Senses of Scripture*, 17.
[73] See Gerlinde Baumann, "JHWH—Ein essender Gott? Ein Menü in wenigen Gängen," in *Essen und Trinken in der Bibel*, ed. Michaela Geiger et al. (Gütersloh: Gütersloher Verlagshaus, 2009), 227–237 (229–230).
[74] See Frevel, *Die Klagelieder*, 155.
[75] See Koenen, *Klagelieder*, 328.
[76] See, e.g., Nicla de Zorzi in this volume.

20a	The breath of our life,	רוח אפינו
	the LORD's anointed,	משיח יהוה
	was taken in their pits,	נלכד בשחיתותם
20b	the one of whom we said,	אשר אמרנו
	"Under his shadow we shall live among the nations."	בצלו נחיה בגוים

The smell of ointment stands in the background of verse 20a that refers to the king with the title "YHWH's anointed," hinting maybe at Zedekia, the last king of Juda.[77] לכד ("was taken, captured") is another verb of touch and contact, the שחיתות ("pits, traps") might hint at prison or at garbage pits. While verse 11 mentioned God's nose ("anger, wrath"), here we find רוח אפינו ("the wind, breath of our wrath, nose"), in the active meaning of the nose as sensual organ.

Touching

The sense of touching in Lam 4 can be approached from three sides: (1) the hands as the body parts responsible for touching; (2) verbs of contact; (3) touching in the context of purity/impurity.

(1) The hands are mentioned three times, verses 2b, 6b and 10a. In verse 2 the hands of the potter serve as an image for uselessness: the children of Zion are compared to earthen pots, the work of a potter's hands. God creating humans as a potter resembles Gen 2:7; Isa 64:7; Jer 18:6. The second time the hands are mentioned, in verse 6b, it is not clear to whom the hands belong. The verb linked with the hands here is חול ("dance, writhe, to be firm"), and the metaphoric expression is quite unclear: Sodom as a symbol for destruction without active hands.[78] The third occurrence of the hands are the mentioned hands of the mothers in verse 10, boiling their children, the cruel climax of the text. These examples show that the touch of the hands, representing power, action, authority, and control can be ambivalent.[79] We find this ambivalence of the hands in other chapters of Lamentations as well: the personified Zion can stretch out her hands, as an appeal for help (Lam 1:17). Often the hands are combined with violence, both of the enemy (Lam 1:10, 14; 2:7) and of God (Lam 2:4).

(2) Verbs of contact and touching in the song are יצר ("form"), דבק ("stick to," of the tongue), חבק ("cling to [NRSV], embrace"), and חול ("dance, writhe, to be firm").

---

[77] See Koenen, *Klagelieder*, 359.

[78] Renkema understands חול in the meaning "to turn oneself against, did not turn herself against her hands"—that is without human agency, the destruction of Sodom was God's work alone. Thus, he translates verse 6b: "without the agency of (human) hand." (*Lamentations*, 509–10).

[79] See Steinert, *Aspekte des Menschseins*, 219.

(3) Verses 14–15: touching in the context of impurity. In Lam 4:14–15, the sense of touching is linked with the priestly concept of purity and impurity.[80]

14a	Blindly they wandered through the streets,	נעו עורים בחוצות
	so defiled with blood	נגאלו בדם
14b	that no one was able	בלא יוכלו
	to touch their garments.	יגעו בלבשיהם
15a	"Away! Unclean!" people shouted at them;	סורו טמא קראו למו
	"Away! Away! Do not touch!"	סורו סורו אל־תגעו
15b	So they became fugitives and wanderers;	כי נצו גם־נעו
	it was said among the nations, "They shall stay here no longer."	אמרו בגוים לא יוסיפו לגור

In these verses, the terms טמא ("impure") and גאל ("defiled, cultic impure") are applied to the citizens of Jerusalem or to their priests and prophets. We find a mixture of ritual and moral impurity here. It is not clear which kind of defilement is at issue and whether it has something to do with touching and contact. Although the words in Lam 4:15 are very general, the concept behind this ritual impurity might be the ritually impure leper: "the ritually impure leper (Lev 13:45) is the symbol of the morally impure leaders. The poet makes this comparison for the purpose of conveying the untouchability—the utter rejection—of those who have sinned."[81] It makes sense to understand טמא and גאל in Lam 4:15 as encompassing various connotations of impurity:

- As a cultic status in which it is not appropriate to approach the sanctuary. This cultic or ritual status is applied to a daily life scene in the streets. The defilement with blood—probably of murdered people—introduces the impurity caused by contact with corpses (Num 19:10–22). Especially priests are not allowed to touch corpses (Lev 21:1).
- Defilement is linked with social borders here: if verse 14 is read in continuation of verse 13, the priests and prophets are described as blind.[82] The nations refuse to allow the exiles to live among them. Boundary maintenance is an aspect of these verses. The authors of the songs in Lamentations use the language of impurity to describe their traumatic experiences during the destruction of Jerusalem and exile. Impurity language is blended with other types of language, including aspects of moral impurity.

---

[80] See Schellenberg, "Ein beschwichtigender Geruch," 138, 152–53.
[81] Berlin, *Lamentations*, 20.
[82] See Koenen, *Klagelieder*, 346.

Ultimately, it is not possible to force these occurrences of purity/impurity into one system. The aforementioned texts in Lam 4 refer to variegated aspects of this notion. Lam 4 can be read as example of the metaphorization of the concept of purity and impurity: ritual impurity, as a state in which it is inappropriate to approach the temple, is on its way to becoming a metaphor for moral impurity. Even if we consider the text as metaphor, the cultic or ritual sense is preserved.

Conclusions

Returning to the questions of the beginning, we can describe the "sensory profile" of Lam 4 in the following way:

The senses emphasized in Lam 4 are vision, taste (in the elementary sense of need for food), and touching. Hearing and smelling play a subordinate role in this text. The sense of vision is central in Lam 4—like in many parts of the Hebrew Bible[83]—but one cannot deduce a hierarchy of senses from one chapter.

Investigating the language of Lam 4 shows that the senses are described in the text in many ways: with nouns, verbs, and imagery. We find many body parts in the text, but not all of them are linked with senses. The sensory organs mentioned are the eye (vision), the tongue and palate (tasting), the hands (touching), and God's nose (symbolizing anger). In addition to that, the multifaceted vocabulary of colors, addressing the sense of vision, is special in the text. We find both senses and their activities in the text and descriptions and imagery especially addressing the senses. The senses are combined, for example, in verse 5b vision, touch, and smell. Verse 14 combines the senses of vision and touch.

The sensory organs do much more than perceiving. The senses stand in a network of different functions and emotions. For example, the hands do more than touching: they can be stretched out for help or even boil children. The nose is combined with anger. The sensory organs are linked with other body parts, with their physical functions, emotions, and the relationship between humans and God and humans. In addition to that, the senses are used as metaphors in this text: for example, "consuming, eating" fire, blindness as a metaphor for not understanding and not knowing what to do, the passing cup in verse 21.

Altogether, we find a converse or inversion of senses in Lam 4: as a consequence of destruction of the city and the temple of Jerusalem and the suffering of the people, the senses do not perceive or function as they should. The eyes become weak and blind, the tongue that is used to taste delicacies sticks to the palate, and the hands of mothers do not touch their children but become violent in their desperation. The senses close and shut down.

---

[83] See Avrahami, *Senses of Scripture*, 224–25.

Bibliography

Avrahami, Yael. *The Senses of Scripture: Sensory Perception in the Hebrew Bible*. LHBOTS 545. New York: T&T Clark, 2012.
Baumann, Gerlinde. "JHWH—Ein essender Gott? Ein Menü in wenigen Gängen." Pages 227–37 in *Essen und Trinken in der Bibel*. Edited by Michaela Geiger et al. Gütersloh: Gütersloher Verlagshaus, 2009.
Berges, Ulrich. *Klagelieder*. HThKAT. Freiburg: Herder, 2002.
Berlin, Adele. *Lamentations: A Commentary*. OTL. Louisville: Westminster John Knox, 2002.
Boman, Thorleif. *Hebrew Thought Compared with Greek*. New York: Norton, 1970.
Bosman, Hendrik Ludolph. "The Function of (Maternal) Cannibalism in the Book of Lamentations (2:20 and 4:10)." *Scriptura* 110 (2012): 152–65.
Cooper, Jerrold S. *The Curse of Agade*. The John Hopkins Near Eastern Studies. Baltimore: Johns Hopkins University Press, 1983.
Dobbs-Allsopp, Fred W. *Weep, O Daughter of Zion: A Study of the City-Lament Genre in the Hebrew Bible*. BibOr 44. Rome: Pontifical Biblical Institute, 1993.
Gabbay, Uri. *Pacifying the Hearts of the Gods: Sumerian Emesal Prayers of the First Millennium BC*. Heidelberger Emesal-Studien 1. Wiesbaden: Harrassowitz, 2014.
Frevel, Christian. "Altes Testament." Pages 38–41 in *Menschsein*. Edited by Christian Frevel and Oda Wischmeyer. Neb.T 11. Würzburg: Echter, 2003.
———. *Die Klagelieder*. NSKAT 20.1. Stuttgart: Katholisches Bibelwerk, 2017.
Hartenstein, Friedhelm. *Das Angesicht "JHWHs": Studien zu einem höfischen und kultischen Bedeutungshintergrund in den Psalmen und in Exodus 32–34*. FAT 55. Tübingen: Mohr Siebeck, 2008.
Helfmeyer, Franz Josef. "בלא." *TDOT* 7:143–64.
Howes, David, and Constance Classen. "Conclusion: Sounding Sensory Profiles." Pages 257–88 in *The Varieties of Sensory Experience: A Sourcebook in the Anthropology of the Senses*. Edited by David Howes. Toronto: University of Toronto Press, 1991.
Jahnow, Hedwig. *Das hebräische Leichenlied im Rahmen der Völkerdichtung*. BZAW 36. Giessen: Töpelmann, 1923.
Kessler, Rainer. *Sozialgeschichte des Alten Israel: Eine Einführung*. Darmstadt: Wissenschaftliche Buchgesellschaft, 2006.
Knohl, Israel. *The Sanctuary of Silence: The Priestly Torah and the Holiness School*. Winona Lake, IN: Eisenbrauns, 2007.
Koenen, Klaus. *Klagelieder (Threni)*. BKAT 20. Neukirchen-Vluyn: Neukirchener Verlag, 2015.
Kraus, Hans-Joachim. *Klagelieder (Threni)*. 3rd ed. BKAT 20. Neukirchen-Vluyn: Neukirchener Verlag, 1968.
Lipschits, Oded. *The Fall and Rise of Jerusalem: Judah under Babylonian Rule*. Winona Lake, IN: Eisenbrauns, 2005.
Parpola, Simo, and Kazuko Watanabe. *Neo-Assyrian Treaties and Loyalty Oaths*. SAA 2. Helsinki: Helsinki University Press, 1988.
Renkema, Johan. *Lamentations*. HCOT. Leuven: Peeters, 1998.

Samet, Nili. *The Lamentation over the Destruction of Ur*. MC 18. Winona Lake, IN: Eisenbrauns, 2014.
Schellenberg, Annette "'Ein beschwichtigender Geruch für JHWH': Zur Rolle der Sinne im Kult." Pages 136–58 in *Anthropologie(n) des Alten Testaments*. Edited by Jürgen van Oorschoot and Andreas Wagner. VWGTh 42. Berlin: Evangelische Verlagsanstalt, 2015.
Smith, Mark M. *Sensing the Past: Seeing, Hearing, Smelling, Tasting, and Touching in History*. Berkeley: University of California Press, 2007.
Staubli, Thomas, and Silvia Schroer. *Menschenbilder der Bibel*. Ostfildern: Patmos Verlag, 2014.
Steinert, Ulrike. *Aspekte des Menschseins im Alten Mesopotamien: Eine Studie zu Person und Identität im 2. und 1. Jt. v. Chr.* CM 44. Leiden: Brill, 2012.
Tiemeyer, Lena-Sofia. "The Question of Indirect Touch: Lam 4,14; Ezek 44,19 and Hag 2,12–13," *Bib* 87 (2006): 64–74.
Wischnowsky, Marc. *Tochter Zion: Aufnahme und Überwindung der Stadtklage in den Prophetenschriften des Alten Testaments*. WMANT 89. Neukirchen-Vluyn: Neukirchener Verlag, 2001.
Zwickel, Wolfgang. "Färben in der Antike." Pages 41–44 in *Edelsteine in der Bibel*. Edited by Wolfgang Zwickel. Mainz: Philipp von Zabern, 2002.

SENSES, SENSUALITY, AND SENSORY IMAGINATION: ON THE ROLE OF THE SENSES IN THE SONG OF SONGS

Annette Schellenberg

> Your lips distill nectar, my bride; honey and milk are under your tongue; the scent of your garments is like the scent of Lebanon.[1] (Song 4:11)

> I say I will climb the palm tree and lay hold of its branches. O may your breasts be like clusters of the vine, and the scent of your breath like apples, and your kisses like the best wine that goes down smoothly, gliding over lips and teeth. (Song 7:9–10)

These and similar sentences explain the Song of Song's fame as the most sensual text of the Bible, and they show that this assessment is true in the double sense of the word: the Song is full both of sensory images (sensual = sensory) and of erotic images (sensual = erotic). In my paper I will primarily focus on the sensory aspect, though in the Song this is not possible without also touching on the connection between sensory experiences and eroticism. I will show how the senses play a role in the Song on different levels—namely, within, before, and after the text—and demonstrate how they build a bridge between the world of the text's protagonists and the world of its recipients.[2]

---

[1] Here and in the following, the Bible is quoted in the translation of the NRSV.

[2] Obviously, not only the Song but all texts can be asked about the role of the senses on these three levels. What makes the Song stand out against most other texts of the Hebrew Bible is the immense importance of the senses within the text (the sensuality of the Song) and after the text (its effect on the recipients). On the importance of the senses in the Song, see also Annette Schellenberg, "Sensuality of the Song of Songs: Another Criterion to Be Considered When Assessing (So-Called) Literal and Allegorical Interpretations of the Song," in *Interpreting the Song: Literal or Allegorical?*, ed. Annette Schellenberg and Ludger Schwienhorst-Schönberger, BTS 26 (Leuven: Peeters, 2016), 103–29, where I focused on the Song's sensuality (and the connection between eroticism and religion) to show that there are some allegorical interpretations that should be appreciated for their sensitivity towards the Song's sensuality.

SENSORY EXPERIENCES AND DESIRES OF THE PROTAGONISTS

The first level to focus on is the text itself, namely, the world of its protagonists. That the senses are important to the protagonists is obvious from the first few verses: "Let him kiss me with the kisses of his mouth! For your love is better than wine, your anointing oils are fragrant, your name is perfume poured out" (1:2–3). The woman's words are full of references to the senses; she is enchanted by her lover's scent, and she wishes to taste his kisses and feel his lips on hers. Throughout the Song, the lovers refer to the senses because they play a crucial role in the way they enjoy their beloved or dream of such joy.[3]

Of all the senses, hearing is the least important for the lovers—probably because hearing (like seeing) is a sense that works over distance and hence is more public and less intimate than smelling, touching, and tasting, which require proximity.[4] A closer look at the two lovers' references to hearing reveals a telling gender-difference: for the woman, hearing her beloved is an indication of his presence. Twice the woman points out that she hears her beloved, a sign that he is approaching (2:8; 5:2). In the first case, the beloved appears and starts talking to the woman (2:10), though probably only in her recollection or imagination.[5] In the second case, however, the woman opens the door and the man is absent. She looks for him, but he is not there; her call remains unanswered (5:6). This last passage especially shows that for the woman hearing her beloved is crucial, because it indicates that he is with her.[6] This is different for the man: unlike the woman, the man is never concerned that he does not know the whereabouts about his beloved. Thus, hearing her is not existential for him but only "sweet" (thus explicitly in 2:14, with the adjective עָרֵב[7]). Twice the man asks the woman to let him hear her voice (2:14; 8:3). For gender-sensitive interpreters today, the contexts of the two verses could give the impression that the man's wish is utter-

---

[3] See Patrick Hunt, *Poetry in the Song of Songs: A Literary Analysis*, StBibLit 96 (New York: Lang, 2008), 83–101; Schellenberg, "Sensuality of the Song of Songs," 113–18.

[4] See 8:13, where the man mentions his companions who can listen to his beloved's voice as well.

[5] The introduction of the man's speech in 2:10 is a clear indication that the woman is only quoting him (indirect speech). Nonetheless, it remains that with her statement about her lover talking to her (and the report of his words) she indicates that she is hearing him, even if only in her recollection or imagination.

[6] See similarly 1:7 where the woman asks her lover about his whereabouts (hoping for an answer that would reveal that he is close).

[7] The adjective derives from the verb ערב, in the meaning of "to be sweet, pleasant." Primarily ערב is connected with the sense of taste (Jer 6:20; Hos 9:4; Prov 20:17) but frequently the root is used in a metaphorical or more abstract way (Ezek 16:37; Ps 104:34; Prov 3:24).

ly patriarchal.[8] However, there is nothing wrong with the request per se—if one is in love it is indeed wonderful to hear the voice of the beloved—and some of the modern irritation might result from misunderstanding the symbolism and context of the request.[9]

Though a "distant" sense like hearing, sight appears plenty of times in the Song. In most cases the focus of sight is on beauty, first and foremost the beauty of the woman (1:5, 8, 10, 15; 2:10, 14; 4:1–7; 6:4; 7:2–7; etc.), but sometimes also the beauty of the man (1:16; 5:10–15) and the beauty of nature (2:12–13; 6:11; 7:13). Frequently beauty is described with general words like "beautiful" (יפה) or "comely" (נאוה); in other cases details like the loveliness of the woman's cheeks (1:10), the black color of the man's hair (5:11), or the blossoming of nature (2:12–13; 6:11; 7:13) are highlighted. Often it is clear that the focus is not solely on visual qualities but also on additional dimensions or the overall impression. For example, in 1:15–16, the two lovers praise each other as "beautiful" (יפה), but most probably they both mean "beautiful" not only in the aesthetic sense but also in an all-compassing sense. Hence, the man compares his beloved's eyes with doves—the symbol of the love goddess[10]—not because they look like doves but because they affect his emotions. In some cases the text makes clear that the lovers' descriptions of beauty go beyond the visual dimension (6:4–5); in other cases it becomes clear through the context, for example, through the description of nonvisual entities as "beautiful" (e.g., "love" in 4:10), the reference or allusion to other senses (like touch and taste in 7:2–3), or the absurdity of statements if interpreted visually. The latter are frequent in the so-called description songs (*waṣfs*), which produce bizarre images of the protagonists if interpreted superficially. 5:10–16 is a good example; when the woman describes her beloved's checks as "bed of spices" (5:13), his lips as "lilies" (5:13), and his legs as "alabaster columns" (5:15), it is clear that the woman not only describes how the body of her beloved looks but also how (she imagines) it smells, tastes (?), and feels. In other descriptions, it is more difficult to get the point of the statements, for example, when the woman's teeth are likened to a "flock of shown ewes that have come up from the washing" (4:2) and her belly

---

[8] In 2:14, the man compares his beloved to a dove (יונה) and implies a similarity between her voice and the voice of the turtle-dove (תור) mentioned in 2:12. In 8:13, he connects his wish to hear her voice with the reference to his companions who listen as well.

[9] The dove is a symbol of the love-goddess (see below with note 10), and the references to the companions might have dramaturgical reasons, namely, to usher in the end of the Song. See Annette Schellenberg, "Boundary Crossings in and through the Song: Observations on the Liminal Character and Function of the Song," in *Reading a Tendentious Bible: Essays in Honor of Robert B. Coote*, ed. Marvin L. Chaney et al., HBM 66 (Sheffield: Sheffield Phoenix, 2014), 151.

[10] See Othmar Keel, *Das Hohelied*, ZBK 18 (Zurich: TVZ, 1986), 71–75, 100–101.

to a "heap of wheat, encircled with lotuses" (7:3). Yet, despite all of the difficulties with the details, it is quite clear that such statements go beyond the visual and reveal at least as much about the emotions and desires of the *describing* protagonist as about the looks of the described.[11] Nonetheless, one cannot deny that the description songs have a strong visual component, namely, in that they sketch mental images of the lovers, describing their bodies upwards or downwards. We will come back to this point later.

Smell is obviously a very important sense in the Song. The text contains many references to fragrant oils, herbs, spices, and the like,[12] and often their fragrancy is pointed out explicitly (see the noun ריח; 1:3, 12; 2:13; 4:10–11; 7:9, 14). For the protagonists, the most important scent is the scent of each other. Repeatedly, they praise each other's fragrance and compare it with well known, and often expensive, scents like oil, myrrh, and balsam (1:3; 3:6; 4:10–11, 13–16; 5:13; 7:9, and below). Like the descriptions of (the beauty of) the body parts, these statements are not objective descriptions of the odors of the described but first and foremost expressions of the emotions and desires of those who describe. And they reveal that the lovers were intimate enough to enjoy each other's scent.[13] In addition, the protagonists of the Song also enjoy the fragrance of nature. Frequently they mention the blooming of nature (2:13, 15; 6:11; 7:13) and plants known for their fragrancy (like the cedar and pine in 1:17, the lotus in 2:16; 6:2–3; balsam in 6:2; and henna in 7:12), and sometimes they specifically point out the scent of these plants or fruits (2:13; 7:14). In most cases, it is clear that places with fragrant plants are of high significance for the lovers, in that they provide space for an intimate rendezvous (1:17; 2:16; 6:2–3; 7:12–13) and/or serve as a symbol that like nature the lovers are "ready" (2:13; 6:11;

---

[11] This has been observed early on by Richard N. Soulen, "The *Waṣfs* of the Song of Songs and Hermeneutic," *JBL* 86 (1967): 187, who has pointed out that the description songs' purpose "is not to provide a parallel to visual appearance" but rather to express "the feelings and sense experiences of the poet himself who then uses a vivid and familiar imagery to present to his hearers knowledge of those feelings in the form of art." Instead of *poet*, I would rather speak of the *protagonist(s)*, whom the authors of the Song characterize as having such feelings and sense experiences.

[12] See "balsam" (בשם; 4:10, 14, 16; 5:1, 13; 6:2; 8:14), "myrrh" (מר; 1:13; 3:6; 4:6, 14; 5:1, 5, 13), "nard" (נרד; 1:12; 4:13–14), "henna" (כפר; 1:14; 4:13; 7:12), "frankincense" (לבונה; 3:6; 4:6, 14), "oil" (שמן; 1:3; 4:10), "scent-powder" (אבקה; 3:6), "safran" (כרכם; 4:14), "cane" (קנה; 4:14), "cinnamon" (קנמון; 4:14), "aloe" (אהלות; 4:14), "spice" (רקח; 8:2), and "aromatic herb" (מרקח; 5:13). For details, see Athalya Brenner, "Aromatics and Perfumes in the Song of Songs," *JSOT* 25 (1983): 75–81; Jill M. Munro, *Spikenard and Saffron: A Study in the Poetic Language of the Song of Songs*, JSOTSup 203 (Sheffield: Sheffield Academic, 1995), 48–52.

[13] 1:2–3 and 4:10 spell out the connection with "love(making)." The closeness of the lovers is also evident in 1:13–14 and 7:10.

7:11–13). Sometimes, the lovers play with this symbolism in that they describe themselves or each other as (places with) fragrant plants/fruits (1:13–14; 2:1–3; 4:12–5:1; 7:9, 14)—often with highly suggestive implications. The identification of plant/perfume and lover (or specific body parts) might be implied in a few other cases as well, but there the statements are less clearly symbolic and could also be interpreted literally (1:12; 4:6; 5:5; 8:14).

Though generally important for lovers, the Song's protagonists seldom focus on touch. Of course, many of the actions described in the text include touch (e.g., "to draw" in 1:4; "to pluck" and "to eat" in 5:1), but in most cases the aspect of touching or being touched does not seem to be relevant. This is different only in a few instances, namely, in verses that allude to intimate touches between the lovers. Most clear in this regard are 2:6 and 8:3, where the woman describes how the man embraces her and thereby points out his right and left arm/hand. Twice touching the beloved is alluded to in description songs, namely, in 7:2 where the man describes her thighs as the "work of a master hand" and thereby triggers erotic images of hands on the woman's thighs, and in 5:14–15 where the woman describes the man as a statue from precious materials like gold, ivory, and alabaster and thereby alludes to the fact that she knows or imagines that his body feels smooth and hard. And in 7:9 the man talks about wanting to "take hold" of the fruit stalks of the palm, namely, the breasts of the woman (7:8). Several other verses describe or allude to erotic situations that include touch, but they highlight either no sense or other senses like smell or taste. For example, in 1:2; 4:11, and 5:16 mentions of or allusions to kissing are accompanied with statements about taste (see also 8:1), and in 1:13 the woman describes how her beloved lies between her breasts but highlights smell and not touch.

The most important sense in the Song is taste, at least if one does not exclude the statements that are metaphorical. As with smell, many of the Song's statements that allude to the sense of taste (or eating and drinking, respectively) blur the lines between literal, symbolic, and metaphorical meanings. The lovers talk about fruits in nature (2:13) and about eating the fruits and drinking the wine produced from them (2:5; 8:2); they describe the taste of kissing with references to fruits, wine, milk, honey, and sweetness (4:11; 5:16; 7:10); they compare love(making) with wine (1:2, 4; 4:10); they compare each other with fruit(tree)s (2:3; 4:3; 4:13; 6:7; 7:8–9); and they employ the metaphor of eating (fruits, etc.) and drinking (wine, etc.) to allude to sex (2:3; 4:16; 5:1; 7:14; see also 2:7, 16; 7:3, 9).[14] Often, the focus is not on taste alone but also on sight,

---

[14] On the sexual metaphor of (fruits and) eating and drinking in the Old Testament and the ancient Near East more generally, see Shalom M. Paul, "Shared Legacy of Sexual Metaphors and Euphemisms in Mesopotamian and Biblical Literature," in *Sex and Gender in the Ancient Near East*, ed. Simo Parpola and Robert M. Whiting, RAI 47.2

smell, and touch (4:10–5:1; 6:11; 7:9–10; 7:13–14). This clustering of senses is one of the reasons why the analogy between eating/drinking (fruits, wine, etc.) and sex works so well: in both cases, different senses are stimulated but the ultimate desire is on consummation. Another reason the analogy works is the involvement of the mouth in both eating/drinking and sex (see most clearly 4:11 and 8:1); and a last reason is the effect of both acts, namely, satisfaction and intoxication (see most clearly 5:1).

DIFFERENCES IN THE CULTURAL PRECONCEPTIONS OF THE SENSES

So far, we did not consider cultural differences. At first glance it is not necessary; most statements of the Song that concern the senses are immediately comprehensible. With that, the Song confirms what we would have expected anyway: that the senses and sensuality were as important for lovers in antiquity as they are for lovers today. Since the senses (and erotic love) are related to the body and the sensations and reactions of the human body did not change fundamentally over the course of time, it is no surprise that much of what is described in the Song sounds most familiar. Nonetheless, there are differences, and studying them is helpful for understanding both the Song and the ancient Israelites' cultural preconceptions about the senses.

Some of these differences become obvious just by comparing the Song's statements with the reality of today. For example, today most of the fragrances mentioned in the Song are not popular scents anymore, at least not in Europe. And in our time "milk and honey" are not ordinarily mentioned in erotic contexts as they are in the Song (see 4:11; 5:1); rather, "milk and honey" are primarily associated with household remedies or the biblical promise of the holy land.

In other cases our general knowledge about the Bible and the ancient Near East helps us to see that some of the Song's references to the senses have implications that go beyond our modern preconceptions. The woman's reference to "(anointing) oil" (שמן) in 1:3 is one example. In a society that used to anoint their kings and fostered the hope for an "anointed one" (משיח), anointing not only serves to describe the man's love(making) and scent as enticing, but also carries the woman's confession that he is her anointed, her "king" (thus explicitly in 1:4, 12; 7:6). Likewise, to better understand the Song's references to myrrh, balsam, frankincense, and other scents, one must remember that in antiquity they were very expensive and had an exotic aura (as clearly mirrored in 1 Kgs 10, the story of the Queen of Sheba, who brought Solomon not only gold but also myrrh).

(Helsinki: Neo-Assyrian Text Corpus Project, 2002), 495–96; Ronald A. Veenker, "Forbidden Fruit: Ancient Near Eastern Sexual Metaphors," *HUCA* 70 (1999): 57–73.

Finally, most interesting in the context of the question about the ancient Israelites' cultural preconceptions of the senses are verses in which sensory vocabulary is used in a way that is uncommon for us. For example, in 1:6 the woman states that the sun had "gazed" (שְׁזָפַתְנִי) on her. Some have explained this anthropomorphism with ancient Near Eastern theology, namely, with the notion that as judge the sun-god watches over everything.[15] The context in 1:6 points in a different direction, namely, a connection between the sun's gazing and the woman's darker skin color. It explains the effect of the sun's heat on humans' skin; it therefore evokes the sense of vision (i.e., the sun looks). Today, many experts consider thermoreception as part of haptic reception,[16] and most lay people would explain the sun's effect on the skin with the sense of touch. Thus, we might ask whether Song 1:6 is an indication that the ancient Israelites understood seeing as some form of touching. This understanding of seeing is well known from the ancient Greeks.[17] However, there were differences in the details. Aristotle and Galen understood sight as a movement from the seen object to the eye; Plato, on the other hand, reckoned movements emitted from both the eye and the object and then met in the middle.[18] If the ancient Israelites indeed had similar ideas, one must conclude from Song 1:6 that for them the movement went from the eye to the object. There are a few other verses in the Hebrew

---

[15] Thus Keel, *Das Hohelied*, 56. In addition to the context (see above), the feminine form of the verb speaks against Keel's thesis, because the sun-god Shamash is a male deity (and with the Hebrew noun שמש the authors would have had the choice to construct it as masculine).

[16] On the discussion, see John Bligh and Karlheinz Voigt, *Thermoreception and Temperature Regulation* (Berlin: Springer, 1990), 9–10.

[17] See Pierre van Hecke, "A New Look at מבט," in *A Pillar of Cloud to Guide: Text-Critical, Redactional, and Linguistic Perspectives on the Old Testament in Honour of Marc Vervenne*, ed. Hans Ausloos and Bénédicte Lemmelijn, BETL 269 (Leuven: Peeters, 2014), 572–73 with n. 22; Robert Jütte, *A History of the Senses: From Antiquity to Cyberspace*, trans. James Lynn (Cambridge: Polity Press, 2005), 31–46; David C. Lindberg, *Theories of Vision from Al-Kindi to Kepler* (Chicago: University of Chicago Press, 1976), 2–8.

[18] Aristotle understood "the process of seeing as a qualitative change caused by a movement that proceeds from the visible object and is transmitted via a transparent medium" (Jütte, *History of the Senses*, 39; see also Lindberg, *Theories of Vision*, 6–9). Galen assumed (in his pneumatic model) "that the pneuma of the eye receives the first optical impression, and that this stimulus is then conveyed to the brain by the nerve fibres situated between the lens and the retina" (Jütte, *History of the Senses*, 44; see also Lindberg, *Theories of Vision*, 10–11). Plato "deals in greatest detail with the sense of sight.... In his view, the act of seeing is based on an interaction between a subject and an object. The movements proceeding from the eye and the object meet at what he calls the middle" (Jütte, *History of the Senses*, 35; see also Lindberg, *Theories of Vision*, 3–6).

Bible that might reflect such an understanding of seeing as well. In Song 4:9 and 6:5, the man talks about the disturbing effect the woman's eyes have on him. Even today many lovers experience the glances of their beloved as most powerful; hence, we can easily understand the man's statement without assuming a special understanding of seeing. Nonetheless, we must also acknowledge that the man's statements imply that the one who looks effects the one looked at.[19] More clearly related with touching is the warning of Num 4:20 that Levites must be careful not to see (ראה) the holy things in the tabernacle, as otherwise they would die—at least if one takes the verse together with the prohibition of Num 4:15 that the Levites must not touch (נגע) the holy, as otherwise they would die. Though it is not spelled out explicitly, the parallel implies that seeing is like touching; and the formulations (highlighting the active role of the Levites) imply that it is the viewing person who "touches" the seen object and not vice versa.[20]

Another verse in the Song that reflects a difference between the ancient Israelites' preconceptions of the senses and ours is 5:4. In this verse, the woman describes her emotional (and/or sexual?) reaction to the man's presence with the verb המה, or more precisely, with the statement, that her מעים ("internal organs," often translated as "heart" or "inmost being") המה on/for him (עליו).[21] From its basic meaning, the root of this verb denotes sound, namely, murmuring, sighing, growling, roaring, and the like (cf. the derivatives המון, המיה). In the Hebrew Bible it is used to describe the sounds of dogs (Ps 59:7, 15), bears (Isa 59:11), doves (Ezek 7:16), musical instruments (Isa 14:11), humans (Ps 55:18; 77:4), armies and other assemblies (Jer 50:42), and waves (Jer 5:22). Often, however, the auditory meaning fades and is complemented (and sometimes replaced) by

---

[19] See also the notion about the evil eye.

[20] See further Hecke, who points out the polysemy of the root נבט, which in addition to "to look" also means "to illuminate," and explains it with the ancient theories of vision and the extramission theory, which in his view was also common in the Levant. "Against the background of this theory, it is perfectly comprehensible that a verb meaning 'to shine, to illumine' also acquired the meaning of 'to watch,' since the intentional act of visual observation was understood as illuminating the object by the light emitted by the eyes" ("New Look," 573).

[21] On המה and derivatives like המון, see Arnulf Baumann, "המה," *ThWAT* 2:444–49; Gillis Gerleman, "Die lärmende Menge: Der Sinn des hebräischen Wortes *hamon*," in *Wort und Geschichte: Festschrift für Karl Elliger zum 70. Geburtstag*, ed. Hartmut Gese and Hans Peter Rüger, AOAT 18 (Neukirchen-Vluyn: Neukirchener Verlag, 1973), 71–75. On the negative assessment of noise in the Hebrew Bible more generally, see further Annette Schellenberg, "Lärm und Stille," in *Handbuch Alttestamentliche Anthropologie*, ed. Jan Dietrich et al. (Tübingen: Mohr Siebeck, forthcoming). Several Hebrew manuscripts have "on, within me" (עלי) instead of "on, for him" (עליו), which is in line with the use in Ps 42:6, 12; 43:5.

meanings that denote turmoil and agitation,[22] be it external or internal. Ordinarily this turmoil and agitation is assessed negatively: with regard to (external) persons, groups, et cetera in the sense of guilt of the acting subject (Ps 46:7; Prov 7:11), with regard to internal organs (which stand for the entire person in his or her inwardness) in the sense of anguish of the acting subject (Jer 4:19; Ps 42:6). We might be tempted to think that these are just nonliteral meanings of המה that have nothing to do with sound anymore. However, several verses show that this would be a misjudgment, that for the ancient Israelites the aspect of sound was still present with the verb המה even if it was used to denote turmoil and agitation: with regard to external turmoil/agitation, passages like Ps 59:7, 15 and Jer 50:42 indicate that there is a connection with (the sound of) roaring and growling; with regard to internal turmoil/agitation, Isa 16:11 and Jer 48:36 make an analogy with musical instruments (of lamenting?), Ezek 7:16 refers to (the sound of) doves, and Ps 77:4 suggests a connection with (the sound of) sighing and moaning.[23] In Song 5:4, the LXX renders המה with θροέω[24] and with that reminds us that the ancient Israelites were not the only ones who assumed a connection between sound and (not only external but also internal) turmoil/agitation. What remains extraordinary in Song 5:4 is the sexually-loaded context, which implies a positive assessment of this internal sound/turmoil.[25]

SENSORY IMAGINATION OF THE (PROTAGONISTS AND) RECIPIENTS

Despite differences in cultural preconceptions about the senses (and other dimensions of life) and many statements that are hard to understand, throughout the ages the Song had a strong appeal on many people. Up to today, many can immediately connect with the Song and feel enchanted by it. For others, howev-

---

[22] Verses like Isa 17:12; Jer 50:42; 51:55 show that an important juncture of the two aspects (noise and turmoil) is the (noise of the) sea (= chaos). Furthermore, the similarity of המה with המם ("to make a noise, move noisily, confuse, discomfit") and נהם ("to growl, groan") probably plays a role as well.

[23] With regard to internal turmoil one might dispute whether the use of המה primarily reflects that the Israelites imagined to hear their own emotional agitation or that their internal organs were groaning. Probably, they did not distinguish the two possibilities. With regard to external turmoil it is clear that the use of המה reflects that agitated waves and crows are loud (and hence can be heard).

[24] In the active, the verb θροέω means "cry aloud"; in the passive (thus in Song 5:4) it means "to be stirred, moved."

[25] Most similarly the verb המה is used in Sir 51:21 (MS B; like in Song 5:4 with המה + מעים in an erotic context), though this verse probably is dependent on the Song; see Annette Schellenberg, "'May Her Breasts Satisfy You at All Times' (Prov 5:19): On the Erotic Passages in Proverbs and Sirach and the Question of How They Relate to the Song of Songs," *VT* 68 (2018): 260.

er, the Song remains a strange text. In my view, this difference primarily is caused by the difference that some recipients only read the text (and try to understand it intellectually), whereas others also picture it mentally (*Kopfkino*) and thus experience the power of imagination.[26]

Philosophers, psychologists, neuroscientists, and others ordinarily distinguish between at least two types of imagination: cognitive (or propositional) imagination and sensory (or perceptual) imagination. Cognitive imagination is imagination that conceptually entertains a possibility (*imagining that p*), whereas sensory imagination is imagination that forms mental images (*imagining X or imagining Y-ing*).[27] Ultimately, the phenomenon of imagination is complex, and many questions remain disputed.[28] What is clear, however, is that the senses are unimportant for cognitive imagination but highly important for sensory imagination—hence the name. Expressions like "visualizing," "seeing in the mind's eye," and "seeing a mental picture" reflect that in sensory imagination ordinarily the sense of sight is most important. However, other senses can be part of the sensory imagination as well[29]—as becomes obvious as soon as we imagine biting into a lemon or kissing the man or woman of our dreams. The bodily (and emotional) reactions to sensory imagination can be nearly as strong as the bodily (and emotional) reactions to real sensory experiences. The difference that is essential is not the grade of reaction but the type of stimulation: whether it is sensory (physically-sensory) or mental (quasi-sensory).

---

[26] See also Melanie Peetz, *Emotionen im Hohelied: Eine literaturwissenschaftliche Analyse hebräischer Liebeslyrik unter Berücksichtigung geistlich-allegorischer Auslegungsversuche*, HBS 81 (Freiburg: Herder, 2015), who focuses on the emotions, but thereby often touches on the senses.

[27] See Tamar Gendler, "Imagination," *The Stanford Encyclopedia of Philosophy* (Winter 2016 ed.), https://plato.stanford.edu/archives/win2016/entries/imagination/; Bence Nanay, "Philosophy of Perception as a Guide to Aesthetics," in *Aesthetics and the Sciences of Mind*, ed. Greg Currie et al. (Oxford: Oxford University Press, 2014), 104.

[28] See Gendler, "Imagination." On sensory imagination, see further Matthew Kieran and Dominic McIver Lopes, eds., *Imagination, Philosophy, and the Arts* (London: Routledge, 2003); Colin McGinn, *Mindsight: Image, Dream, Meaning* (Cambridge: Harvard University Press, 2006); Elisabeth Schellekens and Peter Goldie, eds., *The Aesthetic Mind: Philosophy and Psychology* (Oxford: Oxford University Press, 2011); Nigel J. T. Thomas, "Mental Imagery," *The Stanford Encyclopedia of Philosophy* (Spring 2017 ed.), https://plato.stanford.edu/archives/spr2017/entries/mental-imagery/. On sensory imagination triggered by literature, see further Thor Grünbaum, "Sensory Imagination and Narrative Perspective: Explaining Perceptual Focalization," *Semiotica* 194 (2013): 111–36.

[29] See Simon Lacey and Rebecca Lawson, eds., *Multisensory Imagery* (New York: Springer, 2013); Thomas, "Mental Imagery," 3; Hendrik N. J. Schifferstein, "Comparing Mental Imagery across the Sensory Modalities," *Imagination, Cognition and Personality* 28 (2008–2009): 371–88.

Mental stimulation of quasi-sensory experiences can start in the mind of the imagining person or be triggered from outside. Some of the outside stimuli work as such just by coincidence (e.g., something we see or hear causes us to start daydreaming); others are set on purpose. The latter is the case in commercials (and advertisement in general) and in erotic literature and movies. Those who create these cultural products purposefully include signals that trigger the recipients' imagination and with that cause them to have quasi-sensory (and sensual) experiences. In both cases (advertisement, erotic genres), these signals often directly relate to the senses—think of commercials that highlight the taste, smell, or touch of a product or erotic literature that describes sensory/sensual experiences—but of course other signals can trigger sensory imagination as well.

As the most sensual text of the Bible, the Song is also the biblical text that most easily triggers the sensory imagination of its recipients.[30] The many references to sensory experiences and the vivid descriptions of the protagonists' erotic desires and encounters make it hard not to be affected by this text on a level that goes beyond the cognitive. I suspect that this is on purpose, that those who created the Song were aware of this phenomenon and intentionally made use of it.[31] For the ancient Israelites such a thesis must remain hypothetical. For the ancient Greeks and Romans, however, it is well documented that they reflected on the power of language to trigger the imagination and trained young rhetoricians to use it.[32] Quintillian and others distinguished between "a plain statement of facts ... and a developed account which makes the audience feel present at the events described and emotionally involved in them."[33] To achieve

---

[30] See Athalya Brenner, "An Afterword," in *A Feminist Companion to the Song of Songs*, ed. Athalya Brenner (Sheffield: Sheffield Academic, 1993), 279: "When I read the Song of Songs I do it, first and foremost and mainly, for the delight of translating the text into personal images. My senses are quickly involved, I can smell and see and taste and hear, and yes, almost touch the sometimes elusive referents of the written word. I am deeply affected by it, as I expect to be, in spite of the textual and linguistic difficulties, regardless of the basic problematics of this collection of love lyrics."

[31] See Hunt, *Poetry in the Song of Songs*, 100, who is convinced ("is clear") that "these multiple sensory clusters and intense sensory images are deliberately wrought and compounded together."

[32] See Gabriele Rippl, *Beschreibungs-Kunst: Zur intermedialen Poetik angloamerikanischer Ikontexte (1880–2000)*, Theorie und Geschichte der Literatur und der Schönen Künste 110 (München: Fink Verlag, 2005), 63–72; Ruth Webb, *Ekphrasis, Imagination and Persuasion in Ancient Rhetorical Theory and Practice* (Farnham: Ashgate, 2009); Robyn J. Whitaker, *Ekphrasis, Vision, and Persuasion in the Book of Revelation* (Tübingen: Mohr Siebeck, 2015), 37–60.

[33] Webb, *Ekphrasis*, 89, referring to a passage in Quintillians *Institutio oratoria* (8.3.67–69), which in our context is also noteworthy, as it includes an example with references not only to the visual but also to other senses: "Doubtless, if one says that the

this effect, *enargeia* and *phantasia* are crucial. *Enargeia* ("vividness"; Lat. *evidentia*) is the technique of providing details and vividness, with the effect of bringing the described scenes to life.³⁴ *Phantasia* ("imagination"; Lat. *visiones*) is the power of the mind to visualize mental images.³⁵ It is important for the author, as it enables him to provide descriptions with *enargeia*, and it is important for the recipients, as it enables them to visualize the author's descriptions, so that they do not just hear them with their ears but also visualize them with their "mind's eye," feel present in the described scenes, and are affected by them emotionally.³⁶ Ruth Webb summarizes these connections as follows: "*Enargeia* … is a quality of language that derives from something beyond words: the capacity to visualize a scene. And its effect also goes beyond words in that it sparks a corresponding image, with corresponding emotional associations, in the mind of the listener."³⁷ The respective genre, "the form of speech that brings the subject matter vividly before the eyes," is called *ekphrasis*.³⁸

We do not know whether the authors of the Song knew about the classic discussions on *enargeia* and *phantasia*, but we can observe that their text in-

---

city has been taken one implies everything which such a fate entails, but, like a brief announcement, this penetrates the emotions less. If instead you open up the things which were included within the single phrase, there will appear flames pouring through houses and temples, the crash of roofs falling and the sound made up of the cries of many individuals, some hesitating as they flee, others clinging to their loved ones in a last embrace, the wailing of women and children and old men lamenting that fate has preserved them for such a terrible destiny. Then there will be the plunder of sacred and profane property and people running to and fro carrying booty and prisoners each driven in front of his captor, and a mother trying to keep hold of her child, and fighting among the victors wherever the booty is greatest" (trans. Webb, *Ekphrasis*, 73).

³⁴ See Rippl, *Beschreibungs-Kunst*, 65–72; Webb, *Ekphrasis*, 87–106; Whitaker, *Ekphrasis*, 45–49.

³⁵ See Webb, *Ekphrasis*, 107–30.

³⁶ The English phrase "mind's eye" goes back to the Latin distinction between inner and outer senses of sight (see Webb, *Ekphrasis*, 98). The language of "visualizing" and terms like "mind's eye" indicate that the visual aspect is particularly important, but some of the ancient authors also make clear that all senses can be involved; see Nina Otto, *Enargeia: Untersuchung zur Charakteristik alexandrinischer Dichtung*, Hermes Einzelschriften 102 (Stuttgart: Steiner, 2009), 105, 113, 116, etc.; Courtney Roby, *Technical Ekphrasis in Greek and Roman Science and Literature: The Written Machine between Alexandria and Rome* (Cambridge: Cambridge University Press, 2016), 3 with n. 7; Webb, *Ekphrasis*, 22, 187. On the (emotional) impact of *enargeia* on the recipients, see Otto, *Enargeia*, 108, 128–29; Rippl, *Beschreibungs-Kunst*, 68–69; Webb, *Ekphrasis*, 76, 98–103, 143–45, 161; Whitaker, *Ekphrasis*, 46–47, 58–60.

³⁷ Webb, *Ekphrasis*, 105.

³⁸ Thus the ancient definition of *ekphrasis*; see Webb, *Ekphrasis*, 1, 51, etc. Webb points out that "ekphrasis is defined primarily in terms of its effect on the listener" (51).

cludes passages that can (and have been[39]) classified as *ekphrasis*. A clear case is Song 2:8–9, where the woman describes how her lover approaches over the mountains and glances through her window. Another clear case is 5:10–16, where the woman describes her beloved from head to toes (legs)—as advised by Aphthonius for *ekphrastic* descriptions of statues.[40] There are other description songs (*waṣfs*) in the Song (4:1–7; 6:5–7; 7:2–6), and they all could be classified as (something like) *ekphrasis*.[41] But 5:10–16 is most interesting because its context makes explicit that, indeed, it is meant to trigger the sensory imagination of those who hear it. Unlike the other description songs, this one is not directed to the described lover but to the daughters of Jerusalem who asked the woman what makes her lover so special (5:9). Through her description the woman makes them see her lover before their mental eyes and with that enables them to feel some of her joy of being in love with him.[42] At the same time, of course, the woman's description is also meant to be heard by the text-external audience and have a similar effect on them.[43] Unlike the daughters of Jerusalem, who must be

---

[39] Thus Frederick William Dobbs-Allsopp and Elaine T. James, "The Ekphrastic Figure(s) in Song 5:10–16," *JBL* 138 (2019): 297–323.

[40] "We will begin from first things and then come to the last, so that if we have a bronze man or painted man or whatever is the subject of the ekphrasis we will start from the head and go through the details in order. For thus the speech becomes lively throughout" (Aphthonius, *Progymnasmata* 36–37; trans. Webb, *Ekphrasis*, 202). For the *waṣfs* of the Song, Esther Ramharter has convincingly argued that their form (a two-tiered list, and especially the list of the body parts) might have had a mnemotechnic purpose; see Esther Ramharter, "On Form and Function of the Waṣfs in the Song of Songs" (forthcoming).

[41] I formulate cautiously ("something like") on purpose to reflect the fact that the term *ekphrasis* originated as term to describe a genre (or literary technique) in Greek and Latin literature, whereas the Song (with its description songs) stands in a much older tradition of ancient Near Eastern love lyrics. But see also Akiko Motoyoshi Sumi, *Description in Classical Arabic Poetry: Waṣfs, Ekphrasis, and Interarts Theory*, JALSupp 25 (Leiden: Brill, 2004), passim and especially 92–121, who applies the term *ekphrasis* to Arabic *waṣfs*.

[42] Obviously, "seeing" here is meant in a way that goes beyond the visual: whereas the mention of the body parts indeed are meant to create a (mental) visual image of the beloved, the metaphors with which they are further qualified in most cases are not significant as descriptions of the described lover's looks but, instead, express something of the describing lover's feelings (see next note).

[43] Soulen was (one of?) the first to describe this purpose of the *waṣfs* in detail, and he even pointed out the senses: "What is suggested here then is that that interpretation is most correct which sees the imagery of the *waṣfs* as a means of arousing emotions consonant with those experienced by the suitor as he beholds the fullness of his beloved's attributes (or so the maiden as she speaks of her beloved in 5 10–16). Just as the sensual experiences of love, beauty, and joy are vivid but ineffable, so the description which centers in and seeks to convey these very subjective feelings must for that reason be

careful not to upstage the woman, the text-external audience are free to fully identify with the woman and indulge in the feeling of being attracted to a beautiful man.

How many passages of the Song qualify as *ekphrastic* is hard to determine; the answer depends on the exact definition of *ekphrastic* that one uses and the willingness to classify an Israelite text with a term that originated in a different context. Regardless of exact definitions and classifications, it remains clear that the Song is full of vivid (and often erotic) descriptions, many of which include references to sensory experiences. With that it has the power to trigger the sensory imagination of its recipients so that they can feel the excitement of the protagonists and be affected by it. Whether they have exactly the same preconceptions of the senses as those who wrote the text does not matter at this point. Even if not, the Song's sensuality builds a bridge that allows many recipients to enter its world in their sensory imagination. Though it is likely that with their presence and their preconceptions the external recipients change this world—or phrased differently: that the world of the Song is not exactly the same in the sensory imagination of the authors and the recipients—it remains that through their sensory imagination the external recipients get a taste of it that remains hidden to those who only try to understand the Song intellectually. Of course, this insight does not release scholars from attempting to understand the Song intellectually—it is not a matter of either-or. However, it is a reminder that to understand the Song one must also pay attention to its character as an *ekphrastic* text and react accordingly with *phantasia*.

BIBLIOGRAPHY

Baumann, Arnulf. "המה." *ThWAT* 2:444–49.
Bligh, John, and Karlheinz Voigt. *Thermoreception and Temperature Regulation*. Berlin: Springer, 1990.
Brenner, Athalya. "An Afterword." Pages 279–80 in *A Feminist Companion to the Song of Songs*. Edited by Athalya Brenner. Sheffield: Sheffield Academic, 1993.
———. "Aromatics and Perfumes in the Song of Songs." *JSOT* 25 (1983): 75–81.

---

unanalytical and imprecise. The writer is not concerned that his hearers be able to retell in descriptive language the particular qualities or appearance of the woman described; he is much more interested that they share his joy, awe, and delight.... 'Bowls of wine,' 'hills of myrrh,' 'mountains of frankincense,' 'heaps of wheat'—just as milk, honey, oil and fruit elsewhere in the poems—titillate the senses, not the capacity to reason. Each in its own way triggers the imagination.... 'Meaning' here can refer only to what the images 'effect' or 'set in motion. Most images appeal to sight (4 1, 2, 4 etc.), but some to taste (7 2), some to fragrance (4 6), and, as poetry, all to hearing" ("*Waṣfs* of the Song of Songs," 189–90).

Dobbs-Allsopp, Frederick William, and Elaine T. James, "The Ekphrastic Figure(s) in Song 5:10–16." *JBL* 138 (2019): 297–323.

Gendler, Tamar. "Imagination." *The Stanford Encyclopedia of Philosophy* (Winter 2016 ed.). https://plato.stanford.edu/archives/ win2016/entries/imagination/

Gerleman, Gillis. "Die lärmende Menge: Der Sinn des hebräischen Wortes *hamon*." Pages 71–75 in *Wort und Geschichte: Festschrift für Karl Elliger zum 70. Geburtstag*. Edited by Hartmut Gese and Hans Peter Rüger. AOAT 18. Neukirchen-Vluyn: Neukirchener Verlag, 1973.

Grünbaum, Thor. "Sensory Imagination and Narrative Perspective: Explaining Perceptual Focalization." *Semiotica* 194 (2013): 111–36.

Hecke, Pierre van. "A New Look at מבט." Pages 569–79 in *A Pillar of Cloud to Guide: Text-Critical, Redactional, and Linguistic Perspectives on the Old Testament in Honour of Marc Vervenne*. Edited by Hans Ausloos and Bénédicte Lemmelijn. BETL 269. Leuven: Peeters, 2014.

Hunt, Patrick. *Poetry in the Song of Songs: A Literary Analysis*. StBibLit 96. New York: Lang, 2008.

Jütte, Robert. *A History of the Senses: From Antiquity to Cyberspace*. Translated by James Lynn. Cambridge: Polity Press, 2005.

Keel, Othmar. *Das Hohelied*. ZBK 18. Zurich: TVZ, 1986.

Kieran, Matthew, and Dominic McIver Lopes, eds. *Imagination, Philosophy, and the Arts*. London: Routledge, 2003.

Lacey, Simon, and Rebecca Lawson, eds. *Multisensory Imagery*. New York: Springer, 2013.

Lindberg, David C. *Theories of Vision from Al-Kindi to Kepler*. Chicago: University of Chicago Press, 1976.

McGinn, Colin. *Mindsight: Image, Dream, Meaning*. Cambridge: Harvard University Press, 2006.

Munro, Jill M. *Spikenard and Saffron: A Study in the Poetic Language of the Song of Songs*. JSOTSup 203. Sheffield: Sheffield Academic, 1995.

Nanay, Bence. "Philosophy of Perception as a Guide to Aesthetics." Pages 101–20 in *Aesthetics and the Sciences of Mind*. Edited by Greg Currie et al. Oxford: Oxford University Press, 2014.

Otto, Nina. *Enargeia: Untersuchung zur Charakteristik alexandrinischer Dichtung*. Hermes Einzelschriften 102. Stuttgart: Steiner, 2009.

Paul, Shalom M. "Shared Legacy of Sexual Metaphors and Euphemisms in Mesopotamian and Biblical Literature." Pages 489–98 in *Sex and Gender in the Ancient Near East*. Edited by Simo Parpola and Robert M. Whiting. RAI 47.2. Helsinki: Neo-Assyrian Text Corpus Project, 2002.

Peetz, Melanie. *Emotionen im Hohelied: Eine literaturwissenschaftliche Analyse hebräischer Liebeslyrik unter Berücksichtigung geistlich-allegorischer Auslegungsversuche*. HBS 81. Freiburg: Herder, 2015.

Ramharter, Esther. "On Form and Function of the Waṣfs in the Song of Songs" (forthcoming).

Rippl, Gabriele. *Beschreibungs-Kunst: Zur intermedialen Poetik angloamerikanischer Ikontexte (1880–2000)*. Theorie und Geschichte der Literatur und der Schönen Künste 110. München: Fink Verlag, 2005.

Roby, Courtney. *Technical Ekphrasis in Greek and Roman Science and Literature: The Written Machine between Alexandria and Rome*. Cambridge: Cambridge University Press, 2016.

Schellekens, Elisabeth, and Peter Goldie, eds. *The Aesthetic Mind: Philosophy and Psychology*. Oxford: Oxford University Press, 2011.

Schellenberg, Annette. "Boundary Crossings in and through the Song: Observations on the Liminal Character and Function of the Song." Pages 140–54 in *Reading a Tendentious Bible: Essays in Honor of Robert B. Coote*. Edited by Marvin L. Chaney et al. HBM 66. Sheffield: Sheffield Phoenix, 2014.

———. "Lärm und Stille." In *Handbuch Alttestamentliche Anthropologie*. Edited by Jan Dietrich et al. Tübingen: Mohr Siebeck, forthcoming.

———. "'May Her Breasts Satisfy You at All Times' (Prov 5:19): On the Erotic Passages in Proverbs and Sirach and the Question of How They Relate to the Song of Songs." *VT* 68 (2018): 252–71.

———. "Sensuality of the Song of Songs: Another Criterion to Be Considered When Assessing (So-Called) Literal and Allegorical Interpretations of the Song." Pages 103–29 in *Interpreting the Song: Literal or Allegorical?* Edited by Annette Schellenberg and Ludger Schwienhorst-Schönberger. BTS 26. Leuven: Peeters, 2016.

Schifferstein, Hendrik N. J. "Comparing Mental Imagery across the Sensory Modalities." *Imagination, Cognition and Personality* 28 (2008–2009): 371–88.

Soulen, Richard N. "The Waṣfs of the Song of Songs and Hermeneutic." *JBL* 86 (1967): 183–90.

Sumi, Akiko Motoyoshi. *Description in Classical Arabic Poetry: Waṣfs, Ekphrasis, and Interarts Theory*. JALSupp 25. Leiden: Brill, 2004.

Thomas, Nigel J. T. "Mental Imagery." *The Stanford Encyclopedia of Philosophy* (Spring 2017 ed.). https://plato.stanford.edu/archives/spr2017/entries/mental-imagery/

Veenker, Ronald A. "Forbidden Fruit: Ancient Near Eastern Sexual Metaphors." *HUCA* 70 (1999): 57–73.

Webb, Ruth. *Ekphrasis, Imagination and Persuasion in Ancient Rhetorical Theory and Practice*. Farnham: Ashgate, 2009.

Whitaker, Robyn J. *Ekphrasis, Vision, and Persuasion in the Book of Revelation*. Tübingen: Mohr Siebeck, 2015.

ANCIENT MESOPOTAMIA

"RUDE REMARKS NOT FIT TO SMELL": NEGATIVE VALUE JUDGMENTS RELATING TO SENSORY PERCEPTIONS IN ANCIENT MESOPOTAMIA

Nicla De Zorzi

INTRODUCTION

In an Old Babylonian letter, the sender, a man named Zimri-Eraḫ, states the following: *Nabium-atpalam imqutma ubtazzi'šu u yâšim magriātim ša ana eṣēnim lā naṭâ idbub* ("Nabium-atpalam barged in and proceeded to insult him [i.e., Zimri-Eraḫ's servant], and even to me he made rude remarks that were not fit to smell").[1] In his agitated state, which is obvious from the context, the letter writer makes a creative choice of words by replacing the expected "not fit to hear" with "not fit to smell" (*ana eṣēnim lā naṭâ*). The preference awarded to the sense of smell over hearing, the default choice, is owed to the stronger emotive response triggered by the resulting image.

This quote sets the scene for the topic of this paper: sensory perceptions in ancient Mesopotamian sources that prompt a negative emotional response. The paper is confined mostly to perceptions that elicit disgust.[2] It will be shown that

---

I would like to thank the organizers of the symposium "Sounding Sensory Profiles in Antiquity" for inviting me to present a talk at that event. I am grateful to Yoram Cohen (Tell Aviv University), Donald Lateiner (Ohio Wesleyan University), and Ilan Peled (Universiteit van Amsterdam) for providing me with copies of their contributions, which were relevant to the topic treated in this paper. Finally, I am grateful to Michael Jursa (Universität Wien) for reading and commenting on a final version of the paper.

[1] *AbB* 2.115, obv. 9–14.

[2] This paper has been inspired by the appearance of Donald Lateiner and Dimos Spatharas, eds., *The Ancient Emotion of Disgust* (Oxford: Oxford University Press, 2016). The volume explores the vocabulary and semantics of disgust in Greek and Latin literature and the social use of disgust in these sources as a means of stigmatizing morally or socially condemnable behavior and marginalizing individuals or groups of individuals. As far as I know, no comparable study of disgust based on cuneiform material has ever been attempted. However, interesting insights can be gained by a survey of recent studies

the visceral reaction of disgust, which is both instinctive and socially conditioned, opens up a wide field of emotional responses.

The sources limit the investigation to a certain extent: much of Mesopotamian literature, in particular religious literature, is about praise or about lamenting the absence of what had been praiseworthy; genres that call for negative descriptions and denigration are far less developed. The paper mostly draws on sources belonging to the scholastic or didactic sphere, including wisdom literature, as well as on a certain number of compositions falling within the sphere of what Benjamin Foster calls "effective literature," including incantations, and "expressive literature," that is, "texts that seek to convey a mood or a scene."[3]

---

dedicated to the concept of purity, especially cultic purity, in the ancient Near East, such as Yitzhaq Feder, "The Semantics of Purity in the Ancient Near East: Lexical Meaning as a Projection of Embodied Experience," *JANER* 14 (2014): 87–113; Feder, "Defilement, Disgust, and Disease: The Experiential Basis of Hittite and Akkadian Terms for Impurity," *JAOS* 136 (2016): 99–116; Michaël Guichard and Lionel Marti, "Purity in Ancient Mesopotamia: The Paleo-Babylonian and Neo-Assyrian Periods," in *Purity and the Forming of Religious Traditions in the Ancient Mediterranean and Ancient Judaism*, ed. Christian Frevel and Christophe Nihan (Leiden: Brill, 2013), 47–114. In this context, also the classical study by Karel van der Toorn, *Sin and Sanction in Israel and Mesopotamia: A Comparative Study* (Assen: Van Gorcum, 1985), needs to be mentioned. In recent years, scholarly interest in the study of senses and emotions has gained momentum. Emotion and sensory studies have attracted the attention of scholars who work in a wide spectrum of disciplines, including psychology, neuroscience, philosophy, cultural anthropology, and history. Routledge's series The Senses in Antiquity, edited by Mark Bradley and Shane Butler and volumes such as Jerry Toner, ed., *A Cultural History of the Senses in Antiquity* (London: Bloomsbury, 2016) and Yannis Hamilakis, *Archaeology and the Senses: Human Experience, Memory, and Affect* (Cambridge: Cambridge University Press, 2013) are good examples of the current sensory turn in the study of the textual and archaeological record, especially from classical antiquity. In the field of Assyriology, the scholarly exploration of the sensorium has focused principally on the sensory imagery that is connected with the description of the divine in religious literature; see, most recently, Shawn Z. Aster, *The Unbeatable Light: Melammu and Its Biblical Parallels* (Münster: Ugarit-Verlag, 2012); Anne-Caroline Rendu Loisel, *Les chants du monde: Le paysage sonore de l'ancienne Mésopotamie* (Toulouse: Presse Universitaires du Midi, 2016). One cannot fail to mention also Cassin's ground breaking work on these topics: Elena Cassin, *La Splendeur divine: Introduction à la mentalité mésopotamienne*, Civilisations et Société 8 (Paris: Mouton, 1968). The vocabulary of emotions and emotional displays in Sumerian (and Akkadian) sources is explored by Margaret Jaques, *Le Vocabulaire des sentiments dans les textes sumériens: Recherche sur le lexique sumérien et akkadien* (Münster: Ugarit-Verlag, 2006).

[3] See Benjamin Foster, *Before the Muses: An Anthology of the Akkadian Literature*, 3rd ed. (Bethesda, MD: CDL, 2005), 41–44.

Terminology

Sensory input can be labelled explicitly as unpleasant or disgusting, or it can be described as such indirectly, drawing on culturally conditioned or even universal imagery and concepts that signal the disgusting nature of what is described. We will begin with the explicit terminology. Two Akkadian verbs in particular demand attention: *masāku* ("to be visually unpleasant, to be ugly") and *ba'āšu* ("to be olfactorily unpleasant, to stink"). Both verbs are documented from the beginning of the Middle Bronze Age onwards, even though neither is particularly frequent.[4] The closest match for a verb expressing the idea of "being unpleasant to taste" is *marāru* ("to be bitter").[5] There is, however, no specific Akkadian word to denote the general quality of being unpleasant to hear, or touch. Investigating the values attested to these words, we can hope to gain an insight into the sociology of Mesopotamian aesthetics.

In letters and literature, *masāku* is occasionally used metaphorically, visual unpleasantness standing for moral degradation and reduction of status.[6] A name can be "made to look bad," that is, it can be "reviled" (*mussuku*), as in the following passage taken from an Old Babylonian letter: *aran šumni damqam [in]a ālini um[a]ssaku* ("the guilt for his having re[v]iled our good reputation [i]n our city").[7] A variant of this expression, *šumruṣu* ("to make sickening") is employed in the antiwitchcraft composition Maqlû 4:73 for describing the effects of witchcraft: *eli āmeriya tušamriṣā'inni* ("you have made me sickening in the sight of one who beholds me").[8] The same type of usage can be found for *ba'āšu* ("to be stinking"), which can also give rise to forms meaning "to cause to smell bad" and hence "to besmirch" or "to cast aspersions" (*bu''ušu*),[9] such as in a letter

---

[4] *CAD* 2:4–5 and 10.1:322. Antonyms for both are *banû* (*CAD* 2:90–94), *damāqu* (*CAD* 3:61–64), and *ṭâbu* (*CAD* 19:34–42), "to be pleasant."

[5] *CAD* 10.1:267–68.

[6] For *masāku* and other derivatives of the root *msk*, see Feder, "Defilement, Disgust, and Disease," 114–16.

[7] *AbB* 14.29, lines 38–39.

[8] Tzvi Abusch, *The Magical Ceremony Maqlû: A Critical Edition* (Leiden: Brill, 2016), 122, 323.

[9] Note that *ba'āšu/bu''ušu* ("stink, make stinking") is not only etymologically, but also orthographically and grammatically distinct from *bâšu/buššu* ("to be shameful, put to shame"). See Jean-Marie Durand, "Tabou et transgression: Le sentiment de la honte," in *Tabou et transgression: Actes du colloque organisé par le Collège de France, Paris, les 11–12 avril 2012*, ed. Jean-Marie Durand, Michaël Guichard, and Thomas Römer, OBO 274 (Fribourg: Presses Universitaires; Göttingen: Vandenhoeck & Ruprecht, 2015), 16 and n. 57. On the verb *bâšu* and the terminology related to it, see Ulrike Steinert, *Aspekte des Menschseins im Alten Mesopotamien: Eine Studie zu Person und Identität im*

sent by King Ashurbanipal to the citizens of Babylon: "do not besmirch your reputation, which is good in my eyes and in the eyes of all lands" (*šunkunu ša ina pāniya u ina pān mātāti gabbu banû lā tuba''ašā*).[10] A Neo-Assyrian curse threatens oath breakers with foul breath: *kī ša pispisu bīšuni kī ḫannî ina pān ili šarri amēlūte nipiškunu lib'iš* ("just as [this] bug stinks, just so may your breath stink before god and king [and] mankind").[11] Significantly, this olfactory analogy for expressing a loss of face is much more frequent than the visual one expressed by *masāku*.[12] The unfiltered emotional impact of stinking was more immediate than the more abstract charge of ugliness, and this prompted a particularly close association of olfactory and moral codes.

The physiognomic omen series Alamdimmû offers an approach to unpleasant sensory data that is more carefully crafted than the images based on visceral, spontaneous reactions cited so far. These omens are concerned with a person's external features and behavioral characteristics and provide prognoses about his or her health, life expectancy, character, and social standing.[13] Some of them refer to ugly physical features:

šumma (šārat lēti) masik : [x] x ūmūšu ikarrû : sadāru išakkan[šu]
[šumma šārat qaqqadiš]u kuššât išar[ru] [šumma šārat qaqqadišu] kuššâtma pānū masik išarruma ila[ppin]
šumma pānī bani ūmūšu ikarrû še'a u kaspa irašši : šumma masik mašrâ irašši : mašrâ ušam'ad

---

2. *und 1. Jt. v. Chr.* (Leiden: Brill, 2012), 405–509; and Durand, "Tabou et transgression," 16–17.

[10] *ABL* 3.301, obv. 20–22. For a discussion of this letter with reference to previous bibliography, see Simo Parpola, "Desperately Trying to Talk Sense: A Letter of Assurbanipal Concerning His Brother Šamaš-šumu-ukin," in *From the Upper Sea to the Lower Sea: Studies on the History of Assyria and Babylonia in Honour of A. K. Grayson*, ed. Grant Frame (Istanbul: Nederlands Historisch-Archaelogisch Instituut te Istanbul, 2004), 227–34 (227–29).

[11] SAA 2:55, 6.603–605. Note the paronomasia involving the bug's name, *pispisu* (*p-s*), the verbal forms *bīšuni* and *lib'iš* (*b-š*), and the substantive *nipišu* (*p-š*).

[12] A partial exception is represented by an Old Babylonian letter from Mari. See Nele Ziegler, *Les musiciens et la musique d'après les archives de Mari* (Paris: SEPOA, 2007), 136–38 n. 27. The writer, the musician Rišiya, writes to Yasmaḫ-Addu that he has been accused of teaching *awâtu bīšātu* ("reprehensible things") to apprentices (lines 14–16). In the final part of the letters he refers to these accusations as *maskātu* "ugly" (lines 29–30).

[13] On this series, see Barbara Böck, *Die babylonisch-assyrische Morphoskopie*, AfOB 27 (Vienna: Institut für Orientalistik der Universität Wien, 2000).

If (a man's side buns) are ugly ... his life will be short, [he] will have repetitive tasks.[14]

[If a man ha]s dense [hair], he will become ric[h]; [if a man has] dense [hair] and an ugly face, he will become rich, but (then) he will suffer imp[overishment].[15]

If a man has a beautiful face, his life will be short; he will have grain and silver; if man has an ugly face, he will become rich: he will increase (his) riches.[16]

Masāku ("to be ugly") appears in these texts as an antonym to *banû* ("to be beautiful"). The prediction associated with the description of an ugly physical feature would be expected to be negative, and indeed "ugly side buns" predict "short life and repetitive tasks." A man with dense hair will become rich; a man with dense hair and an ugly face, on the other hand, will become rich, but subsequently he will suffer impoverishment. Other omens, however, are less clear: both an ugly and a beautiful face may predict riches, but the beautiful face also predicts a short life. The first-millennium BCE corpus does not display overall consistency in its aesthetic hermeneutics, possibly because of a confluence of different source texts into the canonical physiognomic omen series. This notwithstanding, the fact remains that we have here some reflection on the values attached to aesthetic judgments.

The deliberate ratiocination on abstract categories of sensory data in the physiognomic omen series Alamdimmû is restricted to the sense of sight, the sense that is most associated with conscious objectification of sensory data. The closest approximation to such an examination of the values of smell comes from bilingual lexical lists. In one instance, the Sumerian root hul, which literally means "bad," is given the following Akkadian correspondences: *lemnu* ("evil"), *masku* ("ugly"), *zēru* ("hated" or "hateful"), *ṣabru* ("false"), *gallû* ("gallû-demon"), *bīšu* ("malodorous"), *pašqu* ("difficult"), *sarru* ("false"), *šulputu* ("ruined" or "to ruin"), and *lapātu ša īni* ("to touch someone [malignantly] with the eyes").[17] So here "smelling badly" is mentioned side by side with ugliness and words that refer to moral or social reprehensiveness. Another lexical passage in the same tradition names the following qualifications of the Akkadian word for "mouth" (*pû*): *masku* ("ugly"), *bīšu* ("malodorous"), *marru* ("bitter"). These unpleasant manifestations of three senses, sight, smell, and taste, are mentioned together with *zēru* ("hated" or "hateful") and *lemnu* ("evil"), and this attests again the interrelation between sensual and moral or social unpleasantness.[18]

---

[14] Alamdimmû, tablet 6, line 64; Böck, *Morphoskopie*, 104–5.

[15] Alamdimmû, tablet 2, lines 63–64; Böck, *Morphoskopie*, 76–77.

[16] Alamdimmû, tablet 8, line 92; Böck, *Morphoskopie*, 113–14.

[17] *MSL* 15:126, lines 132–143; Bruno Meissner, *Studien zur assyrischen Lexikographie* (Leipzig: Harrassowitz, 1929), 8, 50–51, ii.124–34.

[18] *KBo* 1:67, 38.r.12′–16′; *MSL* 13:245.

VISCERAL DISGUST: SMELL AND TASTE

The evidence for the inclusion of the sense of smell in ancient philological investigations into unpleasant sensory perceptions cited above notwithstanding, the Mesopotamian sources clearly give priority to the immediacy of the reaction to olfactory input and to the emotional weight that results from it. This fact explains why the sense of smell is a potent source of figurative language in emotional speech. The quote given at the opening of this paper is a good example: *Nabium-atpalam imqutma ubtazzi'šu u yâšim magriātim ša ana eṣēnim lā naṭâ idbub* ("Nabium-atpalam barged in and proceeded to insult him, and even to me he made rude remarks [*magriātim*] that were not fit to smell").[19] Unsurprisingly therefore, the concept of bad smell is frequently employed for the creation of insults. In early second millennium Sumerian school (*Edubba'a*) literature,[20] we encounter a considerable range of insults that refer to the sense of smell. For instance, in the Sumerian Debate between bird and fish, Bird says to Fish (line 60): ir nu dug$_3$-ga a-ha-an ši-du$_3$-du$_3$ ugu-zu giri$_{17}$ ur$_5$-ur$_5$ ("your smell is awful, you make people throw up, they are wrinkling their nose at you").[21] A collection of insults in Diatribe C (also known as He Is a Good Seed of a Dog) includes (line 2) ir ^{d}nin-kilim ("[he is the] stench of a mongoose")[22]; this is a reference to the fact that mongooses like to explore latrines, as we can read in a description of the behavior of demons who are compared to a mongoose: *kīma šikkê asurrâ uṣṣanū šunu* ("they are the ones who sniff the latrine like a mongoose").[23] The Sumerian composition known as The Father and His Disobedient Son (also known as Der Vater und sein missratener Sohn) contains the following "loving" address directed by a father to his offspring:

---

[19] *AbB* 2.115, obv. 9–14.

[20] On the so-called Edubba'a-literature, see, e.g., Konrad Volk, "Edubba'a und Edubba'a Literatur: Rätsel und Lösungen," *ZA* 90 (2000): 1–30; Andrew R. George, "In Search of the É.DUB.BA.A: The Ancient Mesopotamian School in Literature and Reality," in *An Ancient Scribe Who Neglects Nothing: Ancient Near Eastern Studies in Honor of Jacob Klein*, ed. Yitschak Sefati et al. (Bethesda, MD: CDL, 2005), 127–37; Justin Cale Johnson and Markham Geller, *The Class Reunion: An Annotated Translation and Commentary on the Sumerian Dialogue Two Scribes*, CM 47 (Leiden: Brill, 2015), 1–42.

[21] ETCSL c.5.3.5.

[22] ETCSL c.5.4.12; Åke W. Sjøberg, "'He Is a Good Seed of a Dog' and 'Engardu, the Fool,'" *JCS* 24 (1972): 107–8.

[23] Udug-hul, tablet 6, line 175'; Mark Geller, *Healing Magic and Evil Demons: Canonical Udug-hul Incantations* (Berlin: de Gruyter, 2015), 246. See also Andrew R. George, "On Babylonian Lavatories and Sewers," *Iraq* 77 (2015): 94 n. 32.

saĝ-DU-a lu₂-tumu šu-si ĝiri₃-si lu₂-lul lu₂-tumu lu₂ la-ga e₂ buru₃-buru₃ lu₂ sikil du₃-a lu₂ hab₂-ba-am₃ na-ĝa₂-ah lu₂ mu₂-da eme za₃-ga bar-bar sag šu zi bi₂-ib-du₁₁-ga sag ur₃-ur₃ lu₂ hu-hu-nu ir-ha-an du₁₁-ga ir-hul-a i₃-hab₂ lu₂ hab₂-ba ir-ha-an-di pil₂-pil₂-la₂ x-hul-a ga-an-šub niĝ₂-tur hab₂-ba-am₃ ki-sim gu-du hab₂-ba in-ur₅ in-da-ur₅ ur-gi₇ saĝ us₂-sa si-im-si-im al-ak-e lu₂-tumu

Numbskull,[24] windbag,[25] fingernail, toenail, liar, windbag, burglar, foul-mouthed man, stinking man, rude, rabid man, drooling idiot ... crippled, foul smelling necromancer,[26] stinking oil, stinking man ... stinker, stinking milk, stinking arse that stinks and stinks again, a dog that sniffs the ground, windbag.[27]

In the passage translated as "foul-mouthed person, stinking person" (lu₂ sikil du₃-a lu₂ hab₂-ba-am₃), the first expression corresponds to Akkadian *magrû*:[28] this is a person uttering *magriātu* ("rude remarks"), as translated above in the Old Babylonian letter,[29] utterings said to be "not fit to smell." The underlying association of inappropriate enunciations with bad smell is expressed in English by referring to a person as "foul-mouthed," another transfer from the acoustic to the olfactory sphere. The idea is mirrored precisely in Akkadian, where in Late Babylonian letters "words" can be made "stinking," in the sense of "discredited": *mamma dibbīya ina ekalli lā uba''aš* ("let no one make my words stink [= misrepresent my case] in the palace").[30] In another letter, a man named Nabû-ahu-iddin advises the high priest (*šatammu*) of the Eanna temple as follows: *dibbī lū mādu akanna ina muḫḫini bīšū* ("the talk here is really bad [lit.

---

[24] See Johnson and Geller, *Class Reunion*, 280–81.

[25] For the reading tumu of the sign im, see Johnson and Geller, *Class Reunion*, 104–5 with further bibliographical references.

[26] See Johnson and Geller, *Class Reunion*, 281.

[27] The Father and His Disobedient Son, lines 147–158. The transliteration and translation are based on Åke W. Sjöberg, "Der Vater und sein missratener Sohn," *JCS* 25 (1973): 113; complemented by Bendt Alster, "On the Sumerian Composition 'The Father and His Disobedient Son,'" *RA* 69 (1975): 81–84; Willem H. Ph. Römer, "Der Vater und sein nichtsnutziger Sohn" (*TUAT* 3:77–91); Johnson and Geller, *Class Reunion*. The latter work contains updated translations and detailed discussions of several words belonging to the standard Sumerian repertoire of abusive terms.

[28] Sjöberg, "Der Vater und sein missratener Sohn," 114–15. See also Johnson and Geller, *Class Reunion*, 263.

[29] *AbB* 2.115, obv. 9–14.

[30] SAA 17:49, 53.r.4′–5′.

stinking] for us").[31] Again, the immediate emotional response to the concept of stench trumps the semantic precision of the image. Similarly, an Akkadian proverb associates the verbal outflows erupting from the abusive slandering mouth with flatulence: [*qinna*]*tum ṣurrutam pû babbānûta ublam* ("[the an]us emits flatus, the mouth babbles").[32]

The association between personal odor or stench and shame allows Mesopotamian writers to develop scatological themes for the purpose of insult and ridicule. Here, scatology often goes together with sex, as expected. An Akkadian proverb going back to the Middle Bronze age states: *ša ultu ūm pā*[*nî*] *lā ibaššû ardatum ṣiḫirt*[*um*] *ina sū*[*n*] *mūti*[*ša*] *išr*[*ut*] ("what has never happened since olden da[ys]: a you[ng] woman fart[ed] while having se[x] with [her] husband").[33] This is certainly misogynistic and must be understood as saying: "this is happening all the time," as in fact a Sumerian parallel actually states explicitly: níĝ$_2$ u$_4$-bi-ta la-ba-gal$_2$-la ki-sikil tur ur$_2$ dam-ma-na-ka še$_{10}$ nu-ub-dur$_2$-re ("what has never happened since the olden days: a young woman does not fart while having sex with her husband").[34] This image is also evoked with apparently comical intent in the first millennium composition known as Love Lyrics, a type of ritual drama based on a divine ménage à trois in which the god Marduk cheats on his consort Zarpanītu with Ištar of Babylon.[35]

---

[31] Albert T. Clay, *Neo-Babylonian Letters from Erech*, YOS 3 (New Haven: Yale University Press, 1919), no. 19.r.20–21; Michael Jursa, "Ein Beamter flucht auf Aramäisch: Alphabetschreiber in der spätbabylonischen Epistolographie und die Rolle des Aramäischen in der babylonischen Verwaltung des sechsten Jahrhunderts v. Chr.," in *Leggo! Studies Presented to Frederick Mario Fales on the Occasion of His Sixty-Fifth Birthday*, ed. Giovanni B. Lanfranchi et al. (Wiesbaden: Harrassowitz, 2012), 380.

[32] K 5668.ii.1–4; Wilfred G. Lambert, *Babylonian Wisdom Literature* (Oxford: Oxford University Press, 1960), 251. For the same interweaving of hearing and smell in Greek sources, see Ashley Clemens, "'Looking Mustard': Greek Popular Epistemology and the Meaning of δριμύς," in *Synaesthesia and the Ancient Senses*, ed. Shane Butler and Alex Purves (Durham: Acumen, 2013), 85–86, quoting, among others, a passage from the mimes of the Hellenistic poet Herodas: "Don't get bile in your nose, Koritto, as soon as you hear an unwise word" (*Mime* 6.37).

[33] BM 98743.ii.5–10; Lambert, *Babylonian Wisdom Literature*, 260.

[34] Bendt Alster, *Proverbs of Ancient Sumer* (Bethesda, MD: CDL, 1997), 9 n. 1.12. I think this interpretation is more convincing than Alster's: "Something which has never occurred since time immemorial: Didn't the young girl fart in her husband's lap?" (9); and Jerrold S. Cooper's: "Something that has never occurred since time immemorial: A nubile girl was never [before] flatulent in her husband's lap." See Jerrold S. Cooper, "Virginity in Ancient Mesopotamia," in *Sex and Gender in the Ancient Near East*, ed. Simo Parpola and Robert M. Whiting, RAI 47.2 (Helsinki: Neo-Assyrian Text Corpus Project, 2002), 98.

[35] For editions of these texts, see Wilfred G. Lambert, "The Problem of the Love Lyrics," in *Unity and Diversity: Essays in the History, Literature, and Religion of the*

In a fragmentary speech that is to be attributed to one of two jester figures from Ištar's entourage (*assinnu, kurgarrû*),[36] the speaker's beloved is described as follows: *tappātī āmurma ḫamâku danniš peṣâtima kī pišallurt[i] mašku naqlât kīma diq[āri]* ("I saw my girlfriend and was completely overwhelmed, you are white like a geck[o], you have a carbonized skin like a po[t]")[37]—this is a parody of a loving description: a skin burnt like a pot is hardly attractive.[38] Thereafter, the same lady's behavior is described as follows: *ammēni taṣrutīma tabāšī gišsaparra ša bēliša ammēni taškunī nipiš ri-[x]* ("Why did you fart and were ashamed about it? Why did you make the wagon of her lord a x[x] smell?").[39] Inverting the norms of decency, the speaker is not astonished by his beloved's flatulence, but by her being ashamed of it. In fact, it has been stated with justification that the so-called Love Lyrics are neither lovely nor lyrical.[40]

Ancient Near East, ed. Hans Goedicke and Jimmy J. M. Roberts (Baltimore: John Hopkins University Press, 1975), 98–135; Dietz Otto Edzard, "Zur Ritualtafel der sogenannten 'Love Lyrics,'" in *Language, Literature and History: Philological and Historical Studies Presented to Erica Reiner*, ed. Francesca Rochberg-Halten, AOS 67 (New Haven: American Oriental Society, 1987), 57–69. For a discussion of their content, see Gwendolyn Leick, *Sex and Eroticism in Mesopotamian Literature* (London: Routledge, 1994), 239–46. See also Joan Goodnick Westenholz, "Inanna and Ištar in the Babylonian World," in *The Babylonian World*, ed. Gwendolyn Leick (New York: Routledge, 2007), 342–43; Marten Stol, *Women in the Ancient Near East* (Berlin: de Gruyter, 2016), 435.

[36] These figures and their relationship to Ištar have attracted much scholarly attention. Their religious functions and the question of their sexual orientation are especially debated. This complex subject is beyond the scope of this paper; a recent detailed discussion is offered by Ilan Peled, *Masculinities and Third Gender: The Origins and Nature of an Institutionalized Gender Otherness in the Ancient Near East* (Münster: Ugarit-Verlag, 2016).

[37] K 6082.B.14–16; Lambert, "Problem of the Love Lyrics," 120–21.

[38] See Benjamin R. Foster, "Humor and Cuneiform Literature," *JANES* 6 (1974): 79 and n. 23.

[39] K 6082.B.10–11; Lambert, "Problem of the Love Lyrics," 120–21.

[40] See Edzard, "Zur Ritualtafel der sogenannten 'Love Lyrics,'" 58. In another passage (*LKA* 92 and 81-2-4 294.o.11–17), the speaker, referring to sexual intercourse, calls his penis *kalbu* "dog" and "*ḫaḫḫuru*-bird" (lines 11–12) and alludes to the smell of his partner's private parts: *ḫaḫḫurētiya ṭēma ašakkan addānika ḫaḫḫurtiya ina muḫḫi kamūni lā teqerrub* ("I will tell my *ḫaḫḫuru*-birds: 'Please my *ḫaḫḫuru*-bird, don't go near the fungus!'") (see Lambert, "Problem of the Love Lyrics," 122). For the use of animal names as appellations for human sexual organs, see Nathan Wasserman, *Akkadian Love Literature of the Third and Second Millennium BCE* (Wiesbaden: Harrasowitz, 2016), 38–42.

These topoi belong in the wider context of the motif of female shamelessness, which is frequently encountered in Mesopotamian literature.[41]

The above is thrown into sharp relief by two Assyrian compositions from the seventh century BCE, SAA 3.29 and 30, which preserve a rich range of abusive terminology. They seem to have been styled as parodistic imitations of well-known erudite compositions, an epic poem and an incantation respectively.[42] The main target of the scurrilous invectives is a certain Bēl-ēṭer son of Ibâ. Unfortunately, the context in which these two texts were produced as well as the identity of Bēl-ēṭer and of other individuals bearing non-Assyrian names mentioned in them remain largely unknown.[43] SAA 3.29 is cast as a fictitious stela: *ṭupšinna petēma narâ šit*[*assi*] ("open the tablet box and re[ad] well the stela") (obv. 1).[44] In the first part (obv. 1–6), Bēl-ēṭer is derogatively compared to a dog (*kīma kalbi*),[45] and he is apparently accused of setting himself up as a king. The rest of the main narrative is broken. On the reverse of the tablet the stele-motif is taken up again by parodistically combining traditional elements with clearly ridiculous details—*mā annītu ušmittu ša ḫarimtu tazqupu ana mār Ibâ šarrite* (*blank space*) *tēziba ana aḫrātaš* ("thus this is the stele which the prostitute set up for the son of Ibâ, the farter, [blank space][46] and left for posterity") (lines 4–5)—and Bēl-ēṭer's inflated self-esteem is severely mocked. The beginning of SAA 3.30 offers another whole chain of insults directed at him:[47]

---

[41] See Stol, *Women in the Ancient Near East*, 685–90.

[42] See Foster, *Before the Muses*, 1020.

[43] For a hypothetical historical contextualization, see Simo Parpola, "Assyrian Library Records," *JNES* 42 (1983): 11 and n. 39; Grant Frame, *Babylonia 689–627 BC: A Political History* (Istanbul: Nederlands Historisch-Archaelogisch Instituut te Istanbul, 1992), 118, 156 and n. 107, 174–75.

[44] SAA 3:64, 29.o.1. The same sentence represents the incipit of the Cuthean Legend of Naram-Sin, for which see Christopher B. F. Walker, "The Second Tablet of Tupšenna Pitema, an Old Babylonian Naram-Sin Legend?," *JCS* 33 (1981): 191–95; Joan Goodnick Westenholz, *Legends of the Kings of Akkade: The Texts* (Winona Lake, IN: Eisenbrauns, 1997), 300–301 (Standard Babylonian recension).

[45] On the use of the animal's name to construct derogatory metaphors in ancient Near Eastern texts, see Nicla De Zorzi, "Teratomancy at Tigunāmun: Structure, Hermeneutics and Weltanschauung of a Northern Mesopotamian Omen Corpus," *JCS* 69 (2017): 136–38. The dog is often mentioned in Neo-Assyrian texts as a degrading term of comparison for conquered enemies, see Pierre Villard, "Le chien dans la documentation néo-assyrienne," in *Les animaux et les hommes dans le monde syro-mésopotamien aux époques historiques*, ed. Dominique Parayre et al., Topoi Supp. 2 (Paris: de Boccard, 2000), 246–47.

[46] Foster, *Before the Muses*, 1021 observes: "The blank space was presumably meant to indicate that she had left nothing for the future."

[47] The translation follows principally Foster, *Before the Muses*, 1021.

Bēl-ēṭer ḫibtu nīku aki šinama maḫḫu aki šinama bilṣu aki šinama mār Ibâ adannu lā mēnānu išpīk zê ṣarritim qinnu šapiltu urdu ša ili [m]īte bītu ša kakkabša ina šamê ḫalqu ardatu amīltu urdu ša balīḫīti ziqnu nikâtim

Bēl-ēṭer, you fucked hostage,[48] doubly so, with runny eyes,[49] doubly so, with bulging eyes,[50] doubly so, son of Ibâ, that missed period, that shit bucket of a fart factory,[51] of a vile family, lackey of a [d]ead god, of a house whose star has vanished from the heavens, (and of) a slave girl, a chattel, he, the slave of a Syrian country girl, the (only) bearded one among a pessle of over-fornicated women.[52]

The author pulls out all the stops for his vituperative denigration of Bēl-ēṭer. It is interesting to compare this passage to the quote given above from the Sumerian composition The Father and His Disobedient Son,[53] whose author likewise strives for injurious comprehensiveness. In both texts, the odor theme occurs, but it is clearly more prominent in the earlier, Sumerian text. The Neo-Assyrian composition refers also to ugliness, but its main interest are themes that are not exploited in the Sumerian text: face-threatening issues of status and effeminization.[54] Especially the latter is a theme that is crucial to the Assyrian elite's

---

[48] See also SAA 3:64, 29.o.4: *tappê Nummuraya nīku* ("that fucked comrade of Nummuraya").

[49] Both A. Livingstone (SAA 3:66) and Foster (*Before the Muses*, 1021) derive *maḫḫu* from *maḫāḫu* ("to soak, to soften in a liquid") (*CAD* 10.1:49a; *AHw* 2:577). The term often refers to a disease of the eyes, for which see in detail Jeanette C. Fincke, *Augenleiden nach keilschriftlichen Quellen: Untersuchungen zur altorientalischen Medizin*, Würzburger medizinhistorische Forschungen 70 (Würzburg: Königshausen & Neumann, 2000), 124–25.

[50] The verb *balāṣu* means "to protrude" and is often said of the eyes: see Fincke, *Augenleiden*, 83–85. See also Böck, *Morphoskopie*, 179 n. 620: "mit hervorgetretenen Augen/starren Blickes." Livingstone's (SAA 3:66) and Foster's (*Before the Muses*, 1021) translations of *bilṣu* ("squint-eyed man" and "with shifty eyes"), respectively, emphasize the connection between Bēl-ēṭer's physical ugliness and moral degradation.

[51] See also SAA 3:64, 29.o.4: *išpīk zê Zēru-kīnu* ("the shit bucket of Zēru-kīnu").

[52] SAA 3:66, 30.o.1–4.

[53] Sjøberg, "Der Vater und sein missratener Sohn."

[54] In the main section of SAA 3:65, 29.o.10, 13–14, one finds three broken references to a mare, Akkadian *urītu*. In the first reference someone, probably Bēl-ēṭer, is passing through the street riding a mare. Possibly Bēl-ēṭer's denigration and feminization are emphasized by his choice of a female horse. The motif is used with derogatory intent in an account of Sargon II's campaign against Urartu (714 BCE). The Urartian king Rusa, when attempting to save his life from the approaching Assyrian armies, abandoned his chariot, mounted a mare and fled before his own army. See Walter Mayer, "Sargons

weltanschauung that habitually belittles adversaries and inferiors by attributing them feminine characteristics, in particular a sexually passive role. In Assyrian culture, the impact of such gender-related accusations was clearly stronger and hence more productive for the language of insult and disgust than seemingly comparatively innocent references to bodily odor and bodily waste.[55]

Odor plays an important role in the cultural construction of moral and social disgust, which is used as a mechanism to stigmatize and marginalize people or groups of people representing the Other. Evil-smelling bodily waste and bodily fluids are evinced as tainting the body of an object of disgust and ridicule. Neo-Assyrian royal inscriptions are a fertile ground for research on such constructions of alterity through disgust.[56] Several inscriptions from the reign of

---

Feldzug gegen Urartu 714 v. Chr.: Text und Übersetzung," *MDOG* 115 (1983): 83 line 140. On this episode, see Cynthia R. Chapman, *The Gendered Language of Warfare in the Israelite-Assyrian Encounter* (Winona Lake, IN: Eisenbrauns, 2004), 36–37; Matthias Karlsson, *Relations of Power in Early Neo-Assyrian State Ideology* (Berlin: de Gruyter, 2016), 238; De Zorzi, "Teratomancy at Tigunāmun," 145. Also the Urartian king Sarduri, instead of facing Tiglath-pileser III (745–726 BCE) in battle, rode off alone on a mare during the night. Hayim Tadmor, *The Inscriptions of Tiglath-pileser III, King of Assyria: Critical Edition, with Introductions, Translations and Commentary* (Jerusalem: Israel Academy of Sciences and Humanities, 1994), 64, line 16; 101, lines 33′–37′. See Stefan Zawadzki, "Depicting Hostile Rulers in the Neo-Assyrian Royal Inscriptions," in *From Source to History: Studies on the Ancient Near Eastern Worlds and Beyond Dedicated to Giovanni Battista Lanfranchi on the Occasion of His Sixty-Fifth Birthday on June 23, 2014*, ed. Salvatore Gaspa et al. (Münster: Ugarit-Verlag, 2014), 769–70. The comparison of Bēl-ēṭer with a dog in the initial section of SAA 3:29 may also hint at degrading feminization: the representation of women as dogs is a common misogynistic topos in Neo-Assyrian sources; see Nicla De Zorzi, "Of Raving Dogs and Promiscuous Pigs: Mesopotamian Animal Omens in Context," in *Magikon zoon: Animal et magie / The Animal Magic*, ed. Korshi Dosoo and Jean-Charles Coulon (Turnhout: Brepols, forthcoming).

[55] The topic of gender in Assyrian texts has been recently studied by Karlsson, *Relations of Power*, 228–42. On gender and gender roles in Assyrian royal inscriptions and reliefs, see also Chapman, *Gendered Language of Warfare*; Marc van de Mieroop, "The Madness of King Rusa: The Psychology of Despair in Eighth Century Assyria," *Journal of Ancient History* 4 (2016): 16–39; De Zorzi, "Teratomancy at Tigunāmun," 144–46.

[56] On the construction of the other and the enemy in Mesopotamia, see, e.g., Beate Pongratz-Leisten, "The Other and the Enemy in the Mesopotamian Conception of the World," in *Mythology and Mythologies: Methodological Approaches to Intercultural Influences, Proceedings of the Second Annual Symposium of the Assyrian and Babylonian Intellectual Heritage Project Held in Paris, France, October 4–7, 1999*, ed. Robert M. Whiting, Melammu Symposia 2 (Helsinki: Neo-Assyrian Text Corpus Project, 2001), 195–231; Maria Grazia Masetti-Rouault, "Conceptions de l'autre en Mésopotamie ancienne: Barbarie et différence, entre refus et integration," *Cahiers Kubaba* 7 (2005): 121–41. Karlsson, *Relations of Power*, has a focus on Neo-Assyrian sources.

Sennacherib (704–681 BCE), which detail the events connected with the battle of Halule (691 BCE), report that the Elamite king Ḫumban-menanu and the Babylonian king Mušēzib-Marduk, while fleeing from the Assyrian army, lose control over their bowels and defecate into their chariots:

> *Umman-menanu šar Elamti adi šar Bābili nasikkāni ša māt Kaldi ālikūt idīšu ḫurbāšu tāḫāziya kīmalê zumuršunu isḫup zarātēšun umaššerūma ana šūzub napšātīšunu pagrī ummānātīšunu uda''išū ētiqū kī ša atmi summati kuššudi itarrakū libbūšun šīnātešun uṣarrapū qereb narkabātīšunu umaššerūni zûšun*

(As for) him, Umman-menanu (Ḫumban-menanu), the king of the land Elam, along with the king of Babylon (and) the sheikhs of Chaldea who marched at his side, terror of doing battle with me overwhelmed them like *alû*-demons. They abandoned their tents and, in order to save their lives, they trampled the corpses of their troops as they pushed on. Their hearts throbbed like those of the pursued young of pigeons, they passed their urine hotly (and) shat themselves inside their chariots.[57]

Ḫumban-menanu and Mušēzib-Marduk are described as cowardly escaping the battlefield, the ultimate indignity for proud kings and mighty military commanders. The comparison with the hunted pigeon-chick qualifies them as immature, weak, and helpless in sharp contrast to the attitude befitting successful adult and manly warriors.[58] Precisely as children who cannot control their bodily functions, they are caught in the act of releasing themselves inside their chariots. Adding insult to injury, shameful loss of control over body functions is

---

[57] Sennacherib 22.vi.24–31 (RINAP 3.1:184). See also Sennacherib 34, lines 53b–55a (RINAP 3.1:224); Sennacherib 223, lines 34b–40a (RINAP 3.2:315–16); Sennacherib 230, lines 95b–98a (RINAP 3.2:334).

[58] Quite often in Assyrian texts, enemies act like timid wild animals crawling into holes in the ground or like birds seeking refuge in the mountains or in caves. On animal imagery and the animalization of the enemy in Assyrian royal inscriptions, see, e.g., Mario Fales, "The Enemy in Assyrian Royal Inscriptions: 'The Moral Judgement,'" in *Mesopotamien und seine Nachbarn: Politische und kulturelle Wechselbeziehungen im Alten Vorderasien vom 4. bis 1. Jahrtausend v. Chr.*, ed. Hans J. Nissen and Johannes Renger (Berlin: Reimer, 1982), 425–35; Lucio Milano, "Il nemico bestiale: Su alcune connotazioni animalesche del nemico nella letteratura sumero-accadica," in *Animali tra zoologia, mito e letteratura nella cultura classica e orientale*, ed. Ettore Cingano et al. (Padua: S.A.R.G.O.N, 2005), 57–63; Zawadzki, "Depicting Hostile Rulers," 768–71; Karlsson, *Relations of Power*, 139, 237–38; De Zorzi, "Teratomancy at Tigunāmun," 144–45. On the degrading immaturity motif in these texts, see De Zorzi, "Teratomancy at Tigunāmun," 143–45.

added to military defeat.[59] In an analogous disgust-arousing episode involving the sense of taste as well as that of smell, the enemies of Esarhaddon (680–669 BCE), seized by overpowering fear, vomit bile: *libbašunu itarrakma ima''û marta* ("their hearts were pounding and they were vomiting bile").[60] In an inscription of Ashurbanipal (ca. 669–630 BCE), defeated and fleeing Arabs slit the stomachs of their camels and then proceeded to drink the content: *ana ṣummēšunu ištattû damī u mê paršu* ("against their thirst they drank the blood and liquid from the gore").[61] This is an image of disgusting alterity that is seen as manifesting itself in the revolting sustenance the defeated Arabs take from their beasts. It serves presumably to dehumanize the enemy by referring to their having incorporated the animals' filth.

The interpretation of the Ashurbanipal passage cited above as referring to dehumanization, to a blurring between the lines of (inferior) man and beast, can be corroborated by other sources drawing on animal imagery. Especially domestic animals are regularly used as a *speculum humanitatis* and convey value judgments that may be predicated on visceral, spontaneous feelings of disgust. Imagery can map onto the animal world the social distinction between elites and lowly workers.[62] This is possible because domestic animals are close to us— "us" being male members of the elite—but still clearly different and inferior. Consider these two omens taken from the divinatory series Šumma ālu, tablet 49 omen 4 and tablet 46 omen 10, respectively:

---

[59] On this episode and the incontinence motif, see Eckart Frahm, *Einleitung in die Sanherib-Inschriften*, AfOB 26 (Vienna: Horn, 1997), 263; Frahm, "Humor in assyrischen Königsinschriften," in *Intellectual Life of the Ancient Near East: Papers Presented at the 43rd Rencontre Assyriologique Internationale, Prague, July 1–5, 1996*, ed. Jiří Prosecký (Prague: Oriental Institute, 1998), 159; Frahm, "Family Matters: Psychohistorical Reflections on Sennacherib and His Times," in *Sennacherib at the Gates of Jerusalem*, ed. Isaac Kalimi and Seth Richardson (Leiden: Brill, 2014), 210–13.

[60] Esarhaddon 1.iv.85–v.1 (RINAP 4:21). A similar gloomy expression of distress is attributed to Anatolian merchants in the Amarna recension of the epic tale known as Sargon, King of Battle, lines 16–17: see Westenholz, *Legends of the Kings of Akkade*, 114–15; and Michael Haul, *Stele und Legende: Untersuchungen zu den keilschriftlichen Erzählwerken über die Könige von Akkade* (Göttingen: Universitätsverlag, 2009), 418–19, 431.

[61] Prism A.ix.37; Rykle Borger, *Beiträge zum Inschriftenwerk Assurbanipals* (Wiesbaden: Harrassowitz, 1996), 66, 248. The term *paršu* refers to the undigested content of the stomachs, as well as to the content of the intestines: *CAD* 12:205–6 "excrement, gore," *AHw* 2:836b "Darmhinalt, Kot"; Alexander Militarev and Leonid Kogan, *Anatomy of Man and Animals*, vol. 1 of *Semitic Etymological Dictionary* (Münster: Ugarit-Verlag, 2000), 194–95.

[62] See De Zorzi, "Of Raving Dogs and Promiscous Pigs."

šumma šaḫû ina ribīti iltanassû tīb šāri šumma tibût marri u tupšikki

If pigs run around lively in the main street, (this signifies) rising of [wind], or: calling up of (corvée labourers wielding) spade and basket (for carrying bricks and earth).[63]

šumma kalbānu ina sūqi iltanassumū tibût marri u tupšikki

If dogs run around lively in the street, (this signifies) calling up of (corvée labourers wielding) spade and basket (for carrying bricks and earth).[64]

In these omens, the bustling activity of free-range pigs and dogs in the public square comes to evoke the busy to and fro of corvée laborers. A Hellenistic commentary[65] discusses the first of our two omens, spelling out the underlying association between the confused activity of pigs (or dogs, in the parallel) and the bustle of low status corvée laborers. The commentary quotes the omen verbatim and then adds: *ṣalālu ašar šaḫê : attu ana epēšika k[īma šaḫê lū ṣ]allāt* ("[it means] to sleep where the pig [sleeps] [as in]: 'For doing your work, you shall sleep li[ke a pig]'").[66] The commentary draws on the image of the pig lying or wallowing in mud, which is well attested in cuneiform sources, and thereby offers an unflattering image of corvée laborers: these men are likened to a pig wallowing in mud. Several sources prove the degrading nature of the comparison. An Akkadian spell against stomachache presents the following sequence: *libbi alpi ana tarbaṣi libbi immeri ana supūri libbi šaḫî ana asurrê* ("ox in the pen, sheep in the fold, pig in the sewer").[67] The pig lingers in dirty, foul-smelling places and can be seen eating feces.[68] A Sumerian collection of insults

---

[63] Sally Freedman, *Tablets 41–63*, vol. 3 of *If a City Is Set on a Height: The Akkadian Omen Series Šumma Ālu Ina Mēlê Šakin* (Winona Lake, IN: Eisenbrauns, 2017), 76. A parallel omen appears in Šumma izbu tablet 22, omen 159; Nicla De Zorzi, *La serie teratomantica Šumma izbu: Testo, tradizione, orizzonti culturali*, 2 vols. (Padua: S.A.R.G.O.N, 2014), 881 and 898.

[64] Freedman, *Tablets 41–63*, 52.

[65] CT 41:30–31; Freedman, *Tablets 41–63*, 73–75; CCP 3.5.49.

[66] CT 41:30–31.o.3b–4. This is the reading of the passage proposed and discussed in Nicla De Zorzi, "Of Pigs and Workers: A Note on Lugal-e and a Late Babylonian Commentary on Šumma ālu 49," *NABU* 79 (2016): 131–34.

[67] STT 252.r.23–25; Erica Reiner, "Another Volume of Sultantepe Tablets," *JNES* 26 (1967): 192; Niek Veldhuis, "The Heartgrass and Related Matters," *OLP* 21 (1990): 39. The passage is quoted by George, "On Babylonian Lavatories and Sewers," 95–96 n. 36.

[68] In the Disputation between Bird and Fish, Bird insults Fish calling it: šaḫ$_2$ is-ḫab$_2$ še$_{10}$ ni$_2$-bi gu$_7$-gu$_7$ ("swine, rascal, gorging yourself upon your own excrement") (ETCSL c.5.3.5, line 124). An omen from *Šumma ālu*, tablet 49 refers to a pig entering a man's house and consuming the man's faeces (Freedman, *Tablets 41–63*, 79 omen 77'). A

known as Diatribe B (also known as Diatribe Against Engar-dug and Engardu, the Fool) includes šaḫ₂ lu-ḫu-um-ma sù-a ("pig spattered with filth") (line 8).[69] The Akkadian equivalent of lu-ḫu-um-ma, *luḫummû* ("dirt, filth") is associated with stench in an Old Babylonian chain incantation: *Anu irḫiam šamê šamû erṣetam uld*[*ūn*]*im erṣetam ulid būšam būšum ulid luḫummâm luḫummûm ulid zubba zu*[*b*]*bu ulid tūltam* ("Anu begot the sky, the sky bore the earth, the earth bore the stench, the stench bore the filth, the filth bore the fly, the fly bore the worm").[70] *Luḫummû* describes the dwelling of the pig in a Neo-Assyrian collection of animal anecdotes from Aššur:

šaḫû [*ar*]*šu ul īši ṭēma rabi*[*ṣ ina luḫu*]*mmê ikkala kurummata ... šaḫû lā qašid* [*... mubal*]*il arki mubaḫḫiš sūqāni ʾxʾ* [*mu*]*ṭannipu bītāti šaḫû lā simat ekurri lā amēl* [*ṭ*]*ēme lā kābis agurri ikkib ilāni*

The [dirt]y[71] pig has no sense. It lie[s in fil]th,[72] eating food[73].... The pig is unholy [... bespat]tering his backside, making the street smell, [pol]luting the

---

parallel omen appears in *Šumma izbu*, tablet 22; De Zorzi, *La serie teratomantica Šumma izbu*, 880 omen 153. Note that in both cases the apodosis refers to slander, confirming the association between mouth, anus, and slander in Mesopotamian sources.

[69] ETCSL c.5.4.11; Sjøberg, "'He Is a Good Seed of a Dog,'" 109.o.i.6' and 114 commentary. See also Benjamin Foster and Emmanuelle Salgues, "Everything Except the Squeal: Pigs in Early Mesopotamia," in *De la domestication au tabou: Les cas de suidés dans le Proche-Orient ancient*, ed. Brigitte Lion and Cécile Michel (Paris: de Boccard, 2006), 288–89.

[70] Jan van Dijk, Albrecht Goetze, and Mary I. Hussey, *Early Mesopotamian Incantations and Rituals*, YOS 11 (New Haven: Yale University Press, 1985), 11:5a.o.1–3; Niek Veldhuis, "The Fly, the Worm and the Chain," *OLP* 24 (1993): 45–46; Nathan Wasserman, "On Leeches, Dogs and Gods in Old Babylonian Medical Incantations," *RA* 102 (2008): 73–74). See also the translation in Foster, *Before the Muses*, 180.

[71] The adjective *aršu* is generally used with reference to garments and persons: see *CAD* 1.2:309–10. The semantic range of the term is discussed by Feder, "Defilement, Disgust, and Disease," 104–5. Another attestation of *aršu* in connection with an animal derives from an Akkadian disputation fragment: *ḫulê ša pî aršu* ("dirty-mouthed shrew"). CBS 2266+, line 4; Enrique Jiménez, *The Babylonian Disputation Poems: With Editions of the Series of the Poplar, Palm and Vine, the Series of the Spider, and the Story of the Poor, Forlorn Wren* (Leiden: Brill, 2017), 391 MS NipSchl. The term appears together with three words signifying slander: *pitarru, sullû, sarrātu*.

[72] An unpreserved omen from *Šumma ālu*, Tablet 49; Freedman, *Tablets 41–63*, 71–90 refers to a pig smearing something with filth (*luḫummâ ipšuš*): see the commentary CT 41:30–31.r.14b; Freedman, *Tablets 41–63*, 75; CCP 3.5.49 line 32.

[73] For the restoration of lines 5–6, see Michael Streck, "The Pig and the Fox in Two Popular Sayings from Aššur," in Lanfranchi et al., *Leggo!*, 790.

houses. The pig is not fit for the temple, is not a man with understanding,[74] is not allowed to tread on pavements, an abomination to all gods.[75]

The association of corvée laborers with pigs may have come very naturally to the Hellenistic commentator cited above as the term for corvée laborer in his period was "mud laborer" (*ēpiš dulli ṭiṭṭi*).[76] In his commentary, he refers explicitly to the metonymy underlying the omen (spade and basket representing the workers), basing himself on "mud, filth" as the *tertium comparationis* between the pigs and the wielders of spade and basket. We can conclude from all of this that the lower strata of society from which the workforce for corvée was recruited were derogatorily seen as the "pigs and dogs" of society—they were considered "dirty and disgusting" by the members of the scribal elite.[77]

The image of disgust associated with animals and bodily waste is used also in the context of description of the suffering self and of self-abasement, for instance, in the case of the words put in the mouth of the sufferer in Ludlul Bēl Nēmeqi: *ina rubṣiya abīt kī alpi ubtallil kī immeri ina tabāštāniya* ("I spend the night in my own filth[78] like an ox, and wallow in my own excrement like a sheep") (tablet 2, lines 106–107).[79] In an Old Babylonian letter from Mari (modern Tell Hariri), the writer addresses the king in the following self-denigrating terms: *inanna iâti tu'iltam ša libbi asurrêm bēlī ša ilūtišu suqtī ilput* ("now my lord, as hallmark of his divinity, has touched me [= my chin], a maggot from the sewer").[80] In another Old Babylonian letter from Mari, an *assinnum* named

---

[74] See also Takayoshi Oshima, *Babylonian Poems of Pious Sufferers: Ludlul Bēl Nēmeqi and the Babylonian Theodicy* (Tübingen: Mohr Siebeck, 2014), 189: "It is not a man with reason." This is an explicit reference to the pig's beastliness in contrast to human (male?) nature; Wilfred G. Lambert's translation, "lacks sense," would seem to miss this important point (Lambert, *Babylonian Wisdom Literature*, 215). On this passage, see also Steinert, *Aspekte des Menschseins*, 388.

[75] *KAR* 174.r.iii.5–16; Lambert, *Babylonian Wisdom Literature*, 215.

[76] See De Zorzi, "Of Pigs and Workers."

[77] Note that omens from the northern Mesopotamian city of Tigunānum (ca. 1630 BCE) describe a class of low-level peasants (*ḫupšu*), subject to corvée and military conscription, as pigs. See De Zorzi, "Teratomancy at Tigunānum," 136–38.

[78] According to *CAD* 14:395, *rubṣu* means "litter, lair of cattle and demons." On this passage, see Oshima, *Babylonian Poems of Pious Sufferers*, 263.

[79] Lambert, *Babylonian Wisdom Literature*, 44–45; Amar Annus and Alan Lenzi, *Ludlul Bēl Nēmeqi: The Standard Babylonian Poem of the Righteous Sufferer* (Helsinki: Neo-Assyrian Text Corpus Project: 2010), 37; Oshima, *Babylonian Poems of Pious Sufferers*, 92–93. For parallels in bilingual laments, see Lambert, *Babylonian Wisdom Literature*, 294; Oshima, *Babylonian Poems of Pious Sufferers*, 263.

[80] ARM 26.1:378 n. 13; Klaas R. Veenhof, "Mari A 450: 9 f. (ARM 26/1, p. 378 note 13)," *NABU* (1989): 27. For the meaning of *asurrû* in this letter, see George, "On Babylonian Lavatories and Sewers," 93 n. 28. For the semantic range of *tūltum*, see *CAD*

Šēlebum[81] paints a vivid picture of his current state of destitution (12'–14'): *anāku m[ā]di[š] zê u šināti wašbāku u qa[n] t[e]mēnim akka[l]* ("as for me, I sit in a ma[ss] of excrement and urine and I ea[t] ree[ds] from fu[nd]aments"[82]).

Eating inedible disgusting food, including excrements, and drinking filthy liquids, including urine, belong to the traditional repertoire of ancient Near Eastern curses,[83] as in the treaty between the Assyrian king Aššur-nārārī V (754–745 BCE) and Mati'ilu, king of Arpad: *eprū ana akālišunu qīru ana piššatišunu šīnāt imāri ana šatêšunu niāru ana lubuštišunu liššakin ina tubkinni lū may-*

18:466–67; Wasserman, "On Leeches, Dogs and Gods." The term evokes decay and death, as in a famous passage from Old Babylonian Gilgamesh (ii.9'), in which Gilgamesh refuses to bury Enkidu *adi tūltam imqutma ina appišu* ("until a maggot dropped from his nostril"). See Andrew R. George, *The Babylonian Gilgamesh Epic: Introduction, Critical Edition, and Cuneiform Texts* (Oxford: Oxford University Press, 2003), 278.

[81] Šēlebum appears also in the letters ARM 26.197 and 26.213. He transmits divine messages from Annunītum, a war goddess connected with Ištar, to the queen of Mari. On the prophetic role of the *assinnu*, see, e.g., Jonathan Stöckl, "Gender Ambiguity in Ancient Near Eastern Prophecy? A Reassessment of the Data behind a Popular Theory," in *Prophets Male and Female: Gender and Prophecy in the Hebrew Bible, the Eastern Mediterranean and the Ancient Near East*, ed. Jonathan Stöckl and Corrine L. Carvalho (Atlanta: Society of Biblical Literature, 2013), 59–80; Ilona Zsolnay, "The Misconstrued Role of the Assinnu in Ancient Near Eastern Prophecy," in Stöckl and Carvalho, *Prophets Male and Female*, 81–99.

[82] ARM 26.198; Jean-Marie Durand translates g[i] t[i]-mi-nim as "roseau de l'enceinte" (*Archives épistolaires de Mari*, ARM 26.1 [Paris: Recherche sur les civilisations, 1988], 425). Wolfgang Heimpel translates "the reed of a foundation" and comments "possibly a bulrush is meant. The plant is commonly found on low ground and in abandoned excavations. The lower part of its stalk is edible" (*Letters to the King of Mari: A New Translation, with Historical Introduction, Notes, and Commentary* [Winona Lake, IN: Eisenbrauns, 2003], 252 n. 198). Martti Nissinen leaves the word untranslated ("an inexplicable word": *Prophets and Prophecy in the Ancient Near East*, WAW 12 [Atlanta: Society of Biblical Literature, 2003], 29–30 with n. 8). In view of the context, g[i] t[i]-mi-nim may refer to slimy rotten rushes growing in foul-water drains, maybe a drainage ditch, to be found in connection with foundations or wall footings. Note that the Akkadian word *asurrû*, next to its etymological meaning "sewer," seems to be associated with the idea of "wall footing" (George, "On Babylonian Lavatories and Sewers," 102). The word *temennu* and other Akkadian words for "foundation" are studied by Johanna Tudeau, "Meaning in Perspective: Some Akkadian Terms for 'Foundation' *uššu, temennu, išdu, duruššu*," in *At the Dawn of History: Ancient Near Eastern Studies in Honour of J. N. Postgate*, ed. Yağmur Heffron, Adam Stone, and Martin Worthington (Winona Lake, IN: Eisenbrauns, 2017), 631–50, but this passage from ARM 26.198 is not discussed.

[83] See Hans U. Steymans, *Deuteronomium 28 und die adê zur Thronfolgeregelung Asarhaddons: Segen und Fluch im Alten Orient und in Israel* (Göttingen: Vandenhoeck & Ruprecht, 1995).

yalšunu ("may dust be their food, pitch their ointment, donkey's urine their drink, papyrus their clothing, and may their sleeping place be in the dung heap").[84] In Esarhaddon's Succession Treaty, the oath-breaker is threatened in these words: *qīru kupru lū makalākunu šīnāt imāri lū mašqītkunu napṭu lū piššatkunu elapûa ša nāri lū taktimkunu* ("may tar and pitch be your food, may donkey's urine be your drink, may naphtha be your ointment, may duckweed be your covering").[85] Also the formula *gerdu ekkal kurru išatti* in Neo-Assyrian contracts belongs here. It threatens anyone intending to break the agreement with the obligation of "eating plucked wool" and "drinking sludge from the tannery."[86]

Curses like the one cited above that refer to eating dust draw additional power by evoking death-related imagery: *epru* ("dust, dirt") as well as *ṭiṭṭu* ("clay") and *mû dalḫûtu* ("muddied water") are the sustenance of the dead in the netherworld.[87] Most evocative is a famous passage from the myth of Ištar's Descent to the Netherworld. Somewhat atypically, we encounter the visceral disgust topos in a crafted passage of a highly literary religious text. Our survey of straightforward references to unpleasant odor and to a lesser degree other sensory perceptions based on spontaneous and unconscious responses has drawn heavily on humorous and scatological compositions and other examples of expressive literature. Still, in line with these texts, disgust is evoked also in Ištar's Descent to the Netherworld in the context of an emotional setting. Indeed, it is referred to in a statement made in seething rage. The queen of the netherworld Ereškigal, furious at the *assinnu* Asûšu-namir's request for a waterskin, casts a curse upon him:

aklī epinnēt āli lū akalka ḫabannāt āli lū maltītka ṣilli dūri lū manzāzūka askuppātu lū mušābūka šakru u ṣamû limḫaṣū lētka

---

[84] SAA 2:11, 2.iv.14–16.

[85] SAA 2:49, 6.490–492.

[86] See Karen Radner, *Die neuassyrischen Privatrechtsurkunden als Quelle für Mensch und Umwelt* (Helsinki: Neo-Assyrian Text Corpus Project, 1997), 189–93. The term *kurru* refers to the paste used for the depilation of hides in the preliminary stages of leather manufacture, while *gerdu* refers to the resulting hair tufts. See Jo Ann Scurlock, "On Some Terms for Leatherworking in Ancient Mesopotamia," in *Proceedings of the 51st Rencontre Assyriologique Internationale, Held at the Oriental Institute of the University of Chicago, July 18–22, 2005*, ed. Robert D. Biggs, Jennie Myers, and Martha Tobi Roth (Chicago: Oriental Institute of the University of Chicago, 2008), 171–72. Although the exact content of the depilatory paste is not known, it must have been a vile-smelling concoction.

[87] See Meir Malul, "Eating and Drinking (One's) Refuse," *NABU* 99 (1993): 82–83.

May the city ploughs' 'bread' (= dirt) be your food,[88] may the city sewer pipes be your drinking place, may the shadow of the city wall be your station,[89] may the threshold be your dwelling, may drunk and sober slap your cheek![90]

---

[88] The idea underlying the image is that ploughs "eat" mud and that this food is wished on Aṣûšu-namir. So also Peled, *Masculinities and Third Gender*, 58 n. 137: "clods of earth, as the product of plows ("food of the plows")." The city ploughs' "bread" thus corresponds to *epru* ("dirt") in the curse section of the above mentioned treaty between Aššur-nārārī V and Mati'ilu (SAA 2:11, 2.iv.14–16). The reading of the corresponding line on the Aššur's recension of the myth (see) is debated: [x]x *ana*? *e-pi-<né>-et* uru *lu-ú* šuk-*at-ka* (*KAR* 1.r.20). See Pirjo Lapinkivi, *The Neo-Assyrian Myth of Ištar's Descent and Resurrection* (Helsinki: Neo-Assyrian Text Corpus Project, 2010), xi, 20. The variant *e-pi-et* can be taken as a defective syllabic spelling for the plural of *epinnu* (= *epinnēt* = *e-pi-<né>-et* = ^{giš}*apin.meš*). See Stephanie Dalley, *Myths from Mesopotamia: Creation, the Flood, Gilgamesh, and Others* (Oxford: Oxford University Press, 2000), 161 n. 16. Erica Reiner suggests instead to take it as the plural of *ēpītu* ("woman baker"; *ēpêt*; *epû*, "to bake"); she thus renders the curse as follows: "may the bread of the bakers of the city be your food, may the jugs of the city be your drinking vessel, stay in the protection of the city wall, squat at the threshold of the house" (*Your Thwarts in Pieces, Your Mooring Rope Cut: Poetry from Babylonia and Assyria* [Ann Arbor: H. Rackham School of Graduate Studies at the University of Michigan, 1985], 44–45; Reiner, "City Bread and Bread Baked in Ashes," in *Language and Areas: Studies Presented to George V. Bobrinskoy*, ed. Howard I. Aronson et al. [Chicago: University of Chicago Press, 1967], 117–20). The curse, then, is understood to express antiurban feelings, the attitude "of the noble nomad who despises the effeminate sybaritic city dweller" ("City Bread and Bread Baked in Ashes," 117). Reiner's interpretation, however, does not explain the variant ^{giš}apin.meš (*epinnēt*) in the Nineveh recension and overall fails to convince. See Stefan Maul, "Kurgarrû und Assinnu und ihr Stand in der babylonischen Gesellschaft," in *Aussenseiter und Randgruppen: Beiträge zu einer Sozialgeschichte des Alten Orients*, ed. Volkert Haas (Konstanz: Universitätsverlag, 1992), 168 n. 34; Pongratz-Leisten, "Other and the Enemy," 221–23. I am also not convinced by Maul's suggestion that *epinnu* ("plough") is intended here as a euphemism for the penis and that the first part of the course refers to commercial homosexual activity involving the *assinnu*. See Maul, "Kurgarrû und Assinnu," 162–63, 168 n. 35; see also Martti Nissinen, *Homoeroticism in the Biblical World: A Historical Perspective* (Philadelphia: Fortress, 1998), 28–34. Skepticism regarding this interpretation is expressed also by Peled, *Masculinities and Third Gender*, 58.

[89] In Gilgamesh, tablet 7, line 117, Enkidu curses the prostitute Šamḫat wishing her the "shade of the wall" (*ṣilli dūri*) as her "standing place" (*manzāzu*) (George, *Babylonian Gilgamesh Epic*, 640–41). The two texts use the same range of topoi, as confirmed by the fact that Ištar's Descent to the Netherworld, line 108, corresponds exactly to Gilgamesh, tablet 7, line 119. See Anne D. Kilmer, "How Was Queen Ereshkigal Tricked? A New Interpretation of the Descent of Ishtar," *UF* 3 (1971): 301 n. 17; Jeffrey H. Tigay, *The Evolution of the Gilgamesh Epic* (Philadelphia: University of Philadelphia Press, 1982), 170–73; Lapinkivi, *Ištar's Descent*, 85.

The first two lines of this much-debated passage can be explained in the light of the texts discussed above as a variant of the frequently attested motif of eating and drinking inedible, disgusting food and liquids and even bodily waste as a sign of degradation.[91] The myth suggests that dirt and water from foul-smelling sewage pools are destined to become Aṣûšu-namir's food.[92]

RECHERCHÉ IMAGERY OF DISGUST: THE DOMAIN OF THE VISUAL

Most of the foregoing straightforward references to unpleasant sensory perceptions refer to spontaneous and unconscious responses and are culled from expressive literature, including humorous and scatological compositions. This final section of the paper addresses more carefully crafted, literary descriptions of the unpleasant or disgusting that can be encountered in religious and ritual texts. These descriptions are usually phrased in an indirect manner, that is, they do not normally employ explicit verbs like *masāku* or *ba'āšu*. They also draw on a wider range of sensory experience than expressions of spontaneous disgust for which the sense of smell was predominant, as we have seen.

In expressive literature, the sense of smell is primarily of relevance in fumigation rituals. In general terms, fumigation symbolically invokes the divine.[93]

---

[90] CT 15:45–47.104–107; Lapinkivi, *Ištar's Descent*, 12 and 20.

[91] See Tigay, *Evolution of the Gilgamesh Epic*, 172 n. 31; Malul, "Eating and Drinking (One's) Refuse," 82–83. A connection between the above discussed letter ARM 26.198, lines 12'–14', describing the state of destitution of the *assinnum* Šēlebum, forced to eat slimy rotten rushes, and Ereškigal's curse has been proposed by Heimpel, *Letters to the King of Mari*, 252; Jonathan Stöckl, *Prophecy in the Ancient Near East: A Philological and Sociological Comparison* (Leiden: Brill, 2012), 71 n. 3, 73. Another parallel can be found in the description of the fate awaiting the leper (lu$_2$ sahar šub-ba) in the netherworld in the Sumerian composition known as Gilgamesh, Enkidu, and the Netherworld, lines 285–286a: u$_2$-ni al-bar a-ni a-bar u$_2$ gid$_2$ al-gu$_7$-e a-šeš al-na$_8$-na$_8$ uru bar-ra-a al-tuš ("his food his set aside, his water is set aside, he eats uprooted plants, he drinks bitter water, he lives outside the city"). See Alhena Gadotti, *"Gilgamesh, Enkidu, and the Netherworld" and the Sumerian Gilgamesh Cycle* (Berlin: de Gruyter, 2014), 116 (translation), 231–32 (textual matrix), 293–94 (commentary).

[92] The same idea underlies Robert D. Biggs's proposal that ^{giš}apin.meš and *e-pi-<né>-et* may represent a misinterpretation of the word *tubkinnu* ("dunghill"). See Robert D. Biggs, "Descent of Ištar, line 104," *NABU* 74 (1993): 58–59. This interpretation remains difficult to substantiate, however.

[93] A comprehensive study of fumigation in Mesopotamia in all its attested contexts is absent. See, e.g., Wolfgang Zwickel, *Räucherkult und Räuchergeräte: Exegetische und archäologische Studien zum Räucheropfer im Alten Testament*, OBO 97 (Fribourg: Presses Universitaires; Göttingen: Vandenhoeck & Ruprecht, 1990); Michael Jursa, "Parfüm(rezepte): A. In Mesopotamien," *RlA* 10:335–36; Jursa, "Räucherung, Rauchopfer: A. In Mesopotamien," *RlA* 11:225–29.

We have to make a threefold distinction when it comes to fumigation in religious contexts in Mesopotamia: there is the incense offering—aromatic, fragrant, a call to the gods to attend the offering;[94] there is the fragrant fumigation of purification, intended to signify the dissolution or replacement of a pollutant by the pleasant odor of purity; finally, there is the malodorous fumigation of purification and apotropaic action. In this final type of fumigation, the fetid fumes are meant to disperse and take with them, or symbolize the disappearance of, the miasma, the pollution, the demonic agent of sickness. What the fumes leave behind as a contrast is the absence of stench, understood as the relative fragrance of well-being and purity. An incantation from the antiwitchcraft composition Maqlû spells out the idea underlying the use of fire and smoke in apotropaic rituals. First a long list of afflictions that torment the sufferer is wished on the witch:

> zīru ša tēpušāni tušēpišāni ana muḫḫikun[u ēpuš]a ... utukku lemnu tušaṣbitā'inni utukku lemnu liṣbatku[nūši] ... ašuštu arurtu ḫūṣ ḫīp libbi gilittu piritti u adirti yâši taškunāni ašuštu arurtu ḫūṣ ḫīp libbi gilittu piritti adirti ana kâšunu liššaknakkunūši[sic]

> Hate(-magic) that you have performed against me, have had performed against me, [I perfor]m against you.... An evil demon you have caused to seize me: May an evil demon seize you.... Distress, trembling, depression, fear, and apprehension you have inflicted on me myself: may (the same) be inflicted on you yourselves.[95]

The ritual to which this incantation refers foresees the burning of a figurine of the witch: *aqmūkunūši ina kibrīti elleti u ṭābat amurri alqut quturkunu ikkib šamê epšētēkunu turrānikkunūši* ("I burn you with pure sulphur and the salt of Amurru, I gather up your smoke, an abomination to heaven. Your deeds [of sorcery] are [hereby] turned back to you").[96] When the figurine goes up in smoke, this smoke—"an abomination to heaven"—represents and evokes the evil essence of the witch the fire god is asked to dissolve. This association explains the use of foul ingredients for fumigation, in particular in rituals that are directed against invisible demonic forces. Typical examples are the apotropaic fumigations directed against Lamaštu, perhaps the most horrible demon in the Mesopotamian repertoire of malevolent supernatural beings. The demon

---

[94] The gods were thought to be influenced by odors. Cultic food taboos based on smell (e.g., garlic and leek) depend on the idea that the gods are offended by foul breath: see, e.g., van der Toorn, *Sin and Sanction in Israel and Mesopotamia*, 34–35; Guichard and Marti, "Purity in Ancient Mesopotamia," 84, 87.

[95] Maqlû, tablet 5, lines 57–72; Abusch, *Magical Ceremony Maqlû*, 332–33.

[96] Maqlû, tablet 5, lines 73–75; Abusch, *Magical Ceremony Maqlû*, 333.

Lamaštu not only kills women postpartum and strangles newborn babies but, in the words of Walter Farber, "is an almost satanic force, a personification of evil and aggressiveness."[97] She usually seems to have "a lion's head, a furry or scaly animal's body with big human-like breasts, human hands and big bird of prey feet."[98] A pertinent ritual prescription includes the following list of ingredients:

> *qēma lā napâ qilip šuskilli ina pēnti tuqattaršu qulēpti ṣerri zēr kite ina pēnti tuqattaršu kibrīt saḫlê mušāṭī ina pēnti tuqattaršu*

> (Its ritual:) With unsifted flour (and) peel of šusikillu onions on embers you fumigate him. With snake skin (and) linseed on embers you fumigate him. With sulphur, cress (and) hair combings on embers you fumigate him.[99]

Here, snake skin and hair have the double effect of contributing to the horrible odor of the smoke and of serving as stand-ins for Lamaštu, given her mixed hairy and scaly body. The same principle is at work in the unappealing ointments that are spread on the patient suffering from Lamaštu's ministrations, which include pitch from a boat or boat parts, as well as part of a donkey's hide, because Lamaštu travels by boat or by donkey:[100]

> *kupur eleppi kupur sikkanni kupur gišalli kupur unūt eleppi kalama eper kāri u nēberi nāḫu šaman nūni qīru ḫimētu ankinūtu aktam aprušu azallû mašak imēri kurru ša aškāpi ulāpu lupputu ziqqatû šaman šaḫî pešî napšaltu*

> Pitch from a boat, pitch from the rudder, pitch from an oar, pitch from any other equipment of a boat, dirt from an embankment and a ford, lard, fish train, hot bitumen, ghee, *ankinūtu*-plant, *aktam*-plant, *aprušu*-plant, *anzallû*-plant, a donkey's hide, fuller's paste, a soiled cloth, *ziqqatû*-fish, lard from a white pig: (use as) ointment.[101]

This mixture is clearly supposed to be as revolting as Lamaštu herself, whom it is intended to evoke, just as the eventual removal of the ointment spread on the sufferer evokes the removal of Lamaštu herself.[102]

---

[97] Walter Farber, *Lamaštu: An Edition of the Canonical Series of Lamaštu Incantations and Rituals and Related Texts from the Second and First Millennia B.C.* (Winona Lake, IN: Eisenbrauns, 2014), 3.

[98] Farber, *Lamaštu*, 4.

[99] Lamaštu, series 2, lines 31–33; Farber, *Lamaštu*, 166–67.

[100] The idea must be that these ointments are removed/wiped off, thereby symbolically removing Lamaštu.

[101] Lamaštu, series 3, lines 64–68; Farber, *Lamaštu*, 190–91.

[102] In terms of magical theory, the ritual employs persuasive analogies as described by Stanley J. Tambiah, "Form and Meaning of Magical Acts," in *Culture Thought, and*

Moving from ritual texts to religious compositions such as prayers, myths, and so forth, it appears that smell has no particular role to play in the description of the sensory impact of the divine, as opposed to the gods' symbolic evocation in ritual: a carefully crafted imagery based on sight and sound dominates.

Sensory quality is often represented as context-dependent. Typically, gods are visually overwhelming; this is awe-inspiring, and thus, as in the English term, ambiguous. Much of the vocabulary regarding the radiance and roar of divine beings can be applied to gods and demons alike.[103] It is often entirely owed to the wider context how a given passage is to be understood: as a reference to the awe-inspiring and overwhelming presence of an at least potentially benevolent deity or as a reference to a definitively malevolent being such as a demon. Awesome radiance (*šalummatu*), for instance, is regularly attributed to gods and divine paraphernalia—the god Nergal is enveloped with radiance (*šalummatu*) and clothed in splendor (*namrirru*)—but also kings possess *šalummatu*, as well as temples and lions, and even the semi-human, half demonic, Gutian mountain people can be *šalummat ḫitmuṭ* ("afire with awe-inspiring splendour").[104]

Against this overall trend to describe the numinous as generically awe-inspiring, one can set some descriptions of demons and demonic beings that are clearly intended to cause revulsion, rather than just terror and awe. A case in point is divine Discord, *ṣāltu*. This allegorical figure appears in an exceptional Old Babylonian composition, the hymn known as Aguṣaya A,[105] where Discord is pitched as a rival of warlike Ištar. She is described as follows:

rūšam ša ṣuprīšu adi sebešu iqqur qātīššu ilqe ēpīšu ṣāltam ibtani Ea niššīki ki-ru-gú 4-kam-ma *ilu Ea iḫtīši ištakkan pānīšu ibanni ṣāltam aššūtēṣî itti Ištar*

Social Action: An Anthropological Perspective (Cambridge: Harvard University Press, 1985), 60–86; Tambiah, *Magic, Science and Religion and the Scope of Rationality* (Cambridge: Harvard University Press, 1990).

[103] For a comprehensive treatment of the divine soundscape, see Rendu Loisel, *Les chants du monde*. On the concept of divine radiance, see Cassin, *La Splendeur divine* and, recently, Aster, *Unbeatable Light*.

[104] *CAD* 17.1:283–85; LKA 63.o.13'; Victor Hurowitz and Joan Goodnick Westenholz, "LKA 63: A Heroic Poem in Celebration of Tiglat-pileser I's Muṣru-Qumanu Campaign," *JCS* 42 (1990): 3.

[105] See Brigitte Groneberg, "Philologische Bearbeitung des Aguṣayahymnus," *RA* 75 (1981): 107–25; Groneberg, *Lob der Ištar: Gebet und Ritual an die altbabylonische Venusgöttin "Tanatti Ištar"* (Groningen: Styx, 1997), 75–93. Several passages have been discussed again in Michael Streck, "Notes on the Old Babylonian Hymns of Aguṣaya," *JAOS* 130 (2010): 561–69. A digital edition (transliteration and translation) is available on SEAL (2.1.5.1). My translation follows principally Foster, *Before the Muses*, 96–106.

giš-gi4-gál-bi *abrat šiknassa šunnât miniātim naklat kīma manma[n] lā umaššalū šepṣet ṣāltu šiknassa šunnât miniātim naklat kīma manman lā umaššalū šepṣet šīrūša ṣabā'u ṣēlu šārassa ... ṣāltum kī libši nēzuḫat tuqumtam mār mēli rigmuš nukkurat amāriš palḫat ... [anā]ku arruššêša [a]btani? kâti ... itbukma ṣāltam šūturu biniannim ušāriršī ammagrātim qullulim taršiātim*

(Ea the wise) scraped out seven times the dirt of his nails. He took it in his hand, baked it.[106] Ea the prince has created Discord. The fourth song. God Ea has straightaway set to his task, he is making Discord that she fight with Ištar. Its antiphon. She is powerful in her form, monstrous are her proportions, she is artful as none could rival, she is a fighter. Discord's form is monstrous in proportions. She is artful as none could rival, she is a fighter.[107] Her flesh is battle, the melee her hair.... Discord is girded with combat for clothes, her clamor is born of a deluge, she is strange and terrifying to behold.... (Ea says) To humiliate(?) her, [I, myself] have created you.[108]... So the Extraordinary of Form, dispatched Discord.[109] Drove her to insults, contempt (and) calumny.[110]

Discord is created by wise Ea from the dirt under his nails.[111] The text apparently plays with etymology or at least assonance: dirt is *rūšu*, and Ea tells Discord he had created her for humiliating (*ruššû*) Ištar (vi.29'), and later Discord is said to utter insults (*taršiātum*) (vii.9')—both words phonetically recall Discord's *prima materia*, *rūšu* ("dirt")—and *magrītum* (vii.8'). The description does not get more specific than this. Still, it is revealing for one aspect: the verbal forms that are translated here respectively as "monstrous" (*šunnât*) and "strange" (*nuk-*

---

[106] For this interpretation of *e-pí-i-šu*, see Streck, "Notes on the Old Babylonian Hymns," 565 *ad* v.26'.

[107] SEAL's translation of v.35'–41' is different: "strong is her figure, doubled in shape"; Streck derives *šunnât* from *šanû* ("to do again; D to double") and not from *šanû* ("to become different; D to change") (Streck, "Notes on the Old Babylonian Hymns," 565; thus *AHw* 3:1166 *šanû* IV.D.6; Groneberg, "Philologische Bearbeitung des Agušayahymnus," 144; Groneberg, *Lob der Ištar*, 79; Foster, *Before the Muses*, 100). However, Streck's "doubled in shape" seems doubtful given the absence of a point of reference for the doubling; hence I prefer following Groneberg and Foster in deriving the form from *šanû* ("to become different; D to change").

[108] See Streck, "Notes on the Old Babylonian Hymns," 566 (vi.29').

[109] I connect *šūturu biniannim* to Ea, following Foster, *Before the Muses*, 101. SEAL's translation of the passage, "He led Ṣāltum away, pre-eminent in form," does not explain the masculine form *šūturu*.

[110] Agušaya A v.23'–vii.9'.

[111] In Inanna's Descent to the Netherworld, lines 222–223; William R. Sladek, *Inanna's Descent to the Netherworld* (Ann Arbor: University Microfilms, 1974), 131, 170; ETCSL c.1.4.1. Ea creates from the dirt (mu-dur₇) under his fingernails the *kurgarrû* and the *galaturra* ("young/junior gala"). See Peled, *Masculinities and Third Gender*, 52–53.

kurat) both basically mean "changed"—the underlying idea is a deviation from normality that is automatically and intrinsically negative. This would seem to be typical of the semantics of Mesopotamian aesthetics: features that are described as literally changed are practically always envisaged as having changed to the worse, to the not-normal—hence the translation of "monstrous" for a word that basically means "made different."

Created out of dirt, Discord is so horrible that she strikes dumb a god who sees her (*iqâl elša*, Agušaya B i.18).[112] This terror-induced dumbness leads to a very common feature of the figurative language relating to the unpleasant or disgusting with which this survey will conclude: the recurrence of imagery conveying negative emotions by emphasizing the absence of sensory data. It is a common topos in Akkadian literature to refer to men or gods being shocked into silence or petrified by terror when confronted with some crisis: Akkadian often uses the word *šuḫarruru* ("to become dazed, still, numb with fear") in such contexts.[113] But there is more. Consider these descriptions of Lamaštu, the scaly, lion-headed she-demon, as she comes up from the marshes:[114]

ištu api īlâmma ezzet šamrat gašrat kaṣṣat gapšat ilat namurrat [šēpā]ša Anzû [qāss]a lu'tu ... [ṣilli d]ūri manzāzūša askuppātu mūšabūša [arra]kā? ṣuprāša u[l? gullu]bā šaḫātāša

(Lamaštu) came up from the marshes, being fierce, violent, very strong, raging, overbearing, (of) divine (power), terrifying. Her [feet] (are those of) Anzû (= an eagle), her [hand] (spells) decay[115].... [Dark (corners) of the w]all are her hangouts, on the thresholds she sits around.[116] [Very lo]ng? are her fingernails, u[nsha]ven her armpits.[117]

---

[112] See Groneberg, "Philologische Bearbeitung des Agušayahymnus," 126–34; Groneberg, *Lob der Ištar*, 84–93. Several passages have been discussed again in Streck, "Notes on the Old Babylonian Hymns of Agušaya," 569–70. A digital edition (transliteration and translation) is available on SEAL (2.1.5.2.). For a recent translation, see also Foster, *Before the Muses*, 103–6.

[113] See Erica Reiner, "Dead of Night," in *Studies in Honor of Benno Landsberger on His Seventy-Fifth Birthday, April 21, 1965*, ed. Hans G. Güterbock and Thorkild Jacobsen (Chicago: University of Chicago Press, 1965), 247–51; Cassin, *Splendeur divine*, 37–40; Jaques, *Le Vocabulaires des sentiments*, 205–17.

[114] See Frans Wiggermann, "Lamaštu, Daughter of Anu: A Profile," in *Birth in Babylonia and the Bible: Its Mediterranean Setting*, Marten Stol (Groningen: Styx, 2000), 230; Farber, *Lamaštu*, 3.

[115] On *lu'tu* ("decay"), see Feder, "Semantics of Purity," 103–5.

[116] The "shade of the city wall" (*ṣilli dūri*) is the hangout of the poor and wretched inhabiting the margins of society, such as prostitutes; see Peled, *Masculinities and Third Gender*, 58. Thresholds, sewers, and rubbish heaps are the lair of demons (George, "On Babylonian Lavatories and Sewers," 96) and unsavory animals, such as dogs (George,

This is all pleasingly concrete and lends itself to visualization. However, Lamaštu is also *la[bšat] anqulla umma kuṣṣa ḫalpâ šurīpa* ("cl[ad] in scorching heat, fever, cold, frost and ice").[118] Here, two aspects are of interest. The first is an apparent contradiction: how are we to envisage Lamaštu being clad in scorching heat and frost and ice? This is not actually a problem for a Babylonian speaker, because some of the terms for extreme cold (*šuruppû, šurīpu, ḫimittu*) are derivations from verbal roots that mean "to burn": the two extremes of temperature come down to the same concept. The resulting blurring of the difference between heat and cold is less counterintuitive at a second glance if, for example, the symptoms of high fever are considered—Lamaštu, after all, is mostly an agent of illness.[119] The second aspect of interest here is the effects of Lamaštu's aura of deadly heat/cold. She is not the only demonic being to have such an aura; the Pazuzu demon is also described in similar terms:

iprik qišta iṣṣiša itbuk ūrid ana kirî ittabak inibšu ūrid ina nāri ittabak šurīpa ēlâ ana nābali ḫimitta itbuk ... uššir ana būri ittabak šurīpa

(Pazuzu) beat on the forest, dropped its trees, he passed into the garden, dropped down its fruit, he passed down the river, dropped down ice, he went up into the desert, dropped down frost.... He peered down the well, dropped down ice.[120]

The incantation texts give us sufficient clues as to how we should understand these images: both demons are said to destroy trees and fruit and to cover in ice and frost wherever they pass. Lamaštu turns the water of the river she crosses murky (*dilḫu*) and smears with mud (*luḫummû*) the wall she leans against:

ša š[ūš]i? [i]šissu ša šunî zēršu ša ṣarb[at]i balti ušalli itbuk mutḫummīša ībir nāra dilḫa iškun īmid igāra luḫummâ iptašaš

Babylonian Gilgamesh Epic, 480). The "shade of the city wall" (*ṣilli dūri*) and the "threshold" (*askuppatu*) are the dwelling wished on Aṣûšu-namir in Ištar's Descent to the Netherworld (CT 15:45–47.104–107; Lapinkivi, *Ištar's Descent*, 12 and 20): see above.

[117] Lamaštu, series 1, lines 104–109; Farber, *Lamaštu*, 154–55.

[118] Lamaštu, series 1, line 62; Farber, *Lamaštu*, 152–53.

[119] See Walter Farber, "Lamaštu: Agent of a Specific Disease or a Generic Destroyer of Health?," in *Disease in Babylonia*, ed. Irving L. Finkel and Markham J. Geller (Leiden: Brill, 2007), 137–45; Farber, *Lamaštu*, 3 with n. 11.

[120] Nils P. Heeßel, *Pazuzu: Archäologische und philologische Studien zu einem altorientalischen Dämon* (Leiden: Brill, 2002), 58, lines 37–41; Foster, *Before the Muses*, 977.

The root of the licorice tree, the seed(s) of the chaste tree, the fruit of the poplar, pride of the river meadow, she spoiled. By crossing a river, she makes it murky. By leaning against a wall, she smears (it) with mud.[121]

Muddy water and mud in general are giveaways. These clues are to be connected with Lamaštu's yellowish facial coloring: *kīma kalê lēssa arqat* ("her [Lamaštu] cheek is yellowish pale like ochre").[122] All this recalls death and the netherworld. Death's face is yellow according to a section of the ritual Bīt mēsiri, which refers to a statue of Death, made of lead, *pānūšu kalâ paššū* ("whose face is smeared with yellow paste").[123] The netherworld is consistently described in Mesopotamian sources as a dark pit of clay, its water is muddy, and, as the myth of Ištar's Descent to the Netherworld tells us, its inhabitants cannot find anything to subsist on but mud and clay: *annītūmê anāku itti Anunnakī mê ašatti kīma akli akkal ṭidda kīma šikāri ašatti mê dalḫūte* ("Here [in the netherworld] I drink water with the Anunnaki. I eat clay for bread, I drink muddy water for beer").[124] The beginning of the myth offers a gloomy portrayal of the afterlife, which is characterized by darkness and silence:

> *ana kurnugê qaqqari l[ā târi] Ištar mārat Sîn uzunšu [iškun] iškunma mārat Sîn uzu[nša] ana bīti eṭê šubat Irkalla ana bīti ša ēribūšu lā āṣû ana ḫarrāni ša alaktaša lā tayyārat ana bīti ša ēribūšu zummû nūra ašar epru bubūssunu akalšunu ṭiddu nūra ul immarū ina eṭūti ašbū labšūma kīma iṣṣūri šubāt gappi el dalti u sikkūri šabuḫ epru [el tal]li šuḫarratu tabkat*

> To the Netherworld, the Land of N[o Return], Ištar, the daughter of Sîn, [set] her mind. Indeed, the daughter of Sîn set [her] mi[nd] to the dark house, the dwelling of Irkalla, to the house which none leaves who enters, to the road where traffic is one-way, to the house, whose dwellers thirst for light, where dust is their food (and) their bread, clay. They see no light, they dwell in dark-

---

[121] Lamaštu, series I, lines 63–66; Farber, *Lamaštu*, 152–53.
[122] Lamaštu, series II, line 38; Farber, *Lamaštu*, 168–69.
[123] SBTU 3 n. 69 §30.
[124] CT 15:45–47.32–33; Lapinkivi, *Ištar's Descent*, 17, 25, 30. Similar passages are attested also in Sumerian sources. For instance, in the composition known as Death of Ur-Namma (or Ur-Namma A), line 83: u₂ kur-ra šeš-am₃ a kur-ra mun₄-na-am₃ ("the food of the netherworld is bitter and the drink of the netherworld is salty"). Esther Flückiger-Hawker, *Urnamma of Ur in Sumerian Literary Tradition*, OBO 166 (Fribourg: Presses Universitaires; Göttingen: Vandenhoeck & Ruprecht, 1999), 116. See, in detail, Dina Katz, *The Image of the Netherworld in the Sumerian Sources* (Bethesda, MD: CDL, 2003), 212–33; Katz, "Death They Dispensed to Mankind: The Funerary World of Ancient Mesopotamia," *Historiae* 2 (2005): 67–68.

ness, clothed like birds in garments of feather.[125] Over the door and the bolt dust has settled, [over the door be]am a deathly silence has sunk.[126]

Another bleak description of the netherworld comes from the text known as the Underworld Vision of an Assyrian Prince: *arallu mali puluḫtu ina pān mār rubê nadi šiššu dannu* ("the Netherworld was full of terror; a mighty silence [*šiššu*][127] lay before the crown prince").[128] Also Pazuzu's and Lamaštu's frost and ice evoke the stillness of death: a frozen—or scorched—world is a dead world, and sure enough, once it is said of Pazuzu that [*itta*]*di qūltu* ("[he establish]ed silence"),[129] the silence of death.[130] This is perhaps the most basic negative statement about sensory data to be found in Mesopotamian texts: the worst sensory perception is no sensory perception; and this is exactly what awaits humankind in the netherworld, which is conceived of essentially as a vast grave devoid of sensory stimuli.

---

[125] On the bird imagery related to the description of the afterlife in Akkadian sources, see, e.g., Angelika Berlejung, "Tod und Leben nach den Vorstellungen der Israeliten: Ein ausgewählter Aspekt zu einer Metapher im Spannungsfeld von Leben und Tod," in *Das biblische Weltbild und seine altorientalischen Kontexte*, ed. Bernd Janowski and Beate Ego (Tübingen: Mohr Siebeck, 2001), 473–85.

[126] CT 15:45–47.1–11a; Lapinkivi, *Ištars Descent*, 9, 15–16, 25, 29. Parallel passages can be found in Nergal and Ereškigal, lines 149–157; Simonetta Ponchia and Mikko Lukko, *The Standard Babylonian Myth of Nergal and Ereškigal* (Helsinki: Neo-Assyrian Text Corpus Project, 2013), 16, 26, 46–47; and Gilgamesh, tablet 7, lines 182–192; George, *Babylonian Gilgamesh Epic*, 644–45. See Berlejung, "Tod und Leben nach den Vorstellungen der Israeliten," 481–82.

[127] The term is equated with *qūlu* in the list of synonyms Malku = šarru, tablet 4, line 98. See Ivan Hrůša, *Die akkadische Synonymenliste mallku = šarru: Eine Textedition mit Übersetzung und Kommentar* (Münster: Ugarit-Verlag, 2010), 384.

[128] SAA 3:72, 32.r.13.

[129] Heeßel, *Pazuzu*, 57, line 16.

[130] On this motif, see, e.g., Takayoshi Oshima, "'Let Us Sleep!' The Motif of Disturbing Resting Deities in Cuneiform Texts," *StMes* 1 (2014): 281–83. In Gilgamesh 12, *qūlu* describes in combination with *šuḫarruru* both the stillness of the deluge and the deathly quiet following it, when *kullat tenēšēti itūrā ana ṭiṭṭi* "all people had turned to clay" (George, *Babylonian Gilgamesh Epic*, 710–11, lines 134–135). On the ambiguity of the categories of noise and silence in Mesopotamian sources, see Peter Machinist, "Rest and Violence in the Poem of Erra," *JAOS* 103 (1983): 221–26; Nicla De Zorzi, "Rumori dalla città: La percezione culturale dei suoni nell' Antica Mesopotamia," in *La città: Realtà e valori simbolici*, ed. Alberto Ellero et al. (Padua: S.A.R.G.O.N, 2011), 1–31; Oshima, "'Let Us Sleep!'"

Conclusions

This paper studies negative value judgments related to sensory perceptions as related in Mesopotamian sources. The various senses are attributed unequal emotional impact. Expressive literature and letters, in which imagery aims at immediate emotional responses, display a certain preponderance of references to smell. The sense of smell is therefore a productive vector for creating insults and for shaming. On the other hand, sight and sound are dominant when it comes to the conscious crafting of images and ratiocination on the implications of unpleasant sensory data. In religious literature, smell plays a significant role only in rituals for the symbolic representation of the divine. In descriptions of the divine, a terminology conveying the concept of overwhelming awe—most often conceived of as visual—dominates; the positive or negative evaluation of such descriptions is context-dependent. Explicitly negative descriptions clearly aim at disgust and revulsion through mostly visual imagery. The final point made, in the discussion of the demons Lamaštu and Pazuzu, concerns imagery evoking sense-deprivation or the absence of sensory input. Such concepts are obviously linked to ideas about death and the netherworld and must be considered one of the most basic types of negative imagery related to the senses in ancient Mesopotamian texts.

Bibliography

Abusch, Tzvi. *The Magical Ceremony Maqlû: A Critical Edition*. Leiden: Brill, 2016.
Alster, Bendt. "On the Sumerian Composition 'The Father and His Disobedient Son.'" *RA* 69 (1975): 81–84.
———. *Proverbs of Ancient Sumer*. Bethesda, MD: CDL, 1997.
Annus, Amar, and Alan Lenzi. *Ludlul Bēl Nēmeqi: The Standard Babylonian Poem of the Righteous Sufferer*. Helsinki: Neo-Assyrian Text Corpus Project: 2010.
Aster, Shawn Z. *The Unbeatable Light: Melammu and Its Biblical Parallels*. Münster: Ugarit-Verlag, 2012.
Berlejung, Angelika. "Tod und Leben nach den Vorstellungen der Israeliten: Ein ausgewählter Aspekt zu einer Metapher im Spannungsfeld von Leben und Tod." Pages 465–502 in *Das biblische Weltbild und seine altorientalischen Kontexte*. Edited by Bernd Janowski and Beate Ego. Tübingen: Mohr Siebeck, 2001.
Biggs, Robert D. "Descent of Ištar, line 104." *NABU* 74 (1993): 58–59.
Böck, Barbara. *Die babylonisch-assyrische Morphoskopie*. AfOB 27. Vienna: Institut für Orientalistik der Universität Wien, 2000.
Borger, Rykle. *Beiträge zum Inschriftenwerk Assurbanipals*. Wiesbaden: Harrassowitz, 1996.
Cassin, Elena. *La Splendeur divine: Introduction à la mentalité mésopotamienne*. Civilisations et Société 8. Paris: Mouton, 1968.
Chapman, Cynthia R. *The Gendered Language of Warfare in the Israelite-Assyrian Encounter*. Winona Lake, IN: Eisenbrauns, 2004.

Clay, Albert T. *Neo-Babylonian Letters from Erech*. YOS 3. New Haven, Yale University Press, 1919.
Clemens, Ashley. "'Looking Mustard': Greek Popular Epistemology and the Meaning of δριμύς." Pages 71–88 in *Synaesthesia and the Ancient Senses*. Edited by Shane Butler and Alex Purves. Durham: Acumen, 2013.
Cooper, Jerrold S. "Virginity in Ancient Mesopotamia." Pages 91–112 in *Sex and Gender in the Ancient Near East*. Edited by Simo Parpola and Robert M. Whiting. RAI 47.2. Helsinki: Neo-Assyrian Text Corpus Project, 2002.
Dalley, Stephanie. *Myths from Mesopotamia: Creation, the Flood, Gilgamesh, and Others*. Oxford: Oxford University Press, 2000.
De Zorzi, Nicla. *La serie teratomantica Šumma izbu: Testo, tradizione, orizzonti culturali*. 2 vols. Padua: S.A.R.G.O.N, 2014.
———. "Of Pigs and Workers: A Note on Lugal-e and a Late Babylonian Commentary on Šumma ālu 49." *NABU* 79 (2016): 131–34.
———. "Of Raving Dogs and Promiscuous Pigs: Mesopotamian Animal Omens in Context." In *Magikon zoon: Animal et magie / The Animal Magic*. Edited by Korshi Dosoo and Jean-Charles Coulon. Turnhout: Brepols, forthcoming.
———. "Rumori dalla città: La percezione culturale dei suoni nell' Antica Mesopotamia." Pages 1–31 in *La città: Realtà e valori simbolici*. Edited by Alberto Ellero et al. Padua: S.A.R.G.O.N, 2011.
———. "Teratomancy at Tigunāmun: Structure, Hermeneutics and Weltanschauung of a Northern Mesopotamian Omen Corpus." *JCS* 69 (2017): 125–50.
Dijk, Jan van, Albrecht Goetze, and Mary I. Hussey. *Early Mesopotamian Incantations and Rituals*. YOS 11. New Haven: Yale University Press, 1985.
Durand, Jean-Marie. *Archives épistolaires de Mari*. ARM 26.1. Paris: Recherche sur les civilisations, 1988.
———. "Tabou et transgression: Le sentiment de la honte." Pages 1–18 in *Tabou et transgression: Actes du colloque organisé par le Collège de France, Paris, les 11–12 avril 2012*. Edited by Jean-Marie Durand, Michaël Guichard, and Thomas Römer. OBO 274. Fribourg: Presses Universitaires; Göttingen: Vandenhoeck & Ruprecht, 2015.
Edzard, Dietz Otto. "Zur Ritualtafel der sogenannten 'Love Lyrics.'" Pages 57–70 in *Language, Literature and History: Philological and Historical Studies Presented to Erica Reiner*. Edited by Francesca Rochberg-Halten. AOS 67. New Haven: American Oriental Society, 1987.
Fales, Mario. "The Enemy in Assyrian Royal Inscriptions: 'The Moral Judgement.'" Pages 425–35 in *Mesopotamien und seine Nachbarn: Politische und kulturelle Wechselbeziehungen im Alten Vorderasien vom 4. bis 1. Jahrtausend v. Chr.* Edited by Hans J. Nissen and Johannes Renger. Berlin: Reimer, 1982.
Farber, Walter. "Lamaštu: Agent of a Specific Disease or a Generic Destroyer of Health?" Pages 137–45 in *Disease in Babylonia*. Edited by Irving L. Finkel and Markham J. Geller. Leiden: Brill, 2007.
———. *Lamaštu: An Edition of the Canonical Series of Lamaštu Incantations and Rituals and Related Texts from the Second and First Millennia B.C.* Winona Lake, IN: Eisenbrauns, 2014.

Feder, Yitzhaq. "Defilement, Disgust, and Disease: The Experiential Basis of Hittite and Akkadian Terms for Impurity." *JAOS* 136 (2016): 99–116.

———. "The Semantics of Purity in the Ancient Near East: Lexical Meaning as a Projection of Embodied Experience." *JANER* 14 (2014): 87–113.

Fincke, Jeanette C. *Augenleiden nach keilschriftlichen Quellen: Untersuchungen zur altorientalischen Medizin*. Würzburger medizinhistorische Forschungen 70. Würzburg: Königshausen & Neumann, 2000.

Flückiger-Hawker, Esther. *Urnamma of Ur in Sumerian Literary Tradition*. OBO 166. Fribourg: Presses Universitaires; Göttingen: Vandenhoeck & Ruprecht, 1999.

Foster, Benjamin. *Before the Muses: An Anthology of the Akkadian Literature*. 3rd ed. Bethesda, MD: CDL, 2005.

———. "Humor and Cuneiform Literature." *JANES* 6 (1974): 69–85.

Foster, Benjamin, and Emmanuelle Salgues. "Everything Except the Squeal: Pigs in Early Mesopotamia." Pages 283–91 in *De la domestication au tabou: Les cas de suidés dans le Proche-Orient ancient*. Edited by Brigitte Lion and Cécile Michel. Paris: de Boccard, 2006.

Frahm, Eckart. *Einleitung in die Sanherib-Inschriften*. AfOB 26. Vienna: Horn, 1997.

———. "Family Matters: Psychohistorical Reflections on Sennacherib and His Times." Pages 163–222 in *Sennacherib at the Gates of Jerusalem*. Edited by Isaac Kalimi and Seth Richardson. Leiden: Brill, 2014.

———. "Humor in assyrischen Königsinschriften." Pages 147–62 in *Intellectual Life of the Ancient Near East: Papers Presented at the 43rd Rencontre Assyriologique Internationale, Prague, July 1–5, 1996*. Edited by Jiří Prosecký. Prague: Oriental Institute, 1998.

Frame, Grant. *Babylonia 689–627 BC: A Political History*. Istanbul: Nederlands Historisch-Archaelogisch Instituut te Istanbul, 1992.

Freedman, Sally. *Tablets 41–63*. Vol. 3 of *If a City Is Set on a Height: The Akkadian Omen Series Šumma Ālu Ina Mēlê Šakin*. Winona Lake, IN: Eisenbrauns, 2017.

Gadotti, Alhena. *"Gilgamesh, Enkidu, and the Netherworld" and the Sumerian Gilgamesh Cycle*. Berlin: de Gruyter, 2014.

Geller, Mark. *Healing Magic and Evil Demons: Canonical Udug-hul Incantations*. Berlin: de Gruyter, 2015.

George, Andrew R. *The Babylonian Gilgamesh Epic: Introduction, Critical Edition, and Cuneiform Texts*. Oxford: Oxford University Press, 2003.

———. "In Search of the É.DUB.BA.A: The Ancient Mesopotamian School in Literature and Reality." Pages 127–37 in *An Ancient Scribe Who Neglects Nothing: Ancient Near Eastern Studies in Honor of Jacob Klein*. Edited by Yitschak Sefati, Pinhas Artzi, Chaim Cohen, Barry L Eichler, and Victor Hurowitz. Bethesda, MD: CDL, 2005.

———. "On Babylonian Lavatories and Sewers." *Iraq* 77 (2015): 75–106.

Groneberg, Brigitte. *Lob der Ištar: Gebet und Ritual an die altbabylonische Venusgöttin "Tanatti Ištar."* Groningen: Styx, 1997.

———. "Philologische Bearbeitung des Agušayahymnus." *RA* 75 (1981): 107–34.

Guichard, Michaël, and Lionel Marti. "Purity in Ancient Mesopotamia: The Paleo-Babylonian and Neo-Assyrian Periods." Pages 47–114 in *Purity and the Forming of*

Religious Traditions in the Ancient Mediterranean and Ancient Judaism. Edited by Christian Frevel and Christophe Nihan. Leiden: Brill, 2013.
Hamilakis, Yannis. *Archaeology and the Senses: Human Experience, Memory, and Affect.* Cambridge: Cambridge University Press, 2013.
Haul, Michael. *Stele und Legende: Untersuchungen zu den keilschriftlichen Erzählwerken über die Könige von Akkade.* Göttingen: Universitätsverlag, 2009.
Heeßel, Nils P. *Pazuzu: Archäologische und philologische Studien zu einem altorientalischen Dämon.* Leiden: Brill, 2002.
Heimpel, Wolfgang. *Letters to the King of Mari: A New Translation, with Historical Introduction, Notes, and Commentary.* Winona Lake, IN: Eisenbrauns, 2003.
Hrůša, Ivan. *Die akkadische Synonymenliste malku = šarru: Eine Textedition mit Übersetzung und Kommentar.* Münster: Ugarit-Verlag, 2010.
Hurowitz, Victor, and Joan Goodnick Westenholz. "LKA 63: A Heroic Poem in Celebration of Tiglat-pileser I's Muṣru-Qumanu Campaign." *JCS* 42 (1990): 1–49.
Jaques, Margaret. *Le Vocabulaire des sentiments dans les textes sumériens: Recherche sur le lexique sumérien et akkadien.* Münster: Ugarit-Verlag, 2006.
Jiménez, Enrique. *The Babylonian Disputation Poems: With Editions of the Series of the Poplar, Palm and Vine, the Series of the Spider, and the Story of the Poor, Forlorn Wren.* Leiden: Brill, 2017.
Johnson, Justin Cale, and Markham Geller. *The Class Reunion: An Annotated Translation and Commentary on the Sumerian Dialogue Two Scribes.* CM 47. Leiden: Brill, 2015.
Jursa, Michael. "Ein Beamter flucht auf Aramäisch: Alphabetschreiber in der spätbabylonischen Epistolographie und die Rolle des Aramäischen in der babylonischen Verwaltung des sechsten Jahrhunderts v. Chr." Pages 379–97 in *Leggo! Studies Presented to Frederick Mario Fales on the Occasion of His Sixty-Fifth Birthday.* Edited by Giovanni B. Lanfranchi et al. Wiesbaden: Harrassowitz, 2012.
———. "Parfüm(rezepte): A. In Mesopotamien." *RlA* 10:335–36.
———. "Räucherung, Rauchopfer: A. In Mesopotamien." *RlA* 11:225–29.
Karlsson, Matthias. *Relations of Power in Early Neo-Assyrian State Ideology.* Berlin: de Gruyter, 2016.
Katz, Dina. "Death They Dispensed to Mankind: The Funerary World of Ancient Mesopotamia." *Historiae* 2 (2005): 55–90.
———. *The Image of the Netherworld in the Sumerian Sources.* Bethesda, MD: CDL, 2003.
Kilmer, Anne D. "How Was Queen Ereshkigal Tricked? A New Interpretation of the Descent of Ishtar." *UF* 3 (1971): 299–309.
Lambert, Wilfred G. *Babylonian Wisdom Literature.* Oxford: Oxford University Press, 1960.
———. "The Problem of the Love Lyrics." Pages 98–135 in *Unity and Diversity: Essays in the History, Literature, and Religion of the Ancient Near East.* Edited by Hans Goedicke and Jimmy J. M. Roberts. Baltimore: John Hopkins University Press, 1975.
Lapinkivi, Pirjo. *The Neo-Assyrian Myth of Ištar's Descent and Resurrection.* Helsinki: Neo-Assyrian Text Corpus Project, 2010.
Lateiner, Donald, and Dimos Spatharas, eds. *The Ancient Emotion of Disgust.* Oxford: Oxford University Press, 2016.

Leick, Gwendolyn. *Sex and Eroticism in Mesopotamian Literature*. London: Routledge, 1994.
Machinist, Peter. "Rest and Violence in the Poem of Erra." *JAOS* 103 (1983): 221–26.
Malul, Meir. "Eating and Drinking (One's) Refuse." *NABU* 99 (1993): 82–83.
Masetti-Rouault, Maria Grazia. "Conceptions de l'autre en Mésopotamie ancienne: Barbarie et différence, entre refus et integration." *Cahiers Kubaba* 7 (2005): 121–41.
Maul, Stefan. "Kurgarrû und Assinnu und ihr Stand in der babylonischen Gesellschaft." Pages 159–72 in *Aussenseiter und Randgruppen: Beiträge zu einer Sozialgeschichte des Alten Orients*. Edited by Volkert Haas. Konstanz: Universitätsverlag, 1992.
Mayer, Walter. "Sargons Feldzug gegen Urartu 714 v. Chr.: Text und Übersetzung." *MDOG* 115 (1983): 65–132.
Meissner, Bruno. *Studien zur assyrischen Lexikographie*. Leipzig: Harrassowitz, 1929.
Mieroop, Marc van de. "The Madness of King Rusa: The Psychology of Despair in Eighth Century Assyria." *Journal of Ancient History* 4 (2016): 16–39.
Milano, Lucio. "Il nemico bestiale: Su alcune connotazioni animalesche del nemico nella letteratura sumero-accadica." Pages 47–67 in *Animali tra zoologia, mito e letteratura nella cultura classica e orientale*. Edited by Ettore Cingano et al. Padua: S.A.R.G.O.N, 2005.
Militarev, Alexander, and Leonid Kogan. *Anatomy of Man and Animals*. Vol. 1 of *Semitic Etymological Dictionary*. Münster: Ugarit-Verlag, 2000.
Nissinen, Martti. *Homoeroticism in the Biblical World: A Historical Perspective*. Philadelphia: Fortress, 1998.
———. *Prophets and Prophecy in the Ancient Near East*. WAW 12. Atlanta: Society of Biblical Literature, 2003.
Oshima, Takayoshi. *Babylonian Poems of Pious Sufferers: Ludlul Bēl Nēmeqi and the Babylonian Theodicy*. Tübingen: Mohr Siebeck, 2014.
———. "'Let Us Sleep!' The Motif of Disturbing Resting Deities in Cuneiform Texts." *StMes* 1 (2014): 271–89.
Parpola, Simo. "Assyrian Library Records." *JNES* 42 (1983): 1–29.
———. "Desperately Trying to Talk Sense: A Letter of Assurbanipal Concerning His Brother Šamaš-šumu-ukin." Pages 227–34 in *From the Upper Sea to the Lower Sea: Studies on the History of Assyria and Babylonia in Honour of A. K. Grayson*. Edited by Grant Frame. Istanbul: Nederlands Historisch-Archaelogisch Instituut te Istanbul, 2004.
Peled, Ilan. *Masculinities and Third Gender: The Origins and Nature of an Institutionalized Gender Otherness in the Ancient Near East*. Münster: Ugarit-Verlag, 2016.
Ponchia, Simonetta, and Mikko Lukko. *The Standard Babylonian Myth of Nergal and Ereškigal*. Helsinki: Neo-Assyrian Text Corpus Project, 2013.
Pongratz-Leisten, Beate. "The Other and the Enemy in the Mesopotamian Conception of the World." Pages 195–231 in *Mythology and Mythologies: Methodological Approaches to Intercultural Influences, Proceedings of the Second Annual Symposium of the Assyrian and Babylonian Intellectual Heritage Project Held in Paris, France, October 4–7, 1999*. Edited by Robert M. Whiting. Melammu Symposia 2. Helsinki: Neo-Assyrian Text Corpus Project, 2001.
Radner, Karen. *Die neuassyrischen Privatrechtsurkunden als Quelle für Mensch und Umwelt*. Helsinki: Neo-Assyrian Text Corpus Project, 1997.

Reiner, Erica. "Another Volume of Sultantepe Tablets." *JNES* 26 (1967): 177–200.
———. "City Bread and Bread Baked in Ashes." Pages 117–20 in *Language and Areas: Studies Presented to George V. Bobrinskoy*. Edited by Howard I. Aronson et al. Chicago: University of Chicago Press, 1967.
———. "Dead of Night." Pages 247–51 in *Studies in Honor of Benno Landsberger on His Seventy-Fifth Birthday, April 21, 1965*. Edited by Hans G. Güterbock and Thorkild Jacobsen. Chicago: University of Chicago Press, 1965.
———. *Your Thwarts in Pieces, Your Mooring Rope Cut: Poetry from Babylonia and Assyria*. Ann Arbor: H. Rackham School of Graduate Studies at the University of Michigan, 1985.
Rendu Loisel, Anne-Caroline. *Les chants du monde: Le paysage sonore de l'ancienne Mésopotamie*. Toulouse: Presse Universitaires du Midi, 2016.
Scurlock, Jo Ann. "On Some Terms for Leatherworking in Ancient Mesopotamia." Pages 171–76 in *Proceedings of the 51st Rencontre Assyriologique Internationale, Held at the Oriental Institute of the University of Chicago, July 18–22, 2005*. Edited by Robert D. Biggs, Jennie Myers, and Martha Tobi Roth. Chicago: Oriental Institute of the University of Chicago, 2008.
Sjøberg, Åke W. "Der Vater und sein missratener Sohn." *JCS* 25 (1973): 113–19.
———. "'He Is a Good Seed of a Dog' and 'Engardu, the Fool.'" *JCS* 24 (1972): 107–19.
Sladek, William R. *Inanna's Descent to the Netherworld*. Ann Arbor: University Microfilms, 1974.
Steinert, Ulrike. *Aspekte des Menschseins im Alten Mesopotamien: Eine Studie zu Person und Identität im 2. und 1. Jt. v. Chr*. Leiden: Brill, 2012.
Stöckl, Jonathan. "Gender Ambiguity in Ancient Near Eastern Prophecy? A Reassessment of the Data behind a Popular Theory." Pages 59–80 in *Prophets Male and Female: Gender and Prophecy in the Hebrew Bible, the Eastern Mediterranean and the Ancient Near East*. Edited by Jonathan Stöckl and Corrine L. Carvalho. Atlanta: Society of Biblical Literature, 2013.
———. *Prophecy in the Ancient Near East: A Philological and Sociological Comparison*. Leiden: Brill, 2012.
Stol, Marten. *Women in the Ancient Near East*. Berlin: de Gruyter, 2016.
Streck, Michael. "Notes on the Old Babylonian Hymns of Agušaya." *JAOS* 130 (2010): 561–71.
———. "The Pig and the Fox in Two Popular Sayings from Aššur." Pages 789–92 in *Leggo! Studies Presented to Frederick Mario Fales on the Occasion of His Sixty-Fifth Birthday*. Edited by Giovanni B. Lanfranchi et al. Wiesbaden: Harrassowitz, 2012.
Steymans, Hans U. *Deuteronomium 28 und die adê zur Thronfolgeregelung Asarhaddons: Segen und Fluch im Alten Orient und in Israel*. Göttingen: Vandenhoeck & Ruprecht, 1995.
Tadmor, Hayim. *The Inscriptions of Tiglath-pileser III, King of Assyria: Critical Edition, with Introductions, Translations and Commentary*. Jerusalem: Israel Academy of Sciences and Humanities, 1994.
Tambiah, Stanley J. "Form and Meaning of Magical Acts," Pages 60–86 in *Culture Thought, and Social Action: An Anthropological Perspective*. Cambridge, MA: Harvard University Press, 1985.

———. *Magic, Science and Religion and the Scope of Rationality*. Cambridge, MA: Harvard University Press, 1990.
Tigay, Jeffrey H. *The Evolution of the Gilgamesh Epic*. Philadelphia: University of Philadelphia Press, 1982.
Toner, Jerry, ed. *A Cultural History of the Senses in Antiquity*. London: Bloomsbury, 2016.
Toorn, Karel van der. *Sin and Sanction in Israel and Mesopotamia: A Comparative Study*. Assen: Van Gorcum, 1985.
Tudeau, Johanna. "Meaning in Perspective: Some Akkadian Terms for 'Foundation' *uššu, temennu, išdu, duruššu*." Pages 631–50 in *At the Dawn of History: Ancient Near Eastern Studies in Honour of J. N. Postgate*. Edited by Yağmur Heffron, Adam Stone, and Martin Worthington. Winona Lake, IN: Eisenbrauns, 2017.
Veenhof, Klaas R. "Mari A 450: 9 f. (ARM 26/1, p. 378 note 13)." *NABU* (1989): 27.
Veldhuis, Niek. "The Heartgrass and Related Matters." *OLP* 21 (1990): 27–44.
———. "The Fly, the Worm and the Chain." *OLP* 24 (1993): 41–64.
Villard, Pierre. "Le chien dans la documentation néo-assyrienne." Pages 235–49 in *Les animaux et les hommes dans le monde syro-mésopotamien aux époques historiques*. Edited by Dominique Parayre et al. Topoi Supp. 2. Paris: de Boccard, 2000.
Volk, Konrad. "Edubba'a und Edubba'a Literatur: Rätsel und Lösungen." *ZA* 90 (2000): 1–30.
Walker, Christopher B. F. "The Second Tablet of Tupšenna Pitema, an Old Babylonian Naram-Sin Legend?" *JCS* 33 (1981): 191–95.
Wasserman, Nathan. *Akkadian Love Literature of the Third and Second Millennium BCE*. Wiesbaden: Harrasowitz, 2016.
———. "On Leeches, Dogs and Gods in Old Babylonian Medical Incantations." *RA* 102 (2008): 71–88.
Westenholz, Joan Goodnick. "Inanna and Ištar in the Babylonian World." Pages 332–47 in *The Babylonian World*. Edited by Gwendolyn Leick. New York: Routledge, 2007.
———. *Legends of the Kings of Akkade: The Texts*. Winona Lake, IN: Eisenbrauns, 1997.
Wiggermann, Frans. "Lamaštu, Daughter of Anu: A Profile." Pages 217–52 in *Birth in Babylonia and the Bible: Its Mediterranean Setting*. By Marten Stol. Groningen: Styx, 2000.
Zawadzki, Stefan. "Depicting Hostile Rulers in the Neo-Assyrian Royal Inscriptions." Pages 767–78 in *From Source to History: Studies on the Ancient Near Eastern Worlds and Beyond Dedicated to Giovanni Battista Lanfranchi on the Occasion of His Sixty-Fifth Birthday on June 23, 2014*. Edited by Salvatore Gaspa et al. Münster: Ugarit-Verlag, 2014.
Ziegler, Nele. *Les musiciens et la musique d'après les archives de Mari*. Paris: SEPOA, 2007.
Zsolnay, Ilona. "The Misconstrued Role of the Assinnu in Ancient Near Eastern Prophecy." Pages 81–99 in *Prophets Male and Female: Gender and Prophecy in the Hebrew Bible, the Eastern Mediterranean and the Ancient Near East*. Edited by Jonathan Stöckl and Corrine L. Carvalho. Atlanta: Society of Biblical Literature, 2013.
Zwickel, Wolfgang. *Räucherkult und Räuchergeräte: Exegetische und archäologische Studien zum Räucheropfer im Alten Testament*. OBO 97. Fribourg: Presses Universitaires; Göttingen: Vandenhoeck & Ruprecht, 1990.

Laying Foundations for Eternity: Timing Temple Construction in Assyria

Kiersten Neumann

Introduction

The construction of an Assyrian temple followed a well-organized sequence of actions, each of which was marked by singular materials and activities. For example, an auspicious time had to be determined by way of divination, words were recited in the form of incantations and prayers, liquids were poured as libation, foundation materials were deposited, and monumental doorways and parapets were erected for the superstructure. Such an ambitious project demanded the participation of expert scholars and craftsmen and, at times, the king himself, and it was materialized by the selection of local and exotic raw materials and masterfully crafted works of art. A study of the sensory experience afforded by the amalgamation of these elements, as well as aspects of affectivity within the temple built environment, offers a powerful avenue for exploring the actual mechanisms by which ritualization took place and the way in which sensory experience created an embodied population. In such an exploration, senses ought to first be understood as extending beyond the hierarchical five-sense framework that is rooted in Western philosophy; and second, the senses ought to be considered from a contextual approach, because sense-making experiences are intricately connected and constituted by a person's active cultural and social context and memory. One of the fundamental practices of the Assyrian temple—construction and renovation—is here explored from a less common avenue for investigating the role of the senses in antiquity, the sense of time. Drawing on the preserved material culture and textual evidence, this paper argues that the perception of time associated with temple construction marked this activity as ritualized practice within an Assyrian elite performative landscape.

A Sense of Time

The sense of time—also referred to as time perception or perception of duration—is not dominant in discussions of the sensorium in antiquity. Time is more commonly spoken of as something physical that can be measured chronometrically. Stoic philosophers of the Hellenistic period were among the earliest to leave a written record of ruminations of the lived experience of time and an attempt to develop a theory of time perception.[1] Today perceiving and experiencing time continues as a core discussion in the fields of philosophy, psychology, and cognitive science, where it is understood, on the one hand, as something that is subjectively experienced and perceived—"our senses present their perceptions to us in the order of time; it is through these perceptions that we participate in the general flow of time which passes through the universe, producing event after event"[2]—and, on the other hand, as something that is objectively quantifiable and measurable. Metaphors for time vary across cultures and languages. The conscious here-and-now is a direct experience that is limited to a few seconds; "we thus remain in an eternal Now, perceiving continually its flowing into the past."[3] There is also independent time, which according to Newton is "of itself, and from its own nature, flows equally without relation to anything external."[4] The term Mental Time Travel (MTT) refers to humans' "ability to mentally navigate through time—thinking about the past, present, and future."[5] With the last, time is often envisioned as an arrow, a linear perception of time that is to be distinguished from cyclical time, or the "wheel of time," that is found in many Eastern traditions such as Hinduism, as well as Egyptian and Mayan traditions.[6] Like other sensory stimuli, "time perception is part of our embodied reality, which means

---

[1] Robert Heller, "Innovators in Thought: The Stoics on Time Perception," *Procedia: Social and Behavioral Sciences* 126 (2014): 273–74; Panayiotis Tzamalikos, "Origen and the Stoic View of Time," *JHI* 52 (1991): 535–61.

[2] Sachchidanan Hiranand Vatsyayan, *A Sense of Time: An Exploration of Time in Theory, Experience and Art* (Delhi: Oxford University Press, 1981), 6.

[3] Vatsyayan, *Sense of Time*, 6.

[4] Isaac Newton, *Sir Isaac Newton's Mathematical Principles of Natural Philosophy and His System of the World* (Berkeley: University of California Press, 1962), 6.

[5] Baptiste Gauthier and Virginie van Wassenhove, "Distance Effects in Mental Space and Time Travels," *Procedia: Social and Behavioral Sciences* 126 (2014): 176–77; Thomas Suddendorf and Michael C. Corballis, "The Evolution of Foresight: What Is Mental Time Travel, and Is It Unique to Humans?," *The Behavioral and Brain Sciences* 30 (2007): 299–313.

[6] Gerald James Whitrow, *What Is Time? The Classic Account of the Nature of Time* (Oxford: Oxford University Press, 2004).

humans are able to perceive time in a non-numerical unconscious way."[7] However, since there is no dedicated sensory organ for time perception, our sense of time is relational; it is measured by other sensory phenomena, such as visual, auditory, and emotional states, as the world around us changes.[8] As such, time perception is at home in discussions of the role of the senses in antiquity, and though not directly observable in material culture because it is a cognitive function, it can be discerned through the reconstruction of people's interactions with objects and the environment and, when available, from textual sources.

Discussions of time in ancient Mesopotamia have drawn primarily from this last group—texts written in Akkadian and Sumerian that were primarily recorded on clay tablets using the cuneiform script—with explorations of chronology, calendrical systems, days of labor, astronomical and divinatory compositions, mathematical models, genealogies, and scholarly corpora, to name a few. Ulla Susanne Koch uses the metaphor of a three-dimensional piece of cake for the Mesopotamian conception of time in her study of divinatory texts, finding linear and cyclical metaphors unfitting.[9] Eleanor Robson has explored issues of temporality in scholarly writing from Assyria and Babylonia, showing the importance of temporal qualifications and calendrical systems to the historical record.[10] Both scholars also recognize the importance of subdivisions of time, or "chronometric entities," as demonstrated by Mesopotamian hemerologies—calendar texts concerned with auspicious/inauspicious and prescriptive/prognostic dates for carrying out particular activities—and the creation myth Enuma Elish, in which the divine protagonist—Marduk in Babylonia and Aššur in Assyria—fixes the stars as markers of the year and months, each star representing a god.[11] Taking a

---

[7] Sven Sulzmann, "Time Perception: An Exploration of Time Perception and Possible Applications in Cognitive Archaeology," *UC Merced Undergraduate Research Journal* 6 (2014): 102.

[8] Robin Le Poidevin, "The Experience and Perception of Time," in *The Stanford Encyclopedia of Philosophy* (Summer Edition 2015): https://plato.stanford.edu/entries/time-experience/.

[9] Ulla Susanne Koch, "Concepts and Perception of Time in Mesopotamian Divination," in *Time and History in the Ancient Near East: Proceedings of the Fifty-Sixth Recontre Assyriologique Internationale at Barcelona, 26–30 July, 2010*, ed. L. Feliu, Jaume Llop, and A. Millet Albà (Winona Lake: Eisenbrauns, 2017), 127–42.

[10] Eleanor Robson, "Counting the Days: Scholarly Conceptions and Quantifications of Time in Assyria and Babylonia, c. 750–250 BC," in *Time and Temporality in the Ancient World*, ed. R. M. Rosen (Philadelphia: University Museum Press, 2004), 45–90.

[11] Alasdair Livingstone, *Hemerologies of Assyrian and Babylonian Scholars* (Bethesda: CDL Press, 2013); Leonard William King, *The Seven Tablets of Creation or, The Babylonian and Assyrian Legends Concerning the Creation of the World and of Mankind* (London: Luzac, 1902).

hermeneutical approach, Àngel Rajadell argues that, in contrast to a Cartesian linear time conception with a forward progression (the future in front and the past behind), the Mesopotamian chronological conception of time was sequential ("a character of *consecutiveness*, being the essence of time the one-after-another itself") with the past in front and the future—a thing of mystery and imagination—behind.[12]

With this paper, I hope to build upon this scholarship by appreciating time as a sensory phenomenon and demonstrating how this particular cognitive aspect of the sensorium was one process by which ritualization took place in the ancient world.[13] Using as my case study the construction of the Neo-Assyrian temple, I argue that the sensory experience of time particular to this practice marked it as something Other and meaningful within an Assyrian cultural and social context.

TEMPLE CONSTRUCTION IN ASSYRIA

The Neo-Assyrian Empire of the early first millennium BCE—located in northern Mesopotamia, present day northern Iraq—had an administrative capital that shifted from the city of Assur (modern Qala'at Sherqat) to Kalḫu (modern Nimrud), then Dur-Šarrukin (modern Khorsabad), and Nineveh (modern Mosul including the mounds Kuyunjik and Nebi Yunus), though past capitals remained important for reasons of continuity and their resident divinities. This mix of tradition and development led to the construction of temples—the gods' houses on earth though not places of worship—at a number of imperial cities. As the high-priest of the god Aššur and principle benefactor of the temples of Assyria, the Neo-Assyrian king assumed responsibility for this work. Master craftsmen and scholarly experts (*ummânu*s) helped in this endeavor in order to ensure the king's

---

[12] Àngel Rajadell, "Mesopotamian Idea of Time through Modern Eyes (Disruption and Continuity)," in Feliu, Llop, and Albà, *Time and History in the Ancient Near East*, 211–28. Gonzalo Rubio articulates this orientation of the past and future: "The Akkadian word for 'future' (*warkītu*) derives from the same root of the noun meaning 'back, behind' (*warkatu*).... The noun meaning 'past' (*pānītu*) originates in the word 'front' (*pānu*)." Gonzalo Rubio, "Time before Time: Primeval Narratives in Early Mesopotamian Literature," in Feliu, Llop, and Albà, *Time and History in the Ancient Near East*, 11–12; see further, Christopher Woods, "At the Edge of the World: Cosmological Conceptions of the Eastern Horizon in Mesopotamia," *JANER* 9 (2009): 209–10.

[13] In this study, ritual is approached as a strategic mode of acting that ritualizes and inflects the practice itself and associated materials, drawing on Catherine Bell's notions of ritualization. Catherine M. Bell, *Ritual Theory, Ritual Practice* (New York: Oxford University Press, 1992).

safety and protection, a responsibility that is articulated by the phrase *maṣṣartu ša šarri naṣāru* ("to keep the king's watch").[14]

One concept of time that the practice of temple construction presents is sequential and quantifiable, with an emphasis on the distant postdiluvian past and recent past, and the near and distant future (fig. 1). This time-sense is espoused most articulately by textual sources related to temple construction.

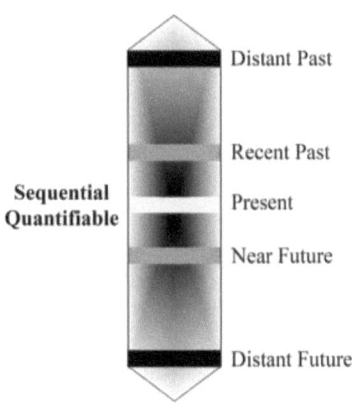

Fig. 1. Illustration of the sequential quantifiable time-sense

Contrasting this sequential time-sense is the way in which the individual experienced time during actual practice. Reconstructed from preserved material culture and texts, this subjective experience of time was shaped by the present—the conscious here-and-now—that simultaneously activated a divine unquantifiable time-

---

[14] Simo Parpola, *Letters from Assyrian and Babylonian Scholars*, SAA 10 (Helsinki: The Neo-Assyrian Text Corpus Project, 1993), XXI–XXII. On the *ummânus*, see Giovanni B. Lanfranchi, "Scholars and Scholarly Tradition in Neo-Assyrian Times: A Case Study," *SAAB* 3.2 (1989): 99–114; Lorenzo Verderame, "Il ruolo degli 'esperti' (*ummânu*) nel periodo neo-assiro" (PhD diss., Università di Roma La Sapienza, 2004); idem, "La formazione dell'esperto (*ummânu*) nel periodo neo-assiro," *Historiae* 5 (2008): 51–67; Verderame, "A Glimpse into the Activities of Experts (*ummânu*) at the Assyrian Court," in *From Source to History: Studies on Ancient Near Eastern Worlds and Beyond, Dedicated to Giovanni Battista Lanfranchi*, ed. Salvatore Gaspa et al., AOAT 412 (Münster: Ugarit-Verlag, 2014), 713–28; Davide Nadali and Lorenzo Verderame, "Experts at War: Masters behind the Ranks of the Assyrian Army," in *Krieg und Frieden im Alten Vorderasien. 52e Rencontre Assyriologique Internationale; International Congress of Assyriology and Near Eastern Archaeology, Münster, 17.–21. Juli 2006*, ed. Hans Neumann et al., AOAT 401 (Münster: Ugarit-Verlag, 2013), 553–66.

sense (fig. 2). I begin with the Assyrian conceptualization of sequential quantifiable time that is presented by the textual sources. In addition to alluding to a sequential time-sense through the very words that are employed, the textual sources allow for the reconstruction of the stages of temple construction into an order of events and actions that in itself is sequential and quantifiable.[15]

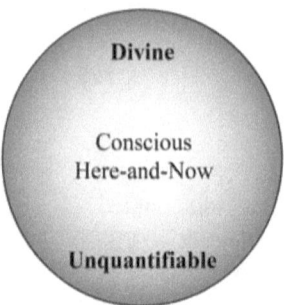

Fig. 2. Illustration of the divine unquantifiable time-sense

Sequential Quantifiable Time

Temple construction began with the king's motivation for the project. Cited reasons include, if a temple could no longer serve its purpose, whether it had suffered intentional destruction, natural disaster, was too small, or too old; if a king wanted to build a temple for the prosperity of the land, for his own life, or for future admiration; if the gods had personally requested temple work to be performed; or simply, if a king's heart moved him to do so—in a boastful manner, certain kings credit "their superior imaginations"[16] as the primary catalyst for their temple work. Such explanatory passages convey a sequential time-sense because of their

---

[15] The following section provides an overview of the stages of temple construction during the Neo-Assyrian period. For more detailed accounts with references to Mesopotamian sources, see Sylvie Lackenbacher, *Le palais sans rival: Le récit de construction en Assyrie* (Paris: La Découverte, 1990); Claus Ambos, "Building Rituals from the First Millennium BC: The Evidence from the Ritual Texts," in *From the Foundations to the Crenellations: Essays on Temple Building in the Ancient Near East and Hebrew Bible*, ed. Mark J. Boda, AOAT 366 (Münster: Ugarit-Verlag, 2010), 221–38; Jamie R. Novotny, "Temple Building in Assyria: Evidence from Royal Inscriptions," in Boda, *From the Foundations to the Crenellations*, 109–40; as well as Richard S. Ellis, *Foundation Deposits in Ancient Mesopotamia* (New Haven: Yale University Press, 1968), 6–7; Brigitte Menzel, *Assyrische Tempel*, StPohl 10 (Rome: Biblical Institute Press, 1981).

[16] Ellis, *Foundation Deposits in Ancient Mesopotamia*, 7.

emphasis on the past and future. An inscription of Sennacherib reads, "May any future ruler, whom (the god) Aššur names for shepherding the land and people (and) during whose reign that temple becomes dilapidated, renovate its dilapidated section(s)."[17]

Next, the king obtained divine consent in order to ensure that the project was in harmony with the plans of the gods. With the aid of the diviner (*bārû*), this approval could be obtained through extispicy, the examination of the entrails of a sacrificial animal; the observation of celestial signs and movements; and less frequently through lecanomancy, the observation of oil in a bowl of water.[18] Divination in Mesopotamia in itself relied upon complex concepts of time.[19] When the construction of a temple was the matter of inquiry, the diviner asked in the present for signs from the gods to appear in the very near future in order to determine if constructing a temple in the more distant near future was a good idea. When rebuilding Ešarra, the temple of the god Aššur in the city of Assur, Esarhaddon (r. 680–669 BCE) makes explicit the divine approval he received: "I was worried, afraid, (and) hesitant about renovating that temple. In the diviner's bowl, the gods Šamaš and Adad answered me a firm 'yes' and they had (their response) concerning the (re)building of that temple (and) the renovation of its cultroom written on a liver."[20] Hemerologies and omen collections were also consulted in order to determine an auspicious time for construction. The series *Iqqur īpuš* ("he demolished, he built") lists favorable times: "If in the month Nisannu the king of the land builds a house of a god, or restores an temple of the land, or gives a gift to a god, or celebrates the *akītu*-festival, or celebrates the *urubātu*-ceremony (of

---

[17] Sennacherib 10.23–25 (RINAP 3.1:82–83).

[18] On the divination corpus associated with the practice of the *bārû*, see Alan Lenzi, *Secrecy and the Gods: Secret Knowledge in Ancient Mesopotamia and Biblical Israel*, SAAS 19 (Helsinki: Neo-Assyrian Text Corpus Project, 2008), 77–84; on extispicy, see Ivan Starr, Jussi Aro, and Simo Parpola, *Queries to the Sungod: Divination and Politics in Sargonid Assyria*, SAA 4 (Helsinki: Helsinki University Press, 1990), XXXVI–LV; see further, Beate Pongratz-Leisten, *Herrschaftswissen in Mesopotamien: Formen der Kommunikation zwischen Gott und König im 2. und 1. Jahrtausend v. Chr.*, SAAS 10 (Helsinki: The Neo-Assyrian Text Corpus Project, 1999), on the modes of communication between the king and gods, which could also include prophecy, dreams, astronomical omens, and hepatoscopy.

[19] "The perception and manipulation of events anywhere in time in the frame of the divinatory process is part of the underlying human cognitive mechanics—detecting agency, reading indexical signs and communicating to gain vital information about events, intentions and actions past, present and future all suspended in time simultaneously. In divination time is not so much perceived as an arrow as a three dimensional piece of cake" (Koch, "Concepts and Perception of Time in Mesopotamian Divination," 220).

[20] Esarhaddon 57.iii.42–iv.6 (RINAP 4:125).

his god's house), the prayers of his land will be in the heart of the god."[21] These listed auspicious times are quantifiable times in the near future, named months and days, that conform to a sequential time-sense. Reaffirming this quality of time is the common expression "in a favorable month, on a propitious day," which is frequently found in passages referencing this stage of temple construction.

Once consent had been obtained and an auspicious time determined, preparations of the building site could begin. This step entailed the identification of preexisting temple architecture and the performance of the ceremony of *libittu maḫrītu* ("first/former brick"). Texts tell of the king locating and removing the *libittu maḫrītu* from the ruins while laments for the destruction of the previous building were recited.[22] As Richard Ellis asserts, "the single brick embodied the essence of the god's home and bridged the gap between the destruction of the old building and the foundation of the next."[23] Considering the material context of a fallen temple, it is reasonable to assume that this practice, which would have taken place many years if not decades after the previous temple's initial construction, would have made use of a former brick, which came to symbolize the true first brick and thus the temple as a whole through the special treatment it received as part of ritualized practice. An inscribed brick of the ninth-century king Shalmaneser III (r. 858–824 BCE) from Ešarra shows that he found a brick of his predecessor Adad-nerari I (r. 1305–1274 BCE), who constructed the same temple in the fourteenth century; the texts are close to verbatim, except for name and genealogy, and were used in the same forecourt of the temple.[24] An excerpt from

---

[21] René Labat, *Un calendrier babylonien des travaux, des signes et des mois (Séries iqqur îpuš)* (Paris: Librairie Honoré Champion, 1965), §32, 1–3. Similarly, *Šumma ālu* ("If a city is situated on a height"), a collection of terrestrial omens that could be observed in a city, including those related to construction; Sally Freedman, *Tablets 1–21*, vol. 1 of *If a City Is Set on a Height: The Akkadian Omen Series Šumma ālu ina mēlê šakin* (Philadelphia: University of Pennsylvania, 1998); Freedman, *Tablets 22–40*, vol. 2 of *If a City Is Set on a Height: The Akkadian Omen Series Šumma ālu ina mēlê šakin* (Philadelphia: University of Pennsylvania, 2006); Nils P. Heeßel, *Divinatorische Texte I: Terrestrische, teratologische, physiognomische und oneiromantische Omina* (Wiesbaden: Harrassowitz Verlag, 2007); Heeßel, *Divinatorische Texte II: Opfershau-Omina* (Wiesbaden: Harrassowitz Verlag, 2012).

[22] Ritual instructions from the Seleucid period give the most detailed account of this practice, for example, Claus Ambos, *Mesopotamische Baurituale aus dem 1. Jahrtausend v. Chr* (Dresden: Islet, 2004), II.D.1.3 (O.174//W.20030/15, BE.13987), though earlier references suggest that it was likely carried out during the Neo-Assyrian period as well (Esarhaddon 57.v.25 [RINAP 4:126]); see further, Ellis, *Foundation Deposits in Ancient Mesopotamia*, 29; Ambos, *Mesopotamische Baurituale*, 66–67, 77–78.

[23] Ellis, *Foundation Deposits in Ancient Mesopotamia*, 29.

[24] Shalmaneser III A.0.102.53 (RIMA 3:133–34); Adad-nerari I A.0.76.35 (RIMA 1:167). Robson notes a similar material connection between foundation inscriptions of

an inscription of Aššurbanipal (r. 668–627 BCE) on his reconstruction of Esagil in Babylon provides a textual parallel for this practice: "If at any time in the future, during the days of the reign of some future prince, this work falls into disrepair, may (that prince) repair its dilapidated state! May he write my name with his (own) name! May he look at my royal inscription, anoint (it) with oil, offer a sacrifice, (and) set (my royal inscription back) in its place! The god Marduk will (then) hearken to his prayers."[25]

The subsequent step in the sequence of construction entailed the removal of all preexisting temple remains; as Aššurnaṣirpal II (r. 883–859 BCE) states regarding his preparations for temples at Kalḫu, "I cleared away the old ruin hill (and) dug down to the water level. I sank (the foundation) 120 layers deep."[26] This activity was both practical and purifying, as it cleansed the space of contamination and evil of the past. Passages in the omen series *Šumma ālu* ("If a city is situated on a height") and *Iqqur īpuš* state that the discovery of prestigious materials in the foundations of a fallen house could result in the new owner's lack of prosperity, poverty, or even death.[27] In order to eliminate their affective quality, ritual experts either scattered preexisting foundation materials in rivers, a liminal and ritually pure space,[28] or carried out apotropaic practices at the site. For example, earlier texts of the Sumerian kings Ur-Bau and Gudea tell of both kings purifying a temple's building site with fire.[29]

The next stage included making offerings to the gods and placing foundation deposits. Royal inscriptions include the types of prestigious and organic substances used as offerings and the reasons for this act, for example, to ensure a successful building for the resident divinity and the safety and eternal recognition

---

Esarhaddon and the thirteenth-century king Shalmaneser I (r. 1273–1244 BCE), which describe their rebuilding of Ešarra (Esarhaddon 57.iii.16–41 [RINAP 4:125]; Shalmaneser I A.0.77.2.5–13, 21–24 (RIMA 1:189); see Robson, "Counting the Days," 58–59.

[25] Ashurbanipal B.6.32.6.26–30 (RIMB 2:207); similarly, Esarhaddon 104.vii.19–29 (RINAP 4:201).

[26] Aššurnaṣirpal II A.0.101.32.9 (RIMA 2:296).

[27] Freedman, *Tablets 1–21*, 83–85; Labat, *Un calendrier babylonien des travaux*, §6; Ambos, "Building Rituals from the First Millennium BC," 230–31.

[28] Ambos, *Mesopotamische Baurituale*, II.A.3 E_1 (*Enūma uššē bīt amēli tanamdû*) (K 3664+); see Ambos, *Mesopotamische Baurituale*, 9 on the use of these ritual instructions for a temple as well as the house of a man.

[29] Ur-Bau E3/1.1.6.5.ii.8–iii.2 (RIM 3.1:19); Gudea E3/1.1.7.StC.iii.6–7 (RIM 3.1:39); see further, Ellis, *Foundation Deposits in Ancient Mesopotamia*, 9–10, 17.

of the king as builder, both directed at the future.³⁰ The text, "Tablet for the materials needed in order to lay the foundations of a house of a god: When you are laying the foundations of a house of a god,"³¹ provides a detailed sequence of actions to be performed for creating and depositing seventeen foundation figurines, including when to obtain the clay and when to recite incantations. Foundation inscriptions similarly embody a sequential time-sense, calling out the past and future. An example is an inscription of Esarhaddon on his rebuilding of Ešarra, in which the king, emulating a text of his predecessor Shalmaneser I (r. 1273–1244), credits the temple's earliest inception to Ušpia, a king of the distant past.³² Robson argues that the inclusion of specific temporal quantifications between reconstructions in royal inscriptions demonstrates the skill with which Assyrian scholars harnessed the historical record.³³ An example of the elongation of the temporal dimension in the opposite direction, with references to future iterations of the building and the king's requisition of respectful treatment of his inscription, is Aššurbanipal's inscription on his rebuilding of Esagil in Babylon, quoted above.

The subsequent stage of construction entailed the manufacturing of bricks and laying of foundations. In general mudbricks were created in Sivan (May–June) following the spring rains and in time for the dry summer months.³⁴ In addition to the basic mixture of soil, water, and organic materials for tampering, some kings claim to have included materials of greater value in their bricks, for example oils, resins, and wine, and of using molds made of prestigious materials

---

[30] For example, "In a favorable month, on a propitious day, I laid its foundations with limestone, a strong mountain stone, over gold, silver, stones, antimony, all kinds of aromatics, *pūru*-oil, fine oil, honey, ghee, beer, (and) wine, (and) laid (them) on bedrock" (Esarhaddon 57.v.3–14 [RINAP 4:126]).

[31] Ambos, *Mesopotamische Baurituale*, II.C.2 (*Ṭuppi ḫišiḫti uššē bīt ili epēšu enūma uššē bīt ili tanamdû*) (K2000+).

[32] Ušpia is among the first group of kings listed in the Assyria King List, who are said to have "lived in tents"; Mogens Trolle Larsen, *The Old Assyrian City-State and Its Colonies* (Copenhagen: Akademisk Forlag, 1976), 34–37.

[33] Robson, "Counting the Days," 61.

[34] Novotny, "Temple Building in Assyria," 119. Sivan is written using the logograph for brick, SIG_4, and is described in an inscription of Sargon as the "month of Kulla, because of the molding of bricks and the building of city and house (which are done then)"; see David G. Lyon, *Keilschrifttexte Sargon's Königs von Assyrien (722–705 v. Chr.)* (Leipzig: Hinrichs, 1883), 9–10, translation in Daniel D. Luckenbill, *Historical Records of Assyria from Sargon to the End*, vol. 2 of *Ancient Records of Assyria and Babylonia* (Chicago: University of Chicago Press, 1927), 64, §120; also, Ellis, *Foundation Deposits in Ancient Mesopotamia*, 18, app. A, no. 14. Kulla was the god of brickmaking and of laying the foundations.

in order to form the bricks.³⁵ Once the building materials were in hand, the first brick (*libittiu maḫrītu*) was placed; as Esarhaddon states: "For the preservation of my life, the lengthening of my days, I carried the first brick on my neck and (then) laid its foundations and secured its brickwork."³⁶ Laying the first brick reinforced continuity with the temple of the recent past through the performance of this same act, while also setting up the opportunity for future rulers to continue this tradition. Though the texts tell of the removal of preexisting architecture, kings nonetheless claim to lay the new foundations in line with those of their predecessors: "I opened up its dirt piles and surveyed (and) examined its layout. I measured its foundation in accordance with its earlier plan. I did not add a single brick more."³⁷

Subsequent activity concentrated on erecting the temple superstructure, stages about which the textual sources are less vocal. The creation of doorways stands as an exception. In the Mesopotamian world doors were places of liminality and vulnerability—the evil and threatening entities of the world could pass through such an "interruption in a wall"³⁸ if the proper measures were not taken to block their entry. To counter this threat, the ritual instructions, "when the doorframe is mounted,"³⁹ prescribe the ritual expert to follow a particular sequence of actions: to cleanse and nourish himself in the evening and the following morning, to make offerings and libations to the gods at the door of the cultroom in preparation for mounting the doorframe. Another text with instructions for rebuilding a door prescribes offerings and libations to be made three times: the night before, the morning of, and after completion. The final lines convey the purpose of this practice: "You will perform these deeds and the god will bring peace to the king, the house (of the god), the land (and) the city. The evil of that door will not approach the king."⁴⁰ These prescribed actions firmly call out a sequential time-sense, referencing the very near future of the ritual expert's activities and the more distant future of the success and life of the temple and its builder, the king. Textual sources also mention a final exorcism and purification of the temple structure

---

³⁵ Esarhaddon 57.iv.16–26 (RINAP 4:125–26); Essad Nassouhi, "Prisme d'Assurbânipal daté de sa trentième année, provenant du temple de Gula à Babylone," *AfK* 2 (1924–1925): 100, I.16–17; also, Shalmaneser III A.0.102.10.iv.51–55 (RIMA 3:56) on Shalmaneser III's work on the walls of Assur. See further, Ellis, *Foundation Deposits in Ancient Mesopotamia*, 30, for references from earlier and later periods in Mesopotamia.

³⁶ Esarhaddon 57.v.23–28 (RINAP 4:126).

³⁷ Esarhaddon 113.24–26 (RINAP 4:230).

³⁸ Damerji's characterization of a door perfectly communicates its vulnerable aspect, as a break within an otherwise solid and secure feature of a building, see Muayad Said Basim Damerji, *The Development of the Architecture of Doors and Gates in Ancient Mesopotamia* (Tokyo: Institute for Cultural Studies of Ancient Iraq, Kokushikan University, 1987), 53.

³⁹ Ambos, *Mesopotamische Baurituale*, II.C.3 (*Enūma sippū kunnū*) (K 3810).

⁴⁰ Ambos, *Mesopotamische Baurituale*, II.D.2, 38–39a (ST II 232).

prior to the (re)installation of the divine images, actions that similarly looked towards the future.[41]

The emphasis of the textual sources on these stages of temple construction suggests that what mattered to the Assyrians, with respect to the idealized recorded practice, was the ordered sequence of actions that promised the future success of the temple while simultaneously grounding it in the recent and distant past. In actual practice this idealized scheme would have been adapted to the immediate context of use; however, the fact that it was intentionally recorded communicates the significance of this time-sense in an Assyrian context of practice. This begs the question, how then was time experienced during actual practice? Though likely aware of the idealized sequence of actions that embodied a sequential quantifiable time-sense, time perception for participants in the actual act of temple construction would have been a subjective experience that entailed the conscious here-and-now and which activated a divine unquantifiable time-sense—a distinct experience that set apart and ritualized this act.

Divine Unquantifiable Time

The divine unquantifiable time-sense draws on the concept from Mesopotamian mythology of an antediluvian time, as presented in the cosmogony Enuma Elish, that at first consisted of the Apsû, freshwater, and Tiamat, salt water, and later included a group of early gods. The Apsû is described as a spatial and temporal domain below the earth, a realm of primeval purity that the god Ea eventually made his home and where his wife gave birth to the god Marduk. While both were underground, the Apsû was distinct from the netherworld, the gloomy domain of the dead. Also belonging to the antediluvian time were the *apkallu*s, primeval sages who "represent the wisdom and magical skills of a vanished cosmos."[42] The *apkallu*s are described as "pure," as is the Apsû that they occupy.[43] From a separate mythical tradition though also of the antediluvian time are the *Mischwesen*, demonic creatures who made up Tiamat's army in the battle against Marduk, when the latter was vying for supremacy of the universe.[44] This battle led to the

---

[41] Ambos, *Mesopotamische Baurituale*, II.A.1, A₁ and B (K 3397+, K 4592+).

[42] Mehmet-Ali Ataç, *The Mythology of Kingship in Neo-Assyrian Art* (Cambridge: Cambridge University Press, 2010), 148.

[43] Luigi Cagni, *The Poem of Erra* (Malibu, CA: Undena, 1977), 34; Ataç, *Mythology of Kingship*, 152.

[44] Dieter Kolbe, *Die Reliefprogramme Religiös-Mythologischen Charakters in Neu-Assyrischen Palästen* (Frankfurt: Lang, 1986); Frans Anton Maria Wiggermann, "Mischwesen. A," *RlA* 8:222–45; Anthony Green, "Mischwesen. B. Archäologie. Mesopotamien," *RlA* 8:246–64; Ataç, *Mythology of Kingship*, 145–202; Karen Sonik, "Mesopotamian Conceptions of the Supernatural: A Taxonomy of *Zwischenwesen*," *Archiv für Religionsgeschichte* 14 (2013): 103–16.

phenomenon of the flood, which in turn brought an end to this primeval time, the cosmic cataclysm or benchmark as termed by Mehmet-Ali Ataç, after which the earth, humans, and quantifiable time were created.[45] In this postdiluvian world order, the *apkallus* passed down their knowledge to a group of human masters, the *ummânus*.[46] As stated by Ataç, "these [*apkallu*s] beings are seemingly dead, but in the mythopoeic imagination, they are alive and active in the cosmos in an invisible manner";[47] passing down their knowledge was one way in which they remained active.

The divine unquantifiable time-sense that was activated in temple construction by way of particular actions and/or divine elements drew on this antediluvian tradition. Like the *apkallu*s and *Mischwesen*, this time was ever-present and independent in the Assyrian conceptualization of the world. Four scenarios from temple construction stand as example of the activation of a divine unquantifiable time-sense: preparing for and laying foundations, foundation deposits, foundation figurines, and the installation of doorways.

Cited above is an inscription of Aššurnaṣirpal in which the king emphasizes the depth to which he sank a temple's foundations. Additional texts speak to the transgression of temple foundations into the Apsû or the domain of the netherworld gods. For example, Sargon II (r. 721–705 BCE) states that when he reconstructed Nergal's temple in Cutha, he laid the foundations on the dais like a mountain, the term for dais, *kigallu*, being used symbolically to mean the netherworld as "the base of the earth."[48] Esarhaddon elaborates by referring both to the heavens and the Apsû: "Ešarra, the residence of the god Assur, my lord, to the sky. I raised its top.... Its top was high (and) reached the heavens; below, its foundations were entwined with the Apsû."[49] When rebuilding Esagil, Esarhaddon acknowledges Nudimmud, an alternate name for Ea, god of the Apsû.[50] Similarly, the netherworld god Enmešarra is included in the ritual instructions, "When you lay the foundations (of a temple)."[51] When digging into the earth in preparation for laying the foundations, workers would have perceived the conscious here-and-now through the change in their surrounding environment: the visual change of the dirt, or increasing lack of dirt, below their feet; their position relative to the surface level and daylight above; the change in smell and temperature due to the

---

[45] Ataç, *Mythology of Kingship*, 151.
[46] See n. 14.
[47] Ataç, *Mythology of Kingship*, 197.
[48] Sargon II B.6.22.3.i.39–40 (RIMB 2:148).
[49] Esarhaddon 57.v.31–38.vi.20–27 (RINAP 4:126–27).
[50] Esarhaddon 105.v.23–28 (RINAP 4:206). On Nudimmud, see Antoine Cavigneaux and Manfred Krebernik, "Nudimmud," *RlA* 9:607.
[51] Ambos, *Mesopotamische Baurituale*, II.A.2 (Enūma IM.DÙ.A tapattiqu) (K 48+).

increasing moisture and humidity as they moved deeper into the earth. The archival photograph of the mudbrick and stone foundations of the Isthar temple in Assur during the excavations of the Deutsche Orient-Gesellschaft relays this sense of depth (fig. 3). These sensory phenomena resonate with Assyrian conceptions of the subterranean realms into which the workmen were transgressing, whether the Apsû, as the ever-present freshwater ocean that lay beneath the earth, or the gloomy depths of the netherworld, thereby activating a divine unquantifiable time-sense.

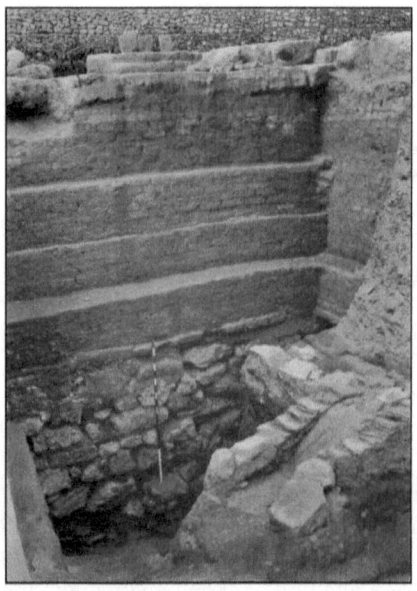

Fig. 3. Stone and mudbrick foundations of the Aššur temple in Assur taken during the excavations of the Deutsche Orient-Gesellschaft. Walter Andrae, *Das wiedererstandene Assur* (Leipzig: Hinrichs, 1938), pl. 41a.

The conceptual association between the depths of the earth and the antediluvian domain is reaffirmed by the use of foundation deposits as a means of pacifying the gods into whose realm the temple foundations penetrated. The selection of what materials to include as offerings was guided by their efficacy to consecrate a site, each raw material having a unique agency within an Assyrian context of practice. In other words, these materials were not placed in the foundations as a reflection of the existing sacredness of a space, but rather, to quote Kim Benzel from her discussion of the Temple Oval foundation material of Khafajah in southern Mesopotamia, as "a perceived means of animating or activating the very foundation of the building to become sacred."⁵² Drawing primarily on evidence from Hittite ritual instructions, Claus Ambos suggests that such materials were intended to embody as a whole the antediluvian primeval temple built by the gods, of which all later temples were reincarnations.⁵³ From the Neo-Assyrian period is a literary text written to the gods Nabu and Tašmetu, in which the scribe refers to a lapis-lazuli door bolt in the goddess Tašmetu's bedroom.⁵⁴ An explanatory work attributed to the ritual expert Kiṣir-Aššur states that the upper, middle, and lower heavens were made of semi-precious stones and that the god Bel sits in a house in the middle heaven upon a dais of lapis-lazuli under the light of a lamp of *elmešu*-stone.⁵⁵ The same text identifies burning *erēnu*-wood as the decaying flesh of evil gods, while another text, similarly attributed to Kiṣir-Aššur, states that the sweetened cake offered by the king to the gods is the heart of Ea.⁵⁶ Another explanatory work, dated to the Seleucid period, ascribes to wood, stone, and plant affective qualities through their association with specific deities, a tradition that stretches back to much earlier periods in Mesopotamia.⁵⁷

Such imaginative, metaphorical, and enlightening texts relay how the materials used in foundation deposits—for example, beads, cylinder seals, and inscriptions crafted from semi-precious stones and precious metals, as well as cakes, incense, and resins—were conceived of as material references to the primeval temple or as representative of aspects of the gods themselves. What is more, in Assyria qualities such as shine, luminosity, and radiance embodied an element of the divine, what is called in Akkadian *melammu*, a "supernatural awe-inspiring sheen."⁵⁸ This vital life-force, as termed by Irene Winter, was "transferred from gods to material and manifest as light" and had "a particular affective emotional impact upon the observer" that likely evoked in the Assyrians states of fear, disorientation, and awe.⁵⁹ Of this synonymity between divine radiance and astral luminosity, Francesca Rochberg cites an address to the god Šamaš: "you, Šamaš,

---

⁵² Kim Benzel, "Puabi's Adornment for the Afterlife: Materials and Technologies of Jewelry at Ur in Mesopotamia" (PhD diss., Columbia University, 2013), 51.
⁵³ Ambos, *Mesopotamische Baurituale*, 50–51.
⁵⁴ SAA 3:14.
⁵⁵ SAA 3:39.
⁵⁶ SAA 3:39, r.24–25; SAA 3:37, 23'.
⁵⁷ Joseph Epping and Johann N. Strassmaier, "Neue babylonische Planetentafeln," *ZA* 6 (1891): 228, 241–44; Alasdair Livingstone, *Mystical and Mythological Explanatory Works of Assyrian and Babylonian Scholars* (Oxford: Clarendon, 1986), 73.
⁵⁸ CAD 10.2:9–12, s.v. "melammu" (ME.LÁM).
⁵⁹ Irene Winter, "Radiance as an Aesthetic Value in the Art of Mesopotamia," in *Art: The Integral Vision; A Volume of Essays in Felicitation of Kapila Vatsyayan*, ed. Madhu Khanna, S. C. Malik, and Baidyanath Saraswati (New Delhi: Printworld, 1994), 124.

have covered the heavens and all the countries with your radiance (*melammu*)."⁶⁰ Of the projection of this radiance to the world, Rochberg continues: "The brilliance and luminosity of a celestial body was seen as emblematic of its divine quality, and as a physical phenomenon such luminosity made the divine manifest in the world." Terms denoting light, shine, brilliance, radiance, and awe, for example, are used in descriptions of heavenly bodies and the gods themselves, while metaphors are used to associate these qualities with raw materials, objects, and temples. Lapis lazuli in particular was associated with divine radiance because of its uniquely dark, lustrous appearance.⁶¹ Gold and silver buttons from a foundation deposit box in Nabu's temple at Kalḫu⁶² and tablets of precious metals from Sargon's palace at Dur-Šarrukin inscribed with the text, "I wrote my name on tablets of gold, silver, copper, tin, lead, lapis lazuli, and alabaster, and I deposited (them) in their (several palaces') foundations"⁶³—these are examples of deposits that would have activated a divine unquantifiable time-sense because of their "supernatural awe-inspiring sheen" for those individuals handling them during temple construction.

Foundation figurines accompanied these deposits in the foundations of a temple (fig. 4). Crafted of various materials, ideally in accordance with prescribed instructions, these figurines took the form of antediluvian *apkallu*s and *Mischwesen*, as well as lesser gods (figs. 5–6).⁶⁴ Interacting with these finished forms—materializations of powerful antediluvian entities—at the time of deposition would

---

⁶⁰ Francesca Rochberg, "'The Stars Their Likeness': Perspectives on the Relation Between Celestial Bodies and Gods in Ancient Mesopotamia," in *What Is a God? Anthropomorphic and Non-Anthropomorphic Aspects of Deity in Ancient Mesopotamia*, ed. Barbara N. Porter (Winona Lake: Eisenbrauns, 2009), 49, citing Stephen Langdon, *Babylonian Penitential Psalms* (Paris: Geuthner, 1927), 52:9.

⁶¹ Irene Winter, "The Aesthetic Value of Lapis Lazuli in Mesopotamia," in *Cornaline et pierres précieuses: La Méditerranée, de l'Antiquité à l'Islam; Actes du colloque organisé au Musée du Louvre par le Service culturel, les 24 et 25 novembre 1995*, ed. Annie Caubet, Conférences et colloques, Musée du Louvre (Paris: La documentation Française, 1999), 49.

⁶² Max Edgar Lucien Mallowan, *Nimrud and Its Remains* (London: British School of Archaeology in Iraq, 1966), 90–91.

⁶³ Victor Place, *Ninive et l'Assyrie* (Paris: Imprimerie impériale, 1867–1870), I, 61–62, III, pl. 77; Ellis, *Foundation Deposits in Ancient Mesopotamia*, 102.

⁶⁴ Frans Anton Maria Wiggermann, *Mesopotamian Protective Spirits: The Ritual Texts* (Groningen: STYX & PP Publications, 1992); Aaron W. Schmitt, "Deponierungen von Figuren bei der Fundamentlegung assyrischer und babylonischer Tempel," in *Mesopotamische Baurituale aus dem 1. Jahrtausend v. Chr*, ed. Claus Ambos (Dresden: Islet, 2004), 229–34; Carolyn Nakamura, "Mastering Matters: Magical Sense and the Figurine Worlds of Neo-Assyria," in *Archaeologies of Materiality*, ed. Lynn Meskell (Oxford: Blackwell, 2005), 18–45.

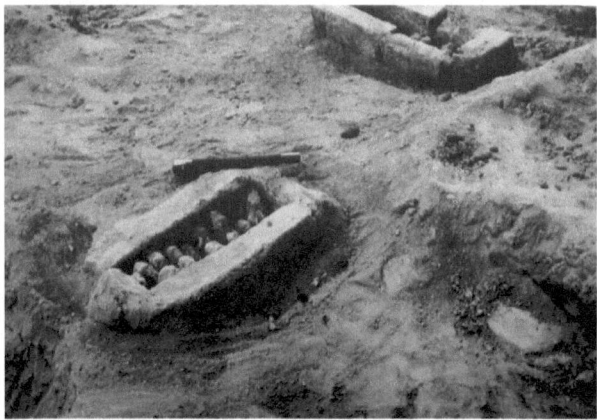

Fig. 4. Brick capsule with fish-*apkallu* figurines from the Haus des Beschwörungspriesters at Assur. Walter Andrae, *Das wiedererstandene Assur* (Leipzig: Hinrichs, 1938), pl. 7.

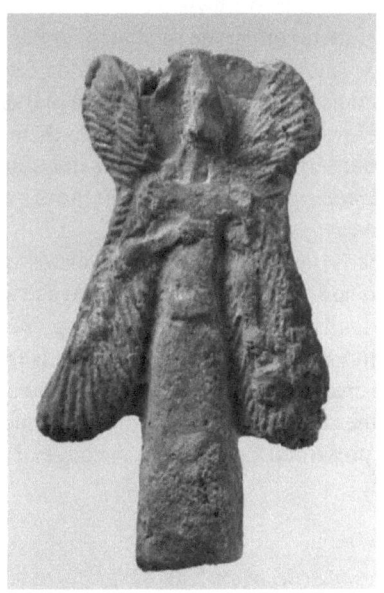
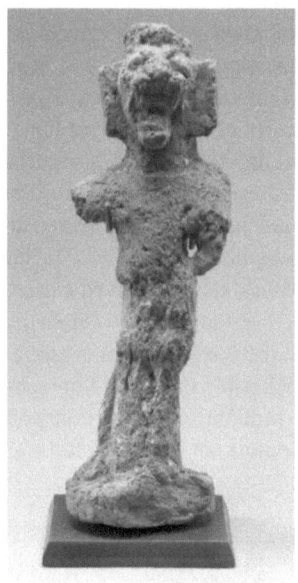

Fig. 5 (left). Bird-headed *apkallu* figurine, Kalḫu (54.117.26). The Metropolitan Museum of Art, New York.

Fig. 6 (right). *ugallu* (lion-headed demon) figurine, Khorsabad (N8287). © Musée du Louvre, dist. RMN-GP / Pierre et Maurice Chuzeville.

have activated in individuals a sense of the divine unquantifiable time; so too during their manufacturing. Ritual instructions ascribe this task to the *ummânu*s, the expert scholars and descendants of the *apkallu*s who acquired their skill and knowledge through "the study and mastery of an extensive technical lore ... the foundations of which were believed to have been laid by the gods themselves."[65] In drawing on this antediluvian wisdom in order to fashion creatures of the Apsû, the *ummânu*s would have activated the divine unquantifiable time-sense that was again evoked when the figurines were placed in subterranean boxes.

The installation of doorways—the last example of a phase of temple construction that activated the divine unquantifiable time-sense—presents similarities to the antediluvian powers of foundation figurines and the *melammu* qualities of materials used in foundation deposits. As noted above, doorways were conceived of as liminal spaces, as vulnerable openings in walls that, if not properly secured, allowed evil influences, demons, and diseases entry into a building. As liminal spaces, doorways existed between time, or rather, were a space where time could be said to stand still, in itself a concept that resonates with an unquantifiable time-sense.

Marking the doorways of Neo-Assyrian temples were visible compliments—mythological guardian figures either cast of metal or carved of stone—to the apotropaic figurines deposited near doorways. An inscription of Esarhaddon reads, "*šēdu*s and *lamassu*s of stone, whose appearance repels the breast of the evil one, protectors of the path, guardians of the walkway of the king, who made them, to the left and the right of its doorjambs, I had installed."[66] Monumental stone carvings of mythological figures, including *lamassu*s (winged bulls or lions) and *apkallu*s, have been excavated at temple doorways at Kalḫu (fig. 7).[67]

As with their smaller figurine counterparts, the creation of these doorway figures would have involved expert craftsmen and scholars who would have drawn on their antediluvian wisdom in order to craft these guardians and to presence within the worked metal or stone the antediluvian entities. A series of panels from Sennacherib's palace at Nineveh depict the creation of a stone *lamassu* at a quarry in the mountains and its transport back to the capital city (fig. 8).[68] Mountains in Mesopotamian literary tradition are often presented as places on the edge of the

---

[65] Parpola, *Letters from Assyrian and Babylonian Scholars*, XIII–XIV.

[66] Esarhaddon 2.v.27–32 (RINAP 4:33–34); further, Esarhaddon 77.10–11 (RINAP 4:155); Sennacherib 17.vi.30–36 (RINAP 3.1:139).

[67] Kiersten Neumann, *Resurrected and Reevaluated: The Neo-Assyrian Temple as a Ritualized and Ritualizing Built Environment* (PhD diss., University of California, Berkeley, 2014), 190, figs. 42–43, 45, 109, 144–45.

[68] John Malcolm Russell, "Bulls for the Palace and Order in the Empire: The Sculptural Program of Sennacherib's Court VI at Nineveh," *Art Bulletin* 69 (1987): 520–39.

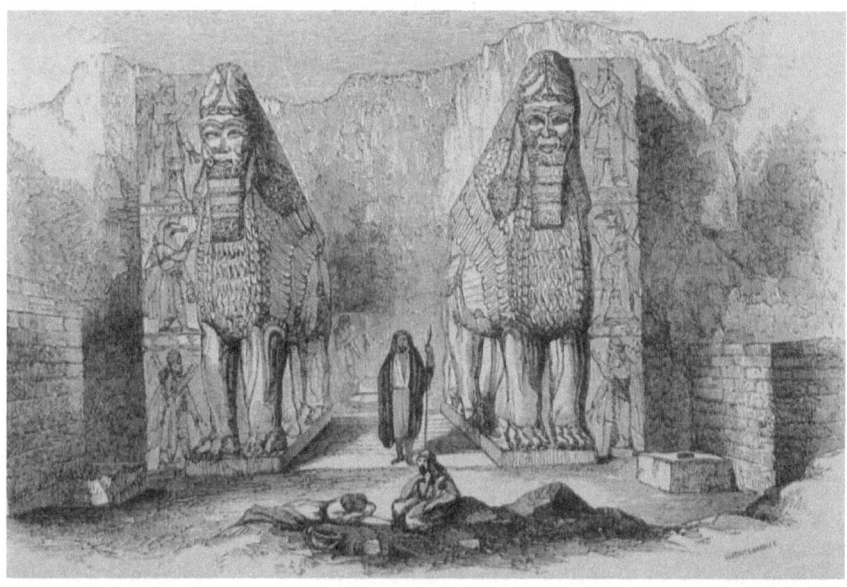

Fig. 7. Drawing of the entrance to the Ninurta temple including stone *lamassu*s and *apkallu*s, Kalḫu. Austen H. Layard, *Discoveries among the Ruins of Nineveh and Babylon* (New York: Harper & Brothers, 1853), 300.

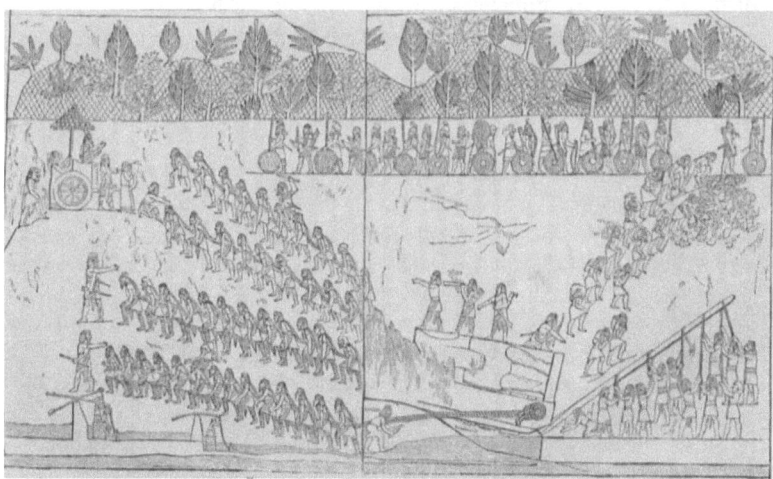

Fig. 8. Drawing of the wall reliefs from Court VI, Southwest Palace of Sennacherib, Nineveh. Austen H. Layard, *Discoveries among the Ruins of Nineveh and Babylon* (New York: Harper & Brothers, 1853), 93.

earth that challenge the sense of cosmic order; for example, the mountainous setting of the battle between the god Ninurta and the demon Asag and his army of stones, or the twin-mountain Mashu to which the epic hero Gilgamesh travels in search of immortality. The crafting of stone *lamassu*s in the mountains, a landscape associated with divine conflict and earth's edge, may well have heightened the experience of the divine unquantifiable time-sense that was already ignited by the very practice of fashioning antediluvian creatures.

Additional architectural components from the doorways of Neo-Assyrian temples contributed to the activation of the divine unquantifiable time-sense. An experientially mindful passage from Esarhaddon's inscriptions reads, "On doors of *šurmēnu*-wood whose fragrance is sweet, I fastened bands of gold, and installed (them) in its doorways."[69] Bronze and gold relief fragments that once decorated wooden door poles and door leaves were recovered in the temples of Dur-Šarrukin and Imgur-Enlil (modern Balawat, fig. 9).[70] Complementing the metal bands at Dur-Šarrukin were polychromatic glazed-brick panels at the base of the temple façades (fig. 10).[71] Similar to certain foundation materials, the awe-inspiring radiance of the metal bands and glazed-brick panels would have manifest divine *melammu*—a modern viewer can well imagine the blinding brilliance of these materials as the sunlight reflected off of their surfaces. Also activating a divine unquantifiable time-sense was the specialized skill of antediluvian origins that would have been called upon in order to create such masterful works, including the chosen imagery.[72] Julian Reade and Irving Finkel proposed a rebus-writing interpretation for the glazed-brick panels from the temples of Dur-Šarrukin with each of the horizontally arranged elements standing for a word: the royal figure for Sargon, the lion for king, the bird for great, the bull for king, the fig-tree for land, the seeder-plough for Assur, and the human figure for the determinative earth, land; the full sequence would read: "Sargon, Great King, King of the Land

---

[69] Esarhaddon 60.22'–23' (RINAP 4:136).

[70] Eleanor Guralnick, "Bronze Reliefs from Khorsabad," in *Proceedings of the 51st Rencontre Assyriologique Internationale*, ed. Robert D. Biggs, Jennie Myers, and Martha Tobi Roth (Chicago: University of Chicago Press), 389–404.

[71] Place, *Ninive et l'Assyrie*; Gordon Loud, *Khorsabad I: Excavations in the Palace and at a City Gate*, OIP 38 (Chicago: University of Chicago Press, 1936); Gordon Loud and Charles B. Altman, *Khorsabad II: The Citadel and the Town*, OIP 40 (Chicago: University of Chicago Press, 1938).

[72] Kiersten Neumann, "Reading the Temple of Nabu as a Coded Sensory Experience," *Iraq* 80 (2018): 181–211. For a scientific study of the raw materials used for pigments, see Vanessa Muros, Vicki Parry, and Alison Whyte, "Conservation Laboratory Research Projects," *The Oriental Institute News & Notes* 175 (2002): 1–8; Alison Whyte, Vanessa Muros, and Sarah Barack, "'Brick by Brick': Piecing Together an Eighth Century B.C. Facade from Iraq," *AIC Objects Speciality Group Postprints* 11 (2004): 172–89.

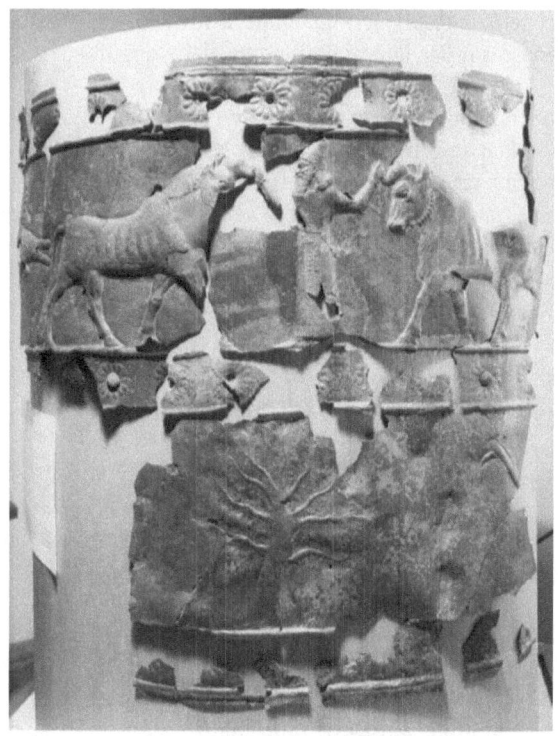

Fig. 9. Embossed bronze bands from the Šamaš temple, Dur-Šarrukin (A12468). Courtesy of the Oriental Institute of the University of Chicago.

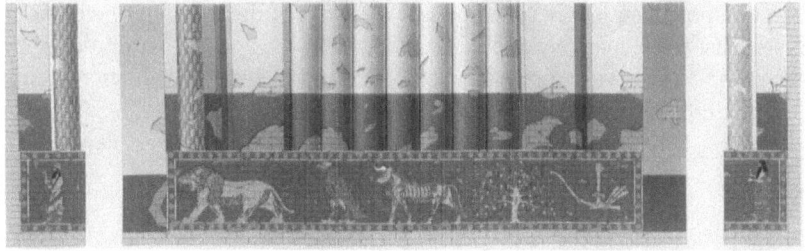

Fig. 10. Drawing of the glazed-brick panels from the Sin temple, Dur-Šarrukin. Victor Place, *Ninive et l'Assyrie* (Paris: Imprimerie impériale, 1867–1870), III, pl. 26.

of Assyria."[73] The color scheme of the yellow astroglyphs against a dark blue background further suggests possible connections with the constellations. Reade and Finkel propose similar interpretations for decoding the designs of the metal relief bands.

Studies from cognitive science have shown that subjective time is affected by emotionality and that fear and awe in particular arouse a person's internal clock. Thinking of this impact with respect to the four scenarios from temple construction here outlined, it would be reasonable to suggest that the experience of awe, wonder, perhaps even fear, related to the activation of a divine unquantifiable time-sense would have had a profound impact on a person's perception of the conscious here-and-now, the experience passing by quicker as one's internal clock sped up. Much more could be said about time perception as experienced during the installation of a divine statue in the temple and subsequent celebrations—a sensorial exploration that is worthy of its own paper.

Conclusion

Questions of the experience and perception of time offer a rich avenue for exploring how people model, interact with, and process the world around them. Investigations of this nature can enrich our understanding of the ways in which the conceptualization and prioritization of this sense-making experience helped to ritualize practice in the ancient world. The elaborate practice of temple construction during the Neo-Assyrian period exhibits, as demonstrated by material and textual evidence, multiple senses of time that together marked this practice as something other and meaningful within the Neo-Assyrian royal landscape. The commonality between the textual sources of different kings and the parallels found in the ritual instructions and omen collections affirm the importance that a sequential quantifiable time-sense had in an idealized conception of temple-construction practices. Yet in actual practice, aspects of the conscious here-and-now experience were complemented and enhanced by the activation of a divine unquantifiable time-sense, presencing the gods and the awe and emotional high of the antediluvian realm in the here-and-now on earth.

---

[73] Julian E. Reade, "The Khorsabad Glazed Bricks and Their Symbolism," in *Khorsabad, le palais de Sargon II, roi d'Assyrie: Actes du colloque organisé au musée du Louvre par le Services culturel les 21 et 22 janvier 1994*, ed. Annie Caubet (Paris: La Documentation française, 1995), 225–51; Irving L. Finkel and Julian E. Reade, "Assyrian Hieroglyphs," *ZA* 86 (1996): 244–68.

BIBLIOGRAPHY

Ambos, Claus. "Building Rituals from the First Millennium BC: The Evidence from the Ritual Texts." Pages 221–38 in *From the Foundations to the Crenellations: Essays on Temple Building in the Ancient Near East and Hebrew Bible*. Edited by Mark J. Boda. AOAT 366. Münster: Ugarit-Verlag, 2010.
Andrae, Walter. *Mesopotamische Baurituale aus dem 1. Jahrtausend v. Chr.* Dresden: Islet, 2004.
———. *Das wiedererstandene Assur*. Leipzig: Hinrichs, 1938.
Ataç, Mehmet-Ali. *The Mythology of Kingship in Neo-Assyrian Art*. Cambridge: Cambridge University Press, 2010.
Bell, Catherine M. *Ritual Theory, Ritual Practice*. New York: Oxford University Press, 1992.
Benzel, Kim. "Puabi's Adornment for the Afterlife: Materials and Technologies of Jewelry at Ur in Mesopotamia." PhD diss., Columbia University, 2013.
Cagni, Luigi. *The Poem of Erra*. Malibu, CA: Undena, 1977.
Cavigneaux, Antoine, and Manfred Krebernik. "Nudimmud." *RlA* 9:607.
Damerji, Muayad Said Basim. *The Development of the Architecture of Doors and Gates in Ancient Mesopotamia*. Tokyo: Institute for Cultural Studies of Ancient Iraq, Kokushikan University, 1987.
Ellis, Richard S. *Foundation Deposits in Ancient Mesopotamia*. New Haven: Yale University Press, 1968.
Epping, Joseph, and Johannes N. Strassmaier. "Neue babylonische Planetentafeln." *ZA* 6 (1891): 217–44.
Finkel, Irving L., and Julian E. Reade. "Assyrian Hieroglyphs." *ZA* 86 (1996): 244–68.
Freedman, Sally. *Tablets 1–21*. Vol. 1 of *If a City Is Set on a Height: The Akkadian Omen Series Šumma ālu ina mēlê šakin*. Philadelphia: University of Pennsylvania, 1998.
———. *Tablets 22–40*. Vol. 2 of *If a City Is Set on a Height: The Akkadian Omen Series Šumma ālu ina mēlê šakin*. Philadelphia: University of Pennsylvania, 2006.
Gauthier, Baptiste, and Virginie van Wassenhove. "Distance Effects in Mental Space and Time Travels." *Procedia: Social and Behavioral Sciences* 126 (2014): 176–77.
Green, Anthony. "Mischwesen. B. Archäologie. Mesopotamien." *RlA* 8:246–64.
Guralnick, Eleanor. "Bronze Reliefs from Khorsabad." Pages 389–404 in *Proceedings of the 51st Rencontre Assyriologique Internationale*. Edited by Robert D. Biggs, Jennie Myers, and Martha Tobi Roth. Chicago: University of Chicago Press.
Heeßel, Nils P. *Divinatorische Texte I: Terrestrische, teratologische, physiognomische und oneiromantische Omina*. Wiesbaden: Harrassowitz Verlag, 2007.
———. *Divinatorische Texte II: Opfershau-Omina*. Wiesbaden: Harrassowitz Verlag, 2012.
Heller, Robert. "Innovators in Thought: The Stoics on Time Perception." *Procedia: Social and Behavioral Sciences* 126 (2014): 273–74.
King, Leonard William. *The Seven Tablets of Creation or, The Babylonian and Assyrian Legends Concerning the Creation of the World and of Mankind*. London: Luzac, 1902.
Koch, Ulla Susanne. "Concepts and Perception of Time in Mesopotamian Divination." Pages 127–42 in *Time and History in the Ancient Near East: Proceedings of the Fifty-*

Sixth Recontre Assyriologique Internationale at Barcelona, 26–30 July, 2010. Edited by L. Feliu, Jaume Llop, and A. Millet Albà. Winona Lake: Eisenbrauns, 2017.
Kolbe, Dieter. *Die Reliefprogramme Religiös-Mythologischen Charakters in Neu-Assyrischen Palästen.* Frankfurt: Lang, 1986.
Labat, René. *Un calendrier babylonien des travaux, des signes et des mois (Séries iqqur îpuš).* Paris: Librairie Honoré Champion, 1965.
Lackenbacher, Sylvie. *Le palais sans rival: Le récit de construction en Assyrie.* Paris: La Découverte, 1990.
Lanfranchi, Giovanni B. "Scholars and Scholarly Tradition in Neo-Assyrian Times: A Case Study." *SAAB* 3.2 (1989): 99–114.
Langdon, Stephen. *Babylonian Penitential Psalms.* Paris: Geuthner, 1927.
Larsen, Mogens Trolle. *The Old Assyrian City-State and Its Colonies.* Copenhagen: Akademisk Forlag, 1976.
Layard, Austen H. *Discoveries among the Ruins of Nineveh and Babylon.* New York: Harper & Brothers, 1853.
Le Poidevin, Robin. "The Experience and Perception of Time." In *The Stanford Encyclopedia of Philosophy* (Summer Edition 2015): https://plato.stanford.edu/entries/time-experience/
Lenzi, Alan. *Secrecy and the Gods: Secret Knowledge in Ancient Mesopotamia and Biblical Israel.* SAAS 19. Helsinki: Neo-Assyrian Text Corpus Project, 2008.
Livingstone, Alasdair. *Hemerologies of Assyrian and Babylonian Scholars.* Bethesda: CDL Press, 2013.
———. *Mystical and Mythological Explanatory Works of Assyrian and Babylonian Scholars.* Oxford: Clarendon, 1986.
Loud, Gordon. *Khorsabad I: Excavations in the Palace and at a City Gate.* OIP 38. Chicago: University of Chicago Press, 1936.
Loud, Gordon, and Charles B. Altman. *Khorsabad II: The Citadel and the Town.* OIP 40. Chicago: University of Chicago Press, 1938.
Luckenbill, Daniel D. *Historical Records of Assyria from Sargon to the End.* Vol. 2 of *Ancient Records of Assyria and Babylonia.* Chicago: University of Chicago Press, 1927.
Lyon, David G. *Keilschrifttexte Sargon's Königs von Assyrien (722–705 v. Chr.).* Leipzig: Hinrichs, 1883.
Mallowan, Max Edgar Lucien. *Nimrud and Its Remains.* London: British School of Archaeology in Iraq, 1966.
Menzel, Brigitte. *Assyrische Tempel.* StPohl 10. Rome: Biblical Institute Press, 1981.
Muros, Vanessa, Vicki Parry, and Alison Whyte. "Conservation Laboratory Research Projects." *The Oriental Institute News & Notes* 175 (2002): 1–8.
Nadali, Davide, and Lorenzo Verderame. "Experts at War: Masters behind the Ranks of the Assyrian Army." Pages 553–66 in *Krieg und Frieden im Alten Vorderasien. 52e Rencontre Assyriologique Internationale; International Congress of Assyriology and Near Eastern Archaeology, Münster, 17.–21. Juli 2006.* Edited by Hans Neumann et al. AOAT 401. Münster: Ugarit-Verlag, 2013.
Nakamura, Carolyn. "Mastering Matters: Magical Sense and the Figurine Worlds of Neo-Assyria." Pages 18–45 in *Archaeologies of Materiality.* Edited by Lynn Meskell. Oxford: Blackwell, 2005.

Nassouhi, Essad. "Prisme d'Assurbânipal daté de sa trentième année, provenant du temple de Gula à Babylone." *AfK* 2 (1924–1925): 97–106.
Neumann, Kiersten. "Reading the Temple of Nabu as a Coded Sensory Experience." *Iraq* 80 (2018): 181–211.
———. *Resurrected and Reevaluated: The Neo-Assyrian Temple as a Ritualized and Ritualizing Built Environment*. PhD diss., University of California, Berkeley, 2014.
Newton, Isaac. *Sir Isaac Newton's Mathematical Principles of Natural Philosophy and His System of the World*. Berkeley: University of California Press, 1962.
Novotny, Jamie R. "Temple Building in Assyria: Evidence from Royal Inscriptions." Pages 109–40 in *From the Foundations to the Crenellations: Essays on Temple Building in the Ancient Near East and Hebrew Bible*. Edited by Mark J. Boda. AOAT 366. Münster: Ugarit-Verlag, 2010.
Parpola, Simo. *Letters from Assyrian and Babylonian Scholars*. SAA 10. Helsinki: The Neo-Assyrian Text Corpus Project, 1993.
Place, Victor. *Ninive et l'Assyrie*. Paris: Imprimerie impériale, 1867–1870.
Pongratz-Leisten, Beate. *Herrschaftswissen in Mesopotamien: Formen der Kommunikation zwischen Gott und König im 2. und 1. Jahrtausend v. Chr.* SAAS 10. Helsinki: The Neo-Assyrian Text Corpus Project, 1999.
Rajadell, Àngel. "Mesopotamian Idea of Time through Modern Eyes (Disruption and Continuity)." Pages 211–28 in *Time and History in the Ancient Near East: Proceedings of the Fifty-Sixth Rencontre Assyriologique Internationale at Barcelona, 26–30 July, 2010*. Edited by L. Feliu, Jaume Llop, and A. Millet Albà. Winona Lake: Eisenbrauns, 2017.
Reade, Julian E. "The Khorsabad Glazed Bricks and Their Symbolism." Pages 225–51 in *Khorsabad, le palais de Sargon II, roi d'Assyrie: Actes du colloque organisé au musée du Louvre par le Services culturel les 21 et 22 janvier 1994*. Edited by Annie Caubet. Paris: La Documentation française, 1995.
Robson, Eleanor. "Counting the Days: Scholarly Conceptions and Quantifications of Time in Assyria and Babylonia, c. 750–250 BC." Pages 45–90 in *Time and Temporality in the Ancient World*. Edited by R. M. Rosen. Philadelphia: University Museum Press, 2004.
Rochberg, Francesca. "'The Stars Their Likeness': Perspectives on the Relation Between Celestial Bodies and Gods in Ancient Mesopotamia." Pages 41–91 in *What Is a God? Anthropomorphic and Non-Anthropomorphic Aspects of Deity in Ancient Mesopotamia*. Edited by Barbara N. Porter. Winona Lake: Eisenbrauns, 2009.
Rubio, Gonzalo. "Time before Time: Primeval Narratives in Early Mesopotamian Literature." Pages 3–17 in *Time and History in the Ancient Near East: Proceedings of the Fifty-Sixth Rencontre Assyriologique Internationale at Barcelona, 26–30 July, 2010*. Edited by L. Feliu, Jaume Llop, and A. Millet Albà. Winona Lake: Eisenbrauns, 2017.
Russell, John Malcolm. "Bulls for the Palace and Order in the Empire: The Sculptural Program of Sennacherib's Court VI at Nineveh." *Art Bulletin* 69 (1987): 520–39.
Schmitt, Aaron W. "Deponierungen von Figuren bei der Fundamentlegung assyrischer und babylonischer Tempel." Pages 229–34 in *Mesopotamische Baurituale aus dem 1. Jahrtausend v. Chr.* Edited by Claus Ambos. Dresden: Islet, 2004.
Sonik, Karen. "Mesopotamian Conceptions of the Supernatural: A Taxonomy of *Zwischenwesen*." *Archiv für Religionsgeschichte* 14 (2013): 103–16.
Starr, Ivan, Jussi Aro, and Simo Parpola. *Queries to the Sungod: Divination and Politics in Sargonid Assyria*. SAA 4. Helsinki: Helsinki University Press, 1990.

Suddendorf, Thomas, and Michael C. Corballis. "The Evolution of Foresight: What Is Mental Time Travel, and Is It Unique to Humans?" *The Behavioral and Brain Sciences* 30 (2007): 299–313.
Sulzmann, Sven. "Time Perception: An Exploration of Time Perception and Possible Applications in Cognitive Archaeology." *UC Merced Undergraduate Research Journal* 6 (2014): 101–9.
Tzamalikos, Panayiotis. "Origen and the Stoic View of Time." *JHI* 52 (1991): 535–61.
Vatsyayan, Sachchidanand Hiranand. *A Sense of Time: An Exploration of Time in Theory, Experience and Art.* Delhi: Oxford University Press, 1981.
Verderame, Lorenzo. "A Glimpse into the Activities of Experts (*ummânu*) at the Assyrian Court." Pages 713–28 in *From Source to History: Studies on Ancient Near Eastern Worlds and Beyond, Dedicated to Giovanni Battista Lanfranchi.* Edited by Salvatore Gaspa et al. AOAT 412. Münster: Ugarit-Verlag, 2014.
———. "Il ruolo degli 'esperti' (*ummânu*) nel periodo neo-assiro." PhD diss., Università di Roma La Sapienza, 2004.
Whitrow, Gerald James. *What Is Time? The Classic Account of the Nature of Time.* Oxford: Oxford University Press, 2004.
Whyte, Alison, Vanessa Muros, and Sarah Barack. "'Brick by Brick': Piecing Together an Eighth Century B.C. Facade from Iraq." *AIC Objects Speciality Group Postprints* 11 (2004): 172–89.
Wiggermann, Frans Anton Maria. *Mesopotamian Protective Spirits: The Ritual Texts.* Groningen: STYX & PP Publications, 1992.
———. "Mischwesen. A." *RlA* 8:222–45.
Winter, Irene. "The Aesthetic Value of Lapis Lazuli in Mesopotamia." Pages 43–58 in *Cornaline et pierres précieuses: La Méditerranée, de l'Antiquité à l'Islam; Actes du colloque organisé au Musée du Louvre par le Service culturel, les 24 et 25 novembre 1995.* Edited by Annie Caubet. Conférences et colloques, Musée du Louvre (Paris: La documentation Française, 1999.
———. "Radiance as an Aesthetic Value in the Art of Mesopotamia." Pages 123–32 in *Art: The Integral Vision; A Volume of Essays in Felicitation of Kapila Vatsyayan.* Edited by Madhu Khanna, S. C. Malik, and Baidyanath Saraswati. New Delhi: Printworld, 1994.
Woods, Christopher. "At the Edge of the World: Cosmological Conceptions of the Eastern Horizon in Mesopotamia." *JANER* 9 (2009): 183–239.

THE DOORS OF PERCEPTION:
SENSES AND THEIR VARIATIONS IN AKKADIAN TEXTS

Anne-Caroline Rendu Loisel

In 1954, for a scientific purpose, Aldous Huxley swallowed a substance called mescaline, a substance extracted from an Indian cactus, a plant called peyotl. He entered into a new reality, characterized with a specific sensorium, full of colors with psychological effects.

Recent archaeological researches conducted in the Near East suggested that sensory phenomena may have been produced to create a particular atmosphere during a ritual, so as to induce a modification of the state of consciousness of the participants: darkness, light, cry, song, music, sweet-smelling smoke, drugs, all these phenomena taking place in a confined space. A kind of *trance* may have been induced.[1] The ritual procedure modified the sensorium of daily life for a community, inviting the living participants to a shared experience that would give them access to a new reality. The individual experienced then a new sensorium with a different aesthetic formation. The number and variety of cuneiform tablets, found in Syria and Iraq and covering more than three millennia of history, seemingly invite us to search for a description of that kind of personal and individual experience. But tablets only transmit to us discourses and cultural representations, so that we can investigate not the personal experience per se but what is culturally accepted and recognized as one. In this paper, my aim is to investigate Akkadian literature (second and first millennia BCE) where we can find a description of such experiences in which the state of consciousness of the individual would be altered. What kind of experiences are we dealing with?

---

[1] For references on the topic, see, e.g., Diana Stein, "The Role of Stimulants in Early Near Eastern Society: Insights through Artifacts and Texts," in *At the Dawn of History, Ancient Near Eastern Studies in Honor of J. N. Postgate*, ed. Yağmur Heffron, Adam Stone, and Martin Worthington, vol. 1 (Winona Lake, IN: Eisenbrauns, 2017), 507–33; and also Stein, "Architecture and Acoustic Resonance: The 'Tholoi' at Arpachiyah Reconsidered in the Context of a Wider Neolithic Horizon," in *Distant Impressions: The Senses in the Ancient Near East*, ed. Ainsley Hawthorn and Anne-Caroline Rendu Loisel (Philadelphia: Penn State University Press, 2019, 125–48).

How different from daily life are they? How can we experience them? What sort of impact do they have on daily life and the normal world? To answer those questions, I selected three different situations in Akkadian cuneiform texts: dreams and near-death experiences, banquets, and ritual procedures. In these particular situations, the modification of the sensorium helps to create a new place, with a particular atmosphere, that the individual will feel in his body through his senses.

ATYPICAL EXPERIENCES: DREAMS AND NEAR-DEATH EXPERIENCES

In the ancient Near East, dreaming was a way to know divine decisions and advices. Oneiromancy is a divinatory practice well attested in the ancient Near East, in both Sumerian and Akkadian sources, from the third to the first millennium BCE.[2] The Assyrian dream-book of the first millennium BCE contains a compendium of omens. Like in other divinatory treaties, each line gives a description of the experience in the protasis—what happened in the dream—and its meaning in the apodosis. Although the Akkadian vocabulary employed to describe an oneiric experience is most of all based on vision, the omens evoke a variety of sensory experiences: one may fly; hear something; eat fruit, bread, and meat; or have forbidden sensory experiences, such as eating human flesh (something that is related to the topic of purity and impurity in daily life).

Narrative texts describe what a dream experience should have been like: the visual aspects are of the utmost importance. The gender and social role, functions, or accessories of the individuals present in the dream—and with whom the dreamer is interacting—are frequently described. Sometimes, the dialogue is reported. When the sensory parameters of the place are described, it is frequently connected to the inner affective and psychological state of the dreamer in his daily life. It is the case in the Epic of Gilgamesh of the first millennium BCE. The king of Uruk has several dreams during his long journey to the Cedar Forest. The dream is a liminal place where human and divine may interact. Dreams may be ritually provoked—it is the case for Gilgamesh—as they may help to know the divine decisions concerning human matters:

---

[2] For a presentation of dreams in the ancient Near East, see: A. Leo Oppenheim, *The Interpretation of Dreams in the Ancient Near East: With a Translation of an Assyrian Dream-Book*, TAPS 46 (Philadelphia: American Philosophical Society, 1956); Sally A. L. Butler, *Mesopotamian Conceptions of Dreams and Dream Rituals*, AOAT 258 (Münster: Ugarit-Verlag, 1998); Annette Zgoll, "Dreams as Gods and Gods in Dreams: Dream-Realities in Ancient Mesopotamia from the Third to the First Millennium B.C.," in *He Has Opened Nisaba's House of Learning: Studies in Honor of Åke Waldemar Sjöberg on the Occasion of His Eighty-Ninth Birthday on August 1st 2013*, ed. Leonhard Sassmannshausen, CM 46 (Leiden: Brill, 2014), 299–313.

My friend, I have seen a third dream, / and the dream I saw was completely confused. / The heavens cried aloud, while the earth was rumbling / the day grew still, darkness went forth. / Lightning flashed down, fire broke out, / [flames] kept flaring up, death kept raining down. / The fire so bright dimmed and went out, / [after] it had diminished little by little, it turned into embers.[3]

This oneiric experience is characterized by a multisensory atmosphere induced by a compendium of negative stimulations. This could be defined as an example of dystopia—that is, the opposite of utopia: sonorous phenomena, rumbling of the earth, luminous instability with flashes. This new sensorium induces an emotional state of fear for Gilgamesh. Enkidu will interpret the dream as a dream of good portent for his forthcoming adventure, basing his interpretation on the inversion principle frequently at stake in divinatory processes.

The substances and material constituting a mythological or atypical place create a particular sensorium: built by the gods, temples in literature are characterized by music, precious stones (lapis lazuli, cornelian), and fruits and animals—I hereby refer to the temple of Eridu in the Sumerian poem Enki's Journey to Nippur.[4] Mythological places follow different rules that human beings may not be aware of. Penetrating in these places without the knowledge of their rules will nullify any attempt to establish a communication between human and divine entities. In one Akkadian myth, Adapa was a priest of the god Enki in the Sumerian city Eridu. Ascending to heaven and dressed like a mourner, he did not eat the bread or drink the beer the great god An was offering him. So, Adapa has to leave the place.[5] The sensorium of these atypical places is frequently characterized by the combination of sensory phenomena at their highest level that can be either positive—such as the divine dwellings—or negative; this is the case with the netherworld, a complete different reality with a specific

---

[3] [i]b-ri a-ta-mar 3ta šu-ut-ta / ʾu₃ʾ šu-ut-ta ša₂ a-mu-ru ka-liš ša₂-ša₂-at₂ / [i]l-su-u₂ AN^{u2} qaq-qa-ru i-ram-mu-um / [u₄]-mu uš-ḫa-ri-ir u₂-ṣa-a ek-le-tum / [ib-r]iq bir-qu in-na-pi-iḫ i-ša₂-a-tum / [nab-l]u iš-tap-pu-u₂ iz-za-nun mu-u₂-tu / [id-ʾ]i-im-ma ne₂-bu-tu₂ ib-te-li i-ša₂-tu / [iš-tu$^?$] im-taq-qu-tu i-tu-ur ana tu-um-ri (Gilgamesh 5:99–106). For the edition of the epic, see Andrew R. George, *The Babylonian Gilgamesh Epic: Introduction, Critical Edition, and Cuneiform Texts*, 2 vols. (Oxford: Oxford University Press, 2003).

[4] For a translation of the text, see Abdul-Hadi A. Al-Fouadi, *Enki's Journey to Nippur: The Journeys of the Gods* (PhD diss., University of Pennsylvania, 1969); online: Jeremy Black et al., eds., *The Electronic Texts Corpus of Sumerian Literature* (Oxford 1998–2006), 1.1.4 (http://etcsl.orinst.ox.ac.uk/cgi-bin/etcsl.cgi?text=c.1.1.4&display=Crit&charenc=gcirc#).

[5] Shlomo Izre'el, *Adapa and the South Wind: Language Has the Power of Life and Death*, MC 10 (Winona Lake, IN: Eisenbrauns, 2001).

sensorium: dead people spend their time in darkness, eating dust. This world may also be accessible with oneiric experience. The Assyrian prince Kummaya experienced it in a night vision (a tablet from the Neo-Assyrian time). After depicting the hybrid demonic entities he saw in the netherworld, he described the frightening atmosphere of this place.

> The netherworld was full of terror, / deathly silence(?) reigned in the presence of the prince. / He seized me by the forelock and dr[ew] me towards him. / When [I] saw him my legs shook, / his wrathful splendor overwhelmed me, / I kissed the feet of his [great] divinity, I knelt. / When I stood up, he was looking at me, shaking his head. / He gave me a fierce [cry and shrieked at me wrathfully, / like a raging storm. / He drew up his scepter, his divine symbol, / ghastly as a serpent, to kill me![6]

The sensory parameters of the place are closely tied to the affective state of the protagonist: his fear is aroused by an acoustic instability that evolves between the two paroxysms, a deathly silence (characterized also with immobility) and a loud and powerful cry, something as violent as the tactile experience he endeavored. The underworld is built in an opposition between its king, sonorous and in movement, and the stillness of the surrounding place and entities. All the descriptions of the netherworld can only be hypothetic as no one has the knowledge of its sensory characteristic: "No one sees death, / no one sees the face [of death,] / no one [hears] the voice of death: / (yet) savage death is the one who hacks man down,"[7] as the Epic of Gilgamesh reminds us.

The sensorium is deeply intertwined with the function of the place. Gilgamesh, the hero who saw the deep and what was hidden, experiences different mythological sensoria, all as fantastic as the hero's accomplishments are. After walking into darkness for a very long time, he arrived in a place, out of the humanly perceived world, the garden of precious stones:

> (The darkness was dense, and light was there none: / it did not allow him to see what was behind him.... He came out before the sun.... There was brilliance).

---

[6] *a-ra-al-lu ma-li pu-luḫ-tu i-na pa-an* DUMU NUN-*e na-di ši-iš$^?$-šu$_2$ dan-nu* [x x x ina] *a-bu-sa-ti-ia iṣ-bat-an-ni-ma a-na maḫ-ri-šu$_2$ u$_2$-qar-*[ri-ba]n$^?$*-ni* / [a]-*mur-šu$_2$-ma i-tar-ru-ra iš-da-a-a me-lam-mu-šu ez-zu-ti is-ḫu-pu-u-ni* GIR$_3$.2 DINGIR-*ti-šu$_2$* [GAL-*t*]*i aš$_2$-šiq-ma ak-mis a-zi-iz$^?$ i-na-ṭa-al-an-ni-ma u$_2$-na-a-š*[*a*$^?$ SAG.D]U$^?$-*s*[*u*] / [*ri-g*]*im-šu u$_2$-dan-nin-am-ma ki-ma* UD-*me š*[*e-g*]*i-i ez-zi-iš e-li-ia i-ša$_2$-as-si šab-bi-ṭu si-mat* DINGIR-*ti-šu$_2$ ša$_2$ ki-ma ba-aš$_2$-me pu-luḫ-tu ma-lu-u$_2$* (The Netherworld Vision of an Assyrian Crown Prince, r. l.13–15 [SAA 3:32 = VAT 10057] [trans. Foster modif.]).

[7] ⸢*ul ma*⸣-*am-ma mu-u$_2$-tu im-mar* / *ul ma-am-m*[*a ša mu-ti i*]*m-*⸢*mar*⸣ *pa-ni-šu$_2$* / ⸢*ul ma-am-ma*⸣ *ša mu-ti rig-*⸢*ma-šu$_2$*⸣ [*i-šem-me*] / *ag-gu* ⸢*mu-tum*⸣ *ḫa-ṣi-pi* LU$_2$(*amēlu*)-*ut-tim* (Gilgamesh 10:304–307).

upon seeing ... the trees of the gods, he went straight (up to them). / A carnelian (tree) was in fruit, / hung with bunches of grapes, lovely to behold. / A lapis-lazuli (tree) bore foliage, / in full fruit and gorgeous to gaze on. / [...] cedar [...] / its leaf-stems were of *pappardilû* [stone and ...] / Sea coral [...] *sāsu*-stone, / instead of thorn and briar [there grew] an-za-gul-me stone. / He touched a carob, [(it was)] *abašmu* stone, / *šubû* stone and haematite [...][8]

This visual experience made Gilgamesh so happy that he laughed (*ṣâḫu*, a verb that is also connected to sexual activities). Colors and brilliance characterize this mythical garden, and taste may be evoked by mentioning literally the fruit (*inbu*) of the trees. The more the journey is exhausted, the more the sensory effects are pleasant. If Gilgamesh can move into this shiny forest, it is only because he travelled the entire world, crossing the borders of the known world, reaching a place never experienced by a human being. The sensorium is here deeply connected to the inner state of the mind of the hero, which has been transformed all through his adventures.

The access to a new reality is only made possible by a modification of the state of consciousness of the individual. The sensorium, characterized by its optima, helps him to recognize the strangeness of the experience. Having the knowledge of this new reality implies to feel it in one's own flesh, in a lonely and individual experience of the surrounding environment. A sensory shared experience will have other consequences, as I will show now very briefly.

EATING AND DRINKING TOGETHER: THE BANQUET IN AKKADIAN LITERATURE

Sumerian and Akkadian literary texts give several examples of banquets. More than a simple narrative anecdote, the banquet is a major social moment where many issues are at stake. The Akkadian term *qerītu* designates a banquet organized in a human community or a banquet owed to the gods in a ritual context. Its Sumerian equivalent kaš de₂-a ("pouring out beer, the poured-out beer") highlights the importance of this alcoholic beverage, which may define the very nature of this social moment.[9]

---

[8] a-x [x x] x x-*ḫi iṣ-ṣi* ⸢*ša*₂⸣ DINGIR$^{?⸢meš}$ *ina a-ma-ri i-ši-ir* / ^{na4}GUG(*sāmtu*) *na-ša*₂-*at i-ni-ib-ša*₂ / *is-ḫu-un-na-tum ul-lu-la-at a-na da-ga-la ḫi-pat* / ^{na4}ZA.GIN *na-ši ḫa-as-ḫal-ta* / *in-ba na-ši-ma a-na a-ma-ri ṣa-a-a-aḫ* / (...) [x x]x *šu*[*r-min*$^?$...] / [x (x)] ^{giš}EREN [...] / ⸢*zi*⸣-*nu-šu* ^{na4}babbar-[dil...]-*ni* / *la-ru-uš* A.AB.BA(*tâmti*) [...^{n}]^{na4}NIR.ZIR(*sāsu*) / GIM ^{giš}DIH₃(*balti*) *u* ^{giš}KI[ŠI₁₆(*ašāgi*) *ibšû*$^?$ ^{na4}]AN.ZA.GUL.ME / *ḫa-ru-bu* ⸢*il*⸣-*p*[*u-ut*$^?$ ^{na4}A]D(*aba*)-*aš*-⸢*mu*⸣ / n^{a4}ŠUBA(*šubû*) ^{na4}K[A.GI.NA(*šadānu*) x (x)] x-*an*-⸢*rat*$^?$⸣ (Gilgamesh 9:172–190).

[9] Jean Bottéro, "Boisson, banquet et vie sociale en Mésopotamie," in *Drinking in Ancient Societies: History and Culture of Drinks in the Ancient Near East; Papers of a Symposium Held in Rome, May 17–19 1990*, ed. Lucio Milano (Padova: Sargon, 1994),

The Babylonian poem called the Enuma Elish, probably written at the end of the second or beginning of the first millennium BCE,[10] narrates how the Babylonian god Marduk became the supreme god, ruling the Babylonian pantheon after defeating the terrible Tiamat. After Marduk created and organized the world, the great gods gathered together in a banquet to celebrate this new state:

> All the great gods who decree destinies, gathered as they went, / They entered the presence of Anšar and became filled with [joy], / They kissed one another as they [...] in the assembly. / They conferred as they [sat] at table, / They ate grain, they drank ale. / They stuffed their bellies with sweet cake, / As they drank beer and felt good, / They became quite carefree, their mood was merry, / And they decreed the destiny for Marduk, their avenger.[11]

Tables are full of sweet and fine goods such as fruits, cakes, bread, and meat. Music, songs, and dance build a pleasant acoustic atmosphere. Touch is also evoked at the beginning of the quote. The banquet is frequently described as a moment and a place where all the senses are combined to create a shared social experience. The Akkadian vocabulary associates the collective drunkenness to a joyful emotional state, physically associated with the idea of "swelling."[12] The verb employed is *ḫabāṣu*, translated as "to be euphoric, to be happy, to be

---

3–13. For an introduction to the topic of the banquet in ancient Mesopotamia, see Maria-Grazia Masetti-Rouault, "Les dangers du banquet en Mésopotamie," in *La fête: La rencontre des dieux et des hommes*, ed. Michel M. Mazoyer et al., Collection Kubaba Série Actes 4 (Paris: L'Harmattan, 2004), 49–66; Piotr Michalowski, "The Drinking Gods: Alcohol in Mesopotamian Ritual and Mythology," in Milano, *Drinking in Ancient Societies*, 27–44; Marvin A. Powell, "Wine and Vine in Ancient Mesopotamia: The Cuneiform Evidence," in *The Origins and Ancient History of Wine*, ed. Patrick E. McGovern, Stuart James Fleming, and Solomon H Katz, Food and Nutrition in History and Anthropology 11 (Luxembourg: Gordon & Breach, 1995), 97–122.

[10] For the editions of the text, see Philippe Talon, *The Standard Babylonian Creation Myth Enūma eliš*, SAACT 4 (Helsinki: Neo-Assyrian Text Corpus Project, 2005); Thomas R. Kammerer and Kai A. Metzler, *Das babylonische Weltschöpfungsepos*, AOAT 375 (Münster: Ugarit-Verlag, 2012); Wilfred G. Lambert, *Babylonian Creation Myths*, MC 16 (Winona Lake, IN: Eisenbrauns, 2013), 3–143.

[11] *ig-gar-šu-nim-ma il-la-[ku-ni] i-ru-bu-ma mut-ti-iš an-šar$_2$ im-lu-u [ḫi-du-ta] / in-niš-qu a-ḫu-u a-ḫi ina* UKKIN [x x x x] / *li-ša$_2$-nu iš-ku-nu ina qe$_2$-re-ti [uš-bu] / aš$_2$-na-an i-ku-lu ip-ti-qu ku-r[u-un-nu] / ši-ri-sa mat-qu u$_2$-sa-an-ni-nu ra-ṭi-šu-[un] / ši-ik-ru ina ša$_2$-te-e ḫa-ba-ṣu zu-um-[ri] / ma-a'-diš e-gu-u$_2$ ka-bat-ta-šu$_2$-un i-te-el-[liš$_x$] / a-na* ^{d}AMAR.UTU *mu-tir gi-mil-li-šu$_2$-nu i-ši-mu šim-[ta]* (Enuma elish 3:129–138 [trans. Lambert]).

[12] Margaret Jaques, *Le vocabulaire des sentiments dans les textes sumériens: Recherche sur le lexique sumérien et akkadien*, AOAT 332 (Münster: Ugarit-Verlag, 2006), 268.

drunk." It also expresses a vocal and collective expression—like a song or an acclamation—in public festival contexts or a prayer to a divine entity. In a prayer devoted to the storm god Adad, fields are said to be "exuberant," "happy" (ḫitbuṣū); in a prayer addressed to the sun god Šamaš, it is said that "all the (foreign) countries are happy because of you, the noisy people [ḫābibu] exult [ḫitbuṣū] because of you."[13] A bilingual text gives also a visual characteristic to this Akkadian term by associating it to the divine splendor (šarūru), a light coming from the body of the goddess Ištar, something that is here similar to the moon light.[14]

The alcoholic substance helps the participants of the banquet to accede to a shared joyful state of mind, in the particular context of an overflowing of positive sensory stimulations. But this modification of the sensorium's parameters may have a terrible impact on the state of the individual's mind, who may lose his own ability to think and his suspicion. In our text, during this banquet, the great gods decided to build—with their own hands—Babylon and its temple, which will be the terrestrial residence of Marduk, a decision that is quite surprising as we know how much Mesopotamian gods hate working in literature. In other literary texts, especially in the Sumerian corpus, the banquet constitutes a major and important moment for the common approval of the divine assembly: it is after a banquet that all the gods accepted and celebrated the construction of the temple in Eridu for the god Enki. It can also be a moment where the alcoholic excesses may lead to a dangerous cosmic situation, in which the balance of the divine powers may be in danger—for example, when Inanna grabbed all the divine powers by taking advantage of Enki's drunkenness—or when atypical beings are created in Enki and Ninmah. More than a drinking session, the banquet is most of all a necessary joyful and festive meeting of a community. Thanks to a modification of the sensory parameters of daily life, the banquet offers a special atmosphere where the minds of the participants may be altered. Alcohol helps to manipulate the individual's ability to think in this shared experience. As it was already suggested by Piotr Michalowski, the banquet has a lot in common with the ritual: it is temporary, it involves the community—or a specific part of it—and leads to a new experience of the surrounding environment.[15] The new sensorium is characterized by an accumulation of various positive sensory phenomena. New social configurations are created in the banquet, as it is the case in the ritual procedure.

---

[13] rīšūnikka KUR.KUR ḫitbuṣūnikka ḫābibu (4R 17.r.11).

[14] si-suḫ-bi ma-az-ma-az: ša-ru-ur-ša ḫi-it-bu-uṣ "Her (Ištar) splendour is as éclatante (as her father's Sîn)" (LKA 23.r.14–15).

[15] Michalowski, "Drinking Gods," 27–44.

Acting on the Sensorium for a New Social Interaction: The Ritual Procedure

Ritual procedures of ancient Mesopotamia are described in cuneiform tablets belonging to the ritual expert (priest, diviner, exorcist, etc.). They give the general instructions concerning the accomplished gestures, the manipulated substances, or the pronounced sentences. Some of them indicate also a modification of the sensorium. The following tw[o texts illustrate two different ritual situations: in the first one, the expert tries to be in a close relationship with the divine realm, and in the second one, someone tries to act on the state of consciousness of someone else.

In one of the well-known prayers to the gods of the night—that is, the Stars—from the beginning of the second millennium BCE, the ritual procedure occurs at night. In his study of these prayers, A. Leo Oppenheim highlighted their poetic content and considered them as certainly one of the most beautiful pieces of the Akkadian literature.[16]

> Text B (Erm 15639): The princes are closely guarded, / the bolts are lowered, rings set in place. The noisy people are silenced, / Gates once opened, are locked. / The gods of the land, goddess of the land, / Šamaš, Sîn, Adad, and Ištar / have gone off into the 'lap of heaven'. / They are not giving judgement, they are not deciding cases. / Veiled is the night. / The palace is still, the fields are in deathly silence. / The wayfarer calls out to (his) god, the petitioner is *hungry for sleep*. / The judge of truth, father of the destitute, / Šamaš has gone into his cella. O great Gods of the Night / Brilliant Girra / Heroic Erra, / Bow, Yoke / Orion, Dragon / Wagon, She-Goat / Bison, Horned-Serpent, / Stand by me. / In the extispicy which I am performing, / In the lamb which I am offering, / Place Truth. / 24 lines. Prayer of the night.[17]

---

[16] A. Leo Oppenheim, "A New Prayer to the 'Gods of the Night,'" *AnBi* 12 (1959): 290, 299; for the bibliographical references and the list of the tablets, see Anne-Caroline Rendu Loisel, "Une nuit, sur un toit, en Babylonie: Recherches sur le silence dans les rituels akkadiens 2ᵉ–1ᵉʳ millénaire av. J.-C.," in *Mille et une empreintes: Un Alsacien en Orient, mélanges en l'honneur de Dominique Beyer à l'occasion de son 65e anniversaire*, ed. Julie Patrier et al. (Paris: Brepols, 2016), 421–34.

[17] *pullulū rubû / wašrū sikkurū šērētum šaknā / ḫabrātum nīšu šaqummâ / petûtum uddulū bābū / ilī mātim ištarāt mātim /* ᵈ*Šamaš* ᵈ*Sîn* ᵈ*Adad u* ᵈ*Ištar / īterbū ana utul šamê / ul idinnū dīnam ul iparrasū awātim / pussumat mušītim* (texte a *mušītim*) */ ekallum šaḫ(r)ur šaqummū adrū / ālik urḫim ilam išassi u ša dīnim ušteberre šittam / dayyān kinātim abi ekiātim /* ᵈ*Šamaš īterub ana kummīšu / rabûtum ilī mušītim / nawārum Girra / qurādum Erra / qaštum nīrum / šitaddarum mušḫuššum / ereqqu inzum / kusarikkum bašmum / lizzizzūma / ina têrti eppušu / ina puḫād akarrabu / kittam šuknan / 24* MU.BI *ikrib mušītim*

This text is recited at night by the diviner, the expert who will submit his oracular request and will accomplish extispicy the following morning. The recitation of the prayer prepares the necessary conditions, so that the oracular inspection will give a clear answer and an unambiguous verdict (*kittam šuknā*, "Place the truth"). The purpose of the recitation is to guarantee a good reading of the entrails. The only gods who are present at night, and to whom the diviner can address his request, are the Stars. The great gods—Sin, Ištar, Šamaš, Adad—revered during the day, have now returned to their private nocturnal chambers. The gods of the night are taking their position in the nocturnal sky,[18] where they keep watch over cities while humankind is surrounded by obscurity, immobility, and silence. The prayer opens with the description of the human city, where everyone has fallen asleep after a hard day of working. The overcrowded places at day—fields, palace—are now extremely silent. For *šuḫarruru* and *šuqammumu*, Wolfram von Soden suggested that these terms with the form *paruss-* belong to the lexical field of the "numinous."[19] With *šuḫarruru* and *šuqammumu*, one may describe a physical and affective silent state, such as dismay, stupor, and awe-inspiring fear. This category characterizes the divine world or when human and divine meet together. Everything is secured, and nobody has a reason to fear.[20] Night is personified as a young bride, donned with her veil, alluding to the sparkling beauty of the starry sky. From the roof of his house, the diviner can see far away in the desert, beyond walls and distances. Just as the obscurity is not complete at all because of the luminosity of the stars, the silence is also not complete. The diviner sees, feels, and hears the lonely traveler crying (*išassi*), in danger because of robbers, animals, or demons. The patient who ordered the extispicy cannot sleep.[21]

Taking the opportunity of the nocturnal modification of the sensorium—with its effective and active silence, the surrounding immobility, and the sparkling obscurity—the expert is in a privileged position as he is the only one who can see the stars moving into the sky. The silence contributes to the secrecy of

---

[18] Wayne Horowitz and Nathan Wasserman. "Another Old Babylonian Prayer to the Gods of the Night," *JCS* 48 (1996): 57–60 (59, n.10).

[19] "Steigerungsadj. mit numinosem Bedeutungsgehalt," (for *namurrum*) "furchtbar glänzend," (for *rašubbum*) "rotgleissend," (and) *da'ummu* "unheimlich dunkel." Wolfram von Soden, *Grundriss der Akkadischen Grammatik* (Rome: Pontifical Biblical Institute, 1952), §55 p. 28 a.III.

[20] Oppenheim, "New Prayer," 298.

[21] For Piotr Steinkeller, the night becomes the Netherworld, where Šamaš judges dead people when he is not visible on earth. Piotr Steinkeller, "Of Stars and Men: The Conceptual and Mythological Setup of Babylonian Extispicy," in *Biblical and Oriental Essays in Memory of William L. Moran*, ed. Augustinus Gianto, BibOr 48 (Rome: Pontifical Biblical Institute, 2005), 11–47.

the meeting. The poet transcends his simple condition and for an ephemeral moment becomes close to the divine entities.

The modification of the daily life sensorium by the ritual procedure may also be effective to act on someone else and modify his/her state of consciousness. In an Old Akkadian incantation,[22] the instructions do not try to help the patient access a new reality. On the contrary, the ritual modifies the parameters of someone else's sensorium. Here I follow the translation of Nathan Wassermann:[23]

> Enki loves the love charm. / The love-charm, Ištar's son, [si]tting in [her?/his? l]ap,
> Turning here through the sap of the incense-tree.
> You, oh two beautiful maiden, are blooming! / To the garden you come down, indeed come down to the garden! / you have drunk the sap of the incense-tree [*ru'ti kanaktim*].
> I have seized now your [f.] drooling mouth [lit. "mouth of sap"], / I have seized your [f.] shining [*burrumāti*] eyes / I have seized you [f.] urinating vulva.
> I leaped to the garden of Sîn, / I cut the poplar-tree for her day / Encircle [f.] me between the boxwood trees, as the shepherd encircles the flock,/ As the goat (encircles) its kid, the sheep its lamb, the mare its foal!
> His arms are adorned: / Oil and (the sound of) harp—his lips. / A cup of oil in his hands, a cup of cedar fragrance on his shoulders. / The love-charms have persuaded her, driven her to ecstasy.
> Now I have seized your [f.] lustful mouth [lit. "mouth of sexual attraction"] / I conjure you [f.] by the name of Ištar and Išḫara: / "Until his neck and your [f.] neck are not entwined—you [f.] shall not find peace![24]

---

[22] Ashm 1930–0143 + Ashm 1930–0175h. First edition by Ignace Gelb, MAD 5.7–12; Joan Goodnick Westenholz and Age Westenholz, "Help for Rejected Suitors: The Old Akkadian Love Incantation MAD V 8," *Or* 46 (1977): 198–219. See also Brigitte Groneberg, "Die Liebesbeschwörung MAD V 8 und ihr literarischer Kontext," *RA* 95 (2001): 97–113; Benjamin R. Foster, *Before the Muses: An Anthology of Akkadian Literature* (Bethesda, MD: CDL, 2005), 66–68; and Nathan Wassermann, *Akkadian Love Literature of the Third and Second Millennium BCE*, LAOS 4 (Wiesbaden: Harrassowitz, 2016).

[23] Wassermann, *Akkadian Love Literature*, 243.

[24] ^{d}EN.KI *ir-e-ma-am* / e_3-*ra*-[...]-*am* / *ir-e-mu-um* DUMU ^{d}INANA / *in za-gi*-[*sa u-ša*]-ʾ*ab*ʾ / *in ru-uḫ$_2$*-ʾ*ti*ʾ [*ga-na*]-*ak-tim* / *u$_2$-da-ra wa-ar-*ʾ*da*ʾ-*ta$_2$* / *da-mi$_3$-iq-ta$_2$ tu-uḫ$_2$-da-na-ma* / *ki-ri$_2$-šum tu-ur$_4$-da* / *tu-ur$_4$-da-ma a-na* ^{giš}KIRI$_6$ / *ru-uḫ$_2$-ti ga-na-ak-tim* / *ti-ib-da-ad-ga* / *a-ḫu-uz$_x$*(EŠ$_5$) *ba-ki ša ru-ga-tim* / *a-ḫu-uz$_x$*(EŠ$_5$) *bu-ra-ma-ti* / *e-ni-ki* / *a-ḫu-uz$_x$*(EŠ$_5$) *ur$_4$-ki* / *ša ši-na-tim* / *a-aš$_2$-ḫi-it ki-ri$_2$-iš* / ^{d}Suen / *ab-dug* ʾ^{geš}ASAL$_2$ʾ / (reverse) *u-me-iš-sa* / *du-ri-ni i-da-az-ga-ri-ni* / *ki* ʾ*sipa*ʾ *i$_3$-du-ru za-nam* / ʾ*ud$_5$*ʾ *ga-lu-ma-sa* ʾ*u$_8$ sila$_3$*ʾ-*za* / *a-da-num$_2$ mu-ra-aš$_2$* / *si-ir-gu-a i-da-su* / ʾ*i$_3$*ʾ *u$_3$ ti-bu-ut-tum* / *sa-ap-da-su* / *a-za-am* ʾ*i$_3$*ʾ *in qa$_2$-ti-su* / *a-za-am i-ri-nim in bu-ti-su* / *ir-e-mu u$_2$-da-bi-bu-si-ma* / *u$_3$ iš-ku-nu-si a-na mu-ḫu-tim* / *a-ḫu-uz$_x$*(EŠ$_5$) *ba-ki ša da-di$_3$* / ^{d}INANA *u$_3$* ^{d}*iš-ḫa-ra* / *u$_3$-dam-me-ki* / *a-ti za-wa-ar-su* / *u$_3$ za-wa-ar-ki* / *la e-dam-da* / *la da-ba-ša-ḫi-ni*

The main purpose of these love charms is to help a man win a woman's favor by magical purposes. It begins with a mythological description of the love charms, a concrete entity sitting on the lap of the goddess of love Ištar (1.1–3). Mentioning the god Ea at the very first beginning of the incantation links the tablet to the magical realm of the god. The scene takes place in a garden, a common literary topic evoking love and sexual desire.

The suitor explains then that he has been attracted by the sweet-smelling sap of an incense-tree, which has been swallowed by two young and attractive girls. Shouting at the woman of his desire, he affirms that he has power over her. At the end of the incantation, the love charms themselves are talking to the beloved woman. They describe the new body of the man: it is now so sensory attractive that the woman cannot ignore it anymore. She will find rest only when she satisfies her sexual desire with him.

A transfer of sensory property and a gender exchange of value seem to be implied between the young women and the male suitor. The sweet-fragrant and moist texture of the sap will be bodily integrated by the male suitor. But the true recipient is the woman, who at the end of the incantation, cannot resist the cedar oil emanating from the man's shoulders. The sensory phenomena are solicited to arouse desire in the sexual partner. The formula recited by the love charms acts in a multisensory way as it suggests visual, gustatory, melodious, scented, and tactile experiences: the body parts of the suitor are associated with fruits and oils; his voice is as sweet as a musical instrument; his arms, hands, and shoulders are as if a sweet-smelling balm has been applied. The state of consciousness of the woman is altered, modified by these ritually effective sensory descriptions.[25] She loses her mind and reason and cannot resist this physical attraction. All of her body is solicited by the love-charm, in a plenitude that is close to a mystical ecstasy, a sensorial utopia. This state of mind should be an everlasting one that nothing could diminish. But, on the opposite side, the man seems to be prisoner of his own sensory experience: he cannot accede to this sensory utopia as he cannot share his love with the woman. The sensory effects have to be felt in interaction with another one, so as to establish a real interaction and communication.

CONCLUSION

By focusing on atypical experiences, my aim was to investigate the role played by the sensorium to define the particular places where sensory experiences occur

---

[25] For a wider development of this topic, see my forthcoming paper: Anne-Caroline Rendu Loisel, "Acting on an Unwilling Partner: Gender and Sensory Phenomena in Old Akkadian and Old Babylonian Love Incantations," in *Gender, Methodology and the Ancient Near East: Proceedings of the Second Workshop held in Barcelona, February 1–3 2017*, ed. S. Budin et al. (Barcelona: Barcino, forthcoming).

and how they affect the relationship established by the individual. Acceding to a new reality—by dreams or journeys—is a way to acquire knowledge, but it is most of all an individual experience of the sensorium. Drinking alcohol, combined with other sensory phenomena, creates a shared experience (something that would be close to the etymology of the term *synaesthesis*, "feeling together") that leads to a modified state of consciousness for all the participants. The various sensoria described in Akkadian texts illustrate the complex relationships established between the individual and his or her society or with members of societies of different natures. Sensorium is a medium to interact with the Other.

BIBLIOGRAPHY

Al-Fouadi, Abdul-Hadi A. *Enki's Journey to Nippur: The Journeys of the Gods*. PhD diss., University of Pennsylvania, 1969.
Black, Jeremy, et al., eds. *The Electronic Texts Corpus of Sumerian Literature*. Oxford 1998–2006. http://etcsl.orinst.ox.ac.uk/cgi-bin/etcsl.cgi?text=c.1.1.4&display=Crit&charenc=gcirc#.
Bottéro, Jean. "Boisson, banquet et vie sociale en Mésopotamie." Pages 3–13 in *Drinking in Ancient Societies: History and Culture of Drinks in the Ancient Near East; Papers of a Symposium Held in Rome, May 17–19 1990*. Edited by Lucio Milano. Padova: Sargon, 1994.
Butler, Sally A. L. *Mesopotamian Conceptions of Dreams and Dream Rituals*. AOAT 258. Münster: Ugarit-Verlag, 1998.
Foster, Benjamin R. *Before the Muses: An Anthology of Akkadian Literature*. Bethesda, MD: CDL, 2005.
George, Andrew R. *The Babylonian Gilgamesh Epic: Introduction, Critical Edition, and Cuneiform Texts*. 2 vols. Oxford: Oxford University Press, 2003.
Groneberg, Brigitte. "Die Liebesbeschwörung MAD V 8 und ihr literarischer Kontext." *RA* 95 (2001): 97–113.
Horowitz, Wayne, and Nathan Wasserman. "Another Old Babylonian Prayer to the Gods of the Night." *JCS* 48 (1996): 57–60.
Izre'el, Shlomo. *Adapa and the South Wind: Language Has the Power of Life and Death*. MC 10. Winona Lake, IN: Eisenbrauns, 2001.
Jaques, Margaret. *Le vocabulaire des sentiments dans les textes sumériens: Recherche sur le lexique sumérien et akkadien*. AOAT 332. Münster: Ugarit-Verlag, 2006.
Kammerer, Thomas R., and Kai A. Metzler. *Das babylonische Weltschöpfungsepos*. AOAT 375. Münster: Ugarit-Verlag, 2012.
Lambert, Wilfred G. *Babylonian Creation Myths*. MC 16. Winona Lake, IN: Eisenbrauns, 2013.
Masetti-Rouault, Maria-Grazia. "Les dangers du banquet en Mésopotamie." Pages 49–66 in *La fête: La rencontre des dieux et des hommes*. Edited by Michel M. Mazoyer et al. Collection Kubaba Série Actes 4. Paris: L'Harmattan, 2004.
Michalowski, Piotr. "The Drinking Gods: Alcohol in Mesopotamian Ritual and Mythology." Pages 27–44 in *Drinking in Ancient Societies: History and Culture of Drinks in*

the Ancient Near East; Papers of a Symposium Held in Rome, May 17–19 1990. Edited by Lucio Milano. Padova: Sargon, 1994.

Oppenheim, A. Leo. *The Interpretation of Dreams in the Ancient Near East: With a Translation of an Assyrian Dream-Book*. TAPS 46. Philadelphia: American Philosophical Society, 1956.

———. "A New Prayer to the 'Gods of the Night.'" *AnBi* 12 (1959): 282–301.

Powell, Marvin A. "Wine and Vine in Ancient Mesopotamia: The Cuneiform Evidence." Pages 97–122 in *The Origins and Ancient History of Wine*. Edited by Patrick E. McGovern, Stuart James Fleming, and Solomon H Katz. Food and Nutrition in History and Anthropology 11. Luxembourg: Gordon & Breach, 1995.

Rendu Loisel, Anne-Caroline. "Acting on an Unwilling Partner: Gender and Sensory Phenomena in Old Akkadian and Old Babylonian Love Incantations." In *Gender, Methodology and the Ancient Near East: Proceedings of the Second Workshop held in Barcelona, February 1–3 2017*. Edited by S. Budin et al. Barcelona: Barcino, forthcoming.

———. "Une nuit, sur un toit, en Babylonie: Recherches sur le silence dans les rituels akkadiens 2e–1er millénaire av. J.-C." Pages 421–34 in *Mille et une empreintes: Un Alsacien en Orient, mélanges en l'honneur de Dominique Beyer à l'occasion de son 65e anniversaire*. Edited by Julie Patrier et al. Paris: Brepols, 2016.

Stein, Diana. "Architecture and Acoustic Resonance: The 'Tholoi' at Arpachiyah Reconsidered in the Context of a Wider Neolithic Horizon." Pages 125–48 in *Distant Impressions: The Senses in the Ancient Near East*. Edited by Ainsley Hawthorn and Anne-Caroline Rendu Loisel. Philadelphia: Penn State University Press, 2019.

———. "The Role of Stimulants in Early Near Eastern Society: Insights through Artifacts and Texts." Pages 507–33 in *At the Dawn of History, Ancient Near Eastern Studies in Honor of J. N. Postgate*. Edited by Yağmur Heffron, Adam Stone, and Martin Worthington. Vol. 1. Winona Lake, IN: Eisenbrauns, 2017.

Steinkeller, Piotr. "Of Stars and Men: The Conceptual and Mythological Setup of Babylonian Extispicy." Pages 11–47 in *Biblical and Oriental Essays in Memory of William L. Moran*. Edited by Augustinus Gianto. BibOr 48. Rome: Pontifical Biblical Institute, 2005.

Talon, Philippe. *The Standard Babylonian Creation Myth Enūma eliš*. SAACT 4. Helsinki: Neo-Assyrian Text Corpus Project, 2005.

Von Soden, Wolfram. *Grundriss der Akkadischen Grammatik*. Rome: Pontifical Biblical Institute, 1952.

Wassermann, Nathan. *Akkadian Love Literature of the Third and Second Millennium BCE*. laos 4. Wiesbaden: Harrassowitz, 2016.

Westenholz, Joan Goodnick, and Age Westenholz. "Help for Rejected Suitors: The Old Akkadian Love Incantation MAD V 8." *Or* 46 (1977): 198–219.

Zgoll, Annette. "Dreams as Gods and Gods in Dreams: Dream-Realities in Ancient Mesopotamia from the Third to the First Millennium B.C." Pages 299–313 in *He Has Opened Nisaba's House of Learning: Studies in Honor of Åke Waldemar Sjöberg on the Occasion of His Eighty-Ninth Birthday on August 1st 2013*. Edited by Leonhard Sassmannshausen. CM 46. Leiden: Brill, 2014.

SENSING NATURE IN THE NEO-ASSYRIAN WORLD

Allison Thomason

The title of this contribution could seem ambiguous, so I aim first to narrow what I mean by *sensing nature*. Nature refers to the animate parts of nature—animals. My project here is to discuss the Assyrian representations of animals acting as they do naturally. Thus, I will touch only briefly on the topographic and floral features—landscapes—of nature in Neo-Assyrian art.[1] Rather, I am more interested in the living, sentient creatures inhabiting those places, including to a lesser

---

I would like to thank the editors of this volume, Annette Schellenberg and Thomas Krueger, as well as the colleagues in attendance at the Vienna conference, whose conversations and insights contributed to this paper. Preliminary ideas for this paper were developed in two papers delivered at conferences in 2016: the Rencontre Assyriologique Internationale (Philadelphia, PA) and the Annual Meetings of ASOR (San Antonio, TX). Therefore, I would also like to thank the organizers of those panels, Marian Feldman and Kiersten Neumann respectively, for the invitation as well as the colleagues from those sessions for their comments and suggestions.

[1] The approaches to landscape in Mesopotamia and Assyria are numerous and varied. Some scholars explore the Mesopotamian construction of landscapes in art as related to ideology; for example, see Michelle I. Marcus, "Geography as Visual Ideology: Landscape, Knowledge and Power in Neo-Assyrian Art," in *Neo-Assyrian Geography*, ed. M. Liverani, Quaderni di Geografia Storica 5 (Rome: Herder, 1995), 193–202; Irene J. Winter, "Tree(s) on the Mountain: Landscape and Territory on the Victory Stele of Naram-Sin of Agade," in *Landscapes: Territories, Frontiers and Horizons in the Ancient Near East*, ed. Lucio Milano, Stefano de Marino, Frederick Mario Fales, and Giovanni B. Lanfranchi, HANE/M 3.1 (Padua: Sargon, 2000), 63–72; Allison Thomason, "Representations of the North Syrian Landscape in Neo-Assyrian Art," *BASOR* 323 (2001): 63–96; Mehmet-Ali Ataç, "'Imaginal' Landscapes in Assyrian Imperial Monuments," in *Experiencing Power, Generating Authority: Cosmos, Politics and the Ideology of Kingship in Ancient Egypt and Mesopotamia*, ed. Jane A. Hill, Philip Jones, and Antonio J. Morales (Philadelphia: University of Pennsylvania Press, 2013), 383–423. Others approach landscapes in Assyria as performative spaces in which the placement of rock reliefs played a role in commensality and memory: see Ann Shafer, "Assyrian Royal Monuments on the Periphery: Ritual and the Making of Imperial Space," in *Ancient Near Eastern Art in Context: Studies in Honor of Irene J. Winter by Her Students*, ed. J. Cheng and M. Feldman (Leiden: Brill, 2007),

degree, humans. Thus, sensing nature can imply humans experiencing the natural, nonhuman world or human representations of the natural world filled with animals as sentient beings.

In a 2016 publication on sensescapes in Assyria, I interrogated the first meaning of sensing nature, that is, understanding humans as sentient beings.[2] Following the seminal work of Yannis Hamilakis and others on sensory experience,[3] I concluded in that article that the Assyrian courtly elites deliberately produced sensory stimuli—sights, sounds, smells, tastes, touches—in their palaces and gardens to control biopolitically the sensory experiences of the inhabitants and visitors to the capitol cities. The elites, too, experienced such stimuli in kinaesthetic and synaesthetic instances. I pointed out that Assyrian palace reliefs and inscriptions (even archival documents such as letters) are rife with references to sensory stimuli and responses of the royal court. They show that the kings were clearly interested in their own sensory experiences within their capital cities, but also determined to produce and inculcate the bodily experiences—whether positive or negative—of the native populations and visitors in the Assyrian heartland. As just one example, in the so-called Banquet Stele of Ashurnasirpal II, the Neo-Assyrian king invited thousands of guests from Assyria and his empire to a consecrating banquet when he built his palace at Nimrud. He plied them with wine, sweets, meats, fruits, vegetables, and aromatics, and then he "sent them back to their lands in peace and joy [*šùlme ù ḫade*]."[4]

I do not intend to reiterate fully the observations and conclusions that I made in that article but to delve further into the topic of sensory experiences in Assyria. I am building from that earlier work to explore the Assyrian sensory interaction with nature. My study of sensing nature would not be complete without a brief nod to an understanding of phenomenology. Recently, colleagues have critiqued the phenomenological understanding of people of the ancient world with respect to self and nature. The idea that nature and culture or nature and humans are separate entities has lived with our modern sensibilities since the creation of what Ömür Harmanşah calls the "Cartesian bifurcation of the world into natural and cultural landscapes" in the seventeenth century.[5] None other than A. Leo Oppenheim, the famous Assyriologist, struggled with this disconnect between modern and ancient views of nature, trying to fit Mesopotamian concepts of the *oikoumene*

133–59; Ömür Harmanşah, "'Source of the Tigris': Event, Place and Performance in the Assyrian Landscapes of the Early Iron Age," *Archaeological Dialogues* 14 (2007): 179–204.

[2] Allison Thomason, "The Sense-Scapes of Neo-Assyrian Capital Cities: Royal Authority and Bodily Experience," *Cambridge Archaeological Journal* 26.2 (2016): 243–64.

[3] Yannis Hamilakis, *Archaeology and the Senses: Human Experience, Memory and Affect* (Cambridge: Cambridge University Press, 2013).

[4] RIMA 2:153, A.0.101.30.

[5] Ömür Harmanşah, ed., *Of Rocks and Water: Towards an Archaeology of Place*, Joukowsky Institute Publications 5 (Oxford: Oxbow, 2014), 4.

and self into a modern dualistic notion of nature versus man (or other similar binaries). In an article completed by his colleague Erica Reiner and published in 2008, nearly two decades after his death, entitled "Man and Nature in the Mesopotamian World," Oppenheim wrote "the data provided to [Mesopotamian man] by his senses were utilized in two essentially different ways by his intellect." And in the next paragraph, he ambiguously concluded, "Mesopotamian man attempted to construct an integrated whole extending beyond the objects he could touch and see, a whole of which he himself was to be an essential part."[6]

I think we are now to the point where we recognize that such phenomenological dichotomies certainly do not exist for all cultures today and did not exist for past civilizations. But because we do live in the present, we are in some ways forced to use the vocabulary we know—the words *nature* and *natural*, which I am defining as everything extrasomatic to humans but especially those spaces that are outside enclosed architectural settings with roofs. Many have argued that gods and humans in Mesopotamia could possess cognitive and sensory essences such as the powerful *melammu* or alluring *kuzbu* that reached out and physically or psychically affected other beings.[7] Or that so-called worshipper statues from Mesopotamia were considered endowed with life and not just inanimate substitutes or representations.[8] Thus, the idea that selves and outside-selves are mutually affective and not separate phenomenological concepts has been advanced repeatedly now for the Mesopotamian world.

In addition, the study of animals in Neo-Assyrian art has caught the attention of scholars, who have tried to discover the real existence of lexically known or pictorially represented creatures—that is, which species were present back then—and their symbolic meanings. For example, Catherine Breniquet, Chiko Watanabe, and Pauline Albenda discuss the anatomical depiction, iconography, and symbolism of different species of animals in Neo-Assyrian art.[9] For specific

---

[6] A. Leo Oppenheim, "Man and Nature in Mesopotamian Civilization," in *The Dictionary of Scientific Biography* 15 (New York: Scribner's Sons, 2008), 634–66, available online at http://www.encyclopedia.com/doc/1G2-2830904949.html.

[7] For *melammu*, see Beate Pongratz-Leisten, "Melammu," in *The Encyclopedia of Ancient History* (Malden, MA: Blackwell, 2012), doi:10.1002/9781444338386.wbeah24143; Irene J. Winter, "Radiance as an Aesthetic Value in the Art of Mesopotamia, with Some Indian Parallels," in *Art, the Integral Vision: A Volume in Felicitation of Kapila Vatsyayan*, ed. Baidyanath M. Saraswati, S. C. Malik, and Madhu Khanna (New Delhi: Printworld, 1994), 123–32. For *kuzbu*, see Zainab Bahrani, *Women of Babylon: Gender and Representation in Mesopotamia* (London: Routledge, 2001), 83–95.

[8] Zainab Bahrani, *The Graven Image: Representation in Babylonia and Assyria* (Philadelphia: University of Pennsylvania Press, 2003); Jean Evans, *The Lives of Sumerian Sculpture* (Cambridge: Cambridge University Press, 2014).

[9] Catherine Breniquet, "Animals in Mesopotamian Art," in *A History of Animals in the Ancient Near East*, ed. Billie Jean Collins, HdO 64 (Leiden: Brill, 2002), 145–68; Chiko

animals or time periods and as just one example: Brent Strawn builds a comparative focus on both the literary and pictorial imagery associated with lions, with an analysis of those animals as tropes for wickedness, ferocity, protection, or raw power.[10]

Clearly, the large-scale hunt cycles and religious or symbolic associations of these animals in Neo-Assyrian art, due to their detail, variety, and ubiquity, have repeatedly drawn scholars to their study. I have always been attracted to little vignettes of the nonhuman world in the later Assyrian reliefs, where the animals are not always the main subject of the relief narratives. Even in those large-scale scenes where animals *are* the main subject, such as the royal hunts, I have wondered about the subtle details that suggest movement and sensory capability. Some examples include lions chasing caprids through various forested landscapes (fig. 1); and a mother sow and her babies nuzzling their way through the marshes, the one baby piglet resting his head on his littermate's back, feet raised, perhaps in a moment of play (fig. 2), both from Sennacherib's Southwest Palace at Nineveh. As another example, a deer with a plain coat grazes through a tall stand of reeds; another deer with a dappled coat rests nearby (fig. 3).[11] A vignette from a hunt preparation scene shows one dog sniffing the hindquarters of another dog (fig. 4). Many of these vignettes appear in the reliefs from the palaces of Sennacherib and Ashurbanipal, but earlier phases of Neo-Assyrian art are not to be ignored. For example, reliefs from Sargon II's palace at Khorsabad show a hunt (without the king) where birds flit through trees, beat their wings, and avidly consume their food (fig. 5).

Why do these vignettes and details exist? They are not inherently necessary to the overall programs or ideological messages related to empire and conquest identified for decades now in the Neo-Assyrian reliefs, so why include them at all? What did they mean to the Assyrian viewers, artisans, and court, and how were they experienced in relation to other reliefs or an entire room of reliefs? Did they have symbolic meaning, as in Egyptian art, or do they represent the artists showing their sense of levity and skill? Are they meant to be breaks from the gnashing intensity of battle and hunts? Certainly, we modern viewers tend to see them as such.

Watanabe, *Animal Symbolism in Mesopotamia: A Contextual Approach* (Vienna: Institut für Orientalistik der Universität Wien, 2002); Pauline Albenda, "Landscape Bas-Reliefs in the Bīt-Hilani of Ashurbanipal," *BASOR* 224 (1976–1977): 49–72; Albenda, "Lions on Assyrian Wall Reliefs," *JANES* 6 (1974): 1–27.

[10] Brent A. Strawn, *What Is Stronger Than a Lion? Leonine Image and Metaphor in the Hebrew Bible and the Ancient Near East*, OBO 212 (Fribourg: Academic Press, 2005).

[11] Julian E. Reade, "The Assyrians as Collectors: From Accumulation to Synthesis," in *From the Upper Sea to the Lower Sea: Studies on the History of Assyrian and Babylonia in Honour of A. K. Grayson*, ed. Grant Frame (Leiden: Nederlands Instituut voor het Nabije Oosten, 2004), 262.

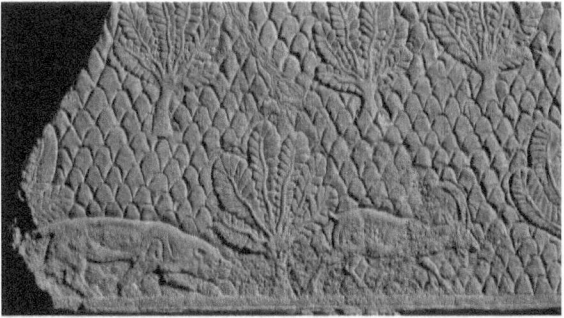

Fig. 1. Lions chasing a caprid through a forested environment. Reign of Ashurbanipal, Southwest Palace, Nineveh. BM 124793. Courtesy of Trustees of the British Museum.

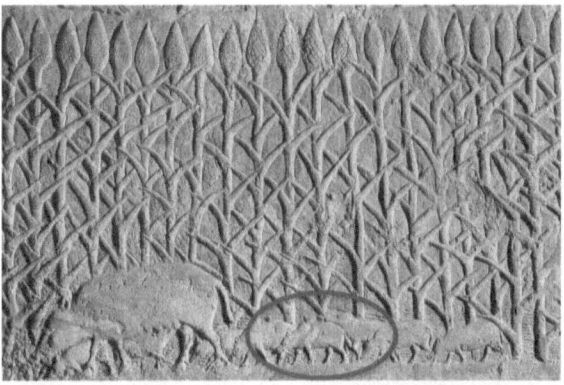

Fig. 2. Pig family in the marshes. Palace of Sennacherib, Nineveh. BM 124824. Courtesy of Trustees of the British Museum.

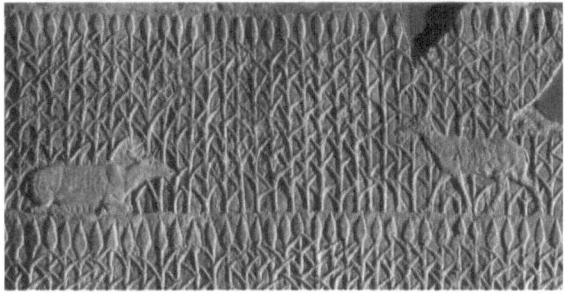

Fig. 3. Deer grazing in the marshes. Palace of Sennacherib, Nineveh. BM 124824. Courtesy of Trustees of the British Museum

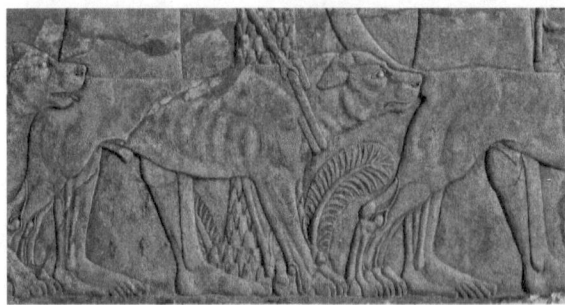

Fig. 4. Dogs processing towards the royal hunt. Palace of Ashurbanipal, Nineveh. BM 118915. Courtesy of Trustees of the British Museum.

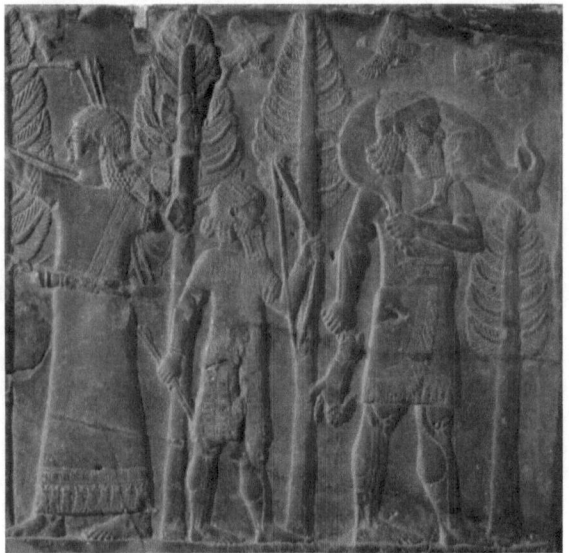

Fig. 5. Hunting scene with birds. Palace of Sargon II, Khorsabad. BM 118829. Courtesy of Trustees of the British Museum.

In fact, the Neo-Assyrians also seemed to appreciate the illustration of animals on portable objects from their west, as they plundered or received as gifts numerous ivory objects showing animal combats, cows suckling calves, and grazing caprids. Assyrian artists of the first millennium might have responded to and transformed these westerly impulses, as they were intent on integrating into their own art these sentient animals responding to their earthly environment.[12] The focus on the narratives and their landscapes, as part of overall palace "programs,"[13] has inexplicitly deemed the animal vignettes secondary or subservient to the action of human activity, and they have received relatively less scholarly attention. Certainly these detailed images of animals doing what they do in their natural habitats could be part of the veracity of the reliefs; imagined or mimetic scenes intended to speak the truth for the viewing audience in the palatial structures for the purpose of geographic specificity, a purpose for the detail that has been identified for the reliefs for decades now.

Animals are also shown in specific landscape settings in the heartland, in an artificially constructed game park or garden, as in Room E of Ashurbanipal's North Palace (fig. 6). There is little doubt that the paired male and female lions within a garden-like setting represent the potential fertility and abundance of the empire brought into the realm by the kings, as argued by Pauline Albenda and Paul Collins, as well as myself.[14] They also fit into the Neo-Assyrian ideological scheme by representing the Assyrian control of nature, known more obviously from the hunting scenes in Neo-Assyrian art and imagery on the royal seal.[15]

Perhaps the most well-known scene with animals is the famous Garden Scene from panels fallen from a second story into Room S of Ashurbanipal's North Palace at Nineveh (fig. 7).[16] The reclining king and seated queen fanned by servants

---

[12] Although I should note images on art dating to the second millennium BCE from Amorite Mari and Ashur show an earlier native interest in animals in nature scenes.

[13] The references on the programs of reliefs in Neo-Assyrian palaces are too numerous to cite. Groundbreaking work includes Irene J. Winter, "Royal Rhetoric and the Development of Historical Narrative in Neo-Assyrian Reliefs," *Studies in Visual Communication* 7 (1981): 2–38; Julian E. Reade, "Ideology and Propaganda in Assyrian Art," in *Power and Propaganda*, ed. Mogens Trolle Larsen (Copenhagen: Akademisk Forlag, 1979), 329–43; John M. Russell, *Sennacherib's Palace without Rival at Nineveh* (Chicago: University of Chicago Press, 1991).

[14] Albenda, "Lions on Assyrian Wall Reliefs"; Paul Collins, "Trees and Gender in Neo-Assyrian Art," *Iraq* 68 (2006): 99–107; Thomason, "Representations of the North Syrian Landscape."

[15] Davide Nadali, "Neo-Assyrian State Seals: An Allegory of Power," *SAAB* XVIII (2009–2010): 215–44.

[16] Richard David Barnett was the first to suggest that these hunt-cycle reliefs fell from an upper story into Room S below. See his *Sculptures from the North Palace of Assurbanipal at Nineveh* (London: British Museum Press, 1976), pl. LVI–LVIX.

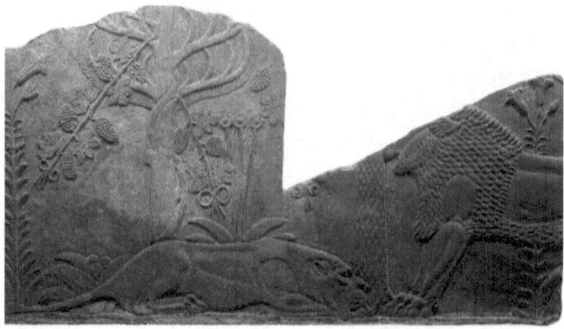

Fig. 6. Lion and lioness in a garden. Palace of Ashurbanipal, Nineveh. BM 118914a. Courtesy of Trustees of the British Museum.

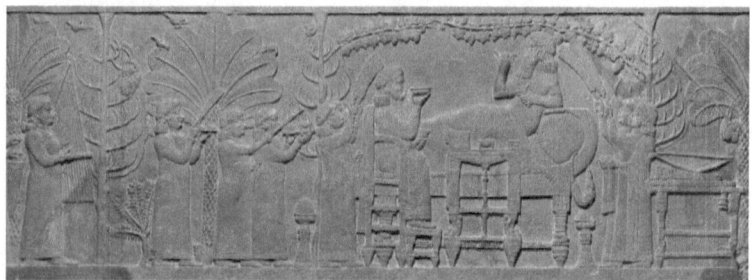

Fig. 7. Garden Scene with king and queen. Palace of Ashurbanipal, Nineveh. BM 124920. Courtesy of Trustees of the British Museum.

in an outdoor garden setting have led scholars to describe this scene as "peaceful," "idyllic," or "pastoral."[17] The landscapes of marshes and conifer trees in the garden show animals making their way habitually among the vegetation. The narratives with these images of animals in gardens might seem to the modern viewer to display relaxation or quietude. Indeed, a *quiet* pastoral environment was desired by nineteenth century European artists escaping industrial cities; however, I suggest that the Assyrian garden with animals invoked rather the busy bustling of life and the possibility of divine presence. Anne-Caroline Rendu Loisel suggests

---

[17] For example, by Karlheinz Deller, "Assurbanipal in der Gartenlaube," *Baghdader Mitteilungen* 18 (1987): 229–38; Pauline Albenda, "Landscape Bas-Reliefs," and myself: Allison Thomason, *Luxury and Legitimation: Royal Collecting in Ancient Mesopotamia* (Aldershot: Ashgate; London: Routledge, 2005).

that the rustling, chewing, calling, and flapping animals and the stimuli they produced for humans to sense might have portended positive or negative future events for the Assyrians as they progressed through quotidian urban life.[18]

That the Mesopotamians were avid consumers of their daily animalscape, and in this case the cries and movement of birds, is clear from a group of omens about city life, the *šumma alū* series, where the gods' intentions for the future were discerned from the movement and noises of birds in the sky outside of houses.[19] Birds were noticed and observed for their divinely-inspired ability to make noise, but also for their constant movement, thus restrictions on their movements were considered ominous or negative. In their royal inscriptions, the Neo-Assyrian kings refer to their cornered or captured enemies as entrapped birds. In one famous prism, Sennacherib claims that he "confined [King Hezekiah] inside the city of Jerusalem, his royal city, like a bird in a cage [GIM.MUŠEN *quppi*]."[20] Conversely, when an enemy king escaped from Sennacherib's grasp in Babylonia, he "flew away like a bird" (*iṣṣuriš ippariš*).[21] In the Garden Scene of Ashurbanipal, the liveliness of the birds contrasts directly with the dead, gaping stillness of Teumman's head. However, while the head is still, it *did* produce numerous other sensory stimuli, such as the smell of decomposing flesh. Furthermore, it could have invoked in a learned Mesopotamian audience an experience of the supernatural or even unnatural. Sarah Graff suggests that Teumman's dismembered and sensing head from the Garden Scene of Ashurbanipal may have invoked the Mesopotamian tradition regarding the demon Humbaba, who was decapitated by Gilgamesh and Enkidu in the Cedar Forest. Ann Guinan observes that the statement "When the severed head laughs …" from the same *šumma ālu* omen texts was interpreted as a horrible omen resulting in the fall of Babylon.[22]

Taking these earlier analyses into consideration, I argue that the vignettes and details of animation, sensing, and being sensed were included by the artisans (and presumably approved by the royal court) to bring the lived sensory experience, wonder, and divinatory revelation or transcendence to Assyrian viewers, learned

---

[18] Anne-Caroline Rendu Loisel, "When Gods Speak to Men: Reading House, Street and Divination from Sound in Ancient Mesopotamia (First Millennium BC)," *JNES* 75.2 (2016): 268.

[19] Akkadian *egirrû*; recently analyzed by Rendu Loisel, "When Gods Speak to Men," 301.

[20] Sennacherib 17.iii.52 (RINAP 3.1:133).

[21] Sennacherib 15.iv.33'–34' (RINAP 3.1:98). Or "they flew away alone like bats living in crevices to inaccessible places" (Sennacherib 16.i.25–26 [RINAP 3.1:111]).

[22] Sarah B. Graff, "The Head of Humbaba," *AR* 14 (2013): 129–44. For discussion of the relevance and experiences of severed heads in omens and literature, see Ann Guinan, "A Severed Head Laughed: Stories of Divinatory Interpretation," in *Magic and Divination in the Ancient World*, ed. Leda Ciraolo and Jonathan Seidel, Ancient Magic and Divination 2 (Groningen: Styx, 2002), 13–40.

or not. These details exhibit what I call "transcendent naturalism." The Assyrians were naturalists, I think, but not for the sake of scientific rationalism. Oppenheim has already warned us against such assumptions, writing:

> It cannot and should not be claimed, of course, that the word lists containing, for example, the names of plants, animals, or stones constitute the beginnings of botany, zoology, or mineralogy in Mesopotamia. They are not a scientific (not even a prescientific) achievement.[23]

Like Oppenheim, I realize these terms are situated in specific times and space, and originated with the age of scientific reasoning in Europe. The anachronism risk may rear its ugly head, but even if the word *naturalism* did not exist in the Assyrian period, it is possible that the habit, feeling, or behavior existed in its own time and space. The term naturalism today refers to both a philosophical stance and an empirical method.[24] Today, philosophers distinguish between ontological and methodological naturalism. Ontological naturalism holds that the supernatural is not rational, as it cannot be observed or explained in the physical reality of nature, and therefore it does not really exist, as everything can and should be explained through observation of natural laws. Methodological naturalism is a bit different. According to the philosophical theorist Barbara Forrest, "methodological naturalism allows us to accumulate substantial knowledge about the cosmos from which ontological categories may be constructed."[25] Certainly, we cannot deny that the Assyrians (and indeed many Mesopotamian scholars and writers) were keen empiricists and observers, noting and categorizing difference and details in the variety and different states of motion and sensing in their environment.[26] As Oppenheim noted, the lexicographic habit of Mesopotamian scribes shows this taxonomic tendency. Marc Van de Mieroop follows this argument and concludes that interpretations of astronomical events as omens by the Babylonians "were highly systematized but they fit quite perfectly within Babylonian philosophy in general."[27] In Babylonian philosophy, the *supernatural* in fact imbued *everything* natural, as it did for Galileo and Newton, who at the inception of the Age of Reason, still ascribed supernatural causes to natural events.

---

[23] Oppenheim, "Man and Nature in Mesopotamian Civilization," 635.

[24] For a recent summary of the term, see David Papineau, "Naturalism," in *The Stanford Encyclopedia of Philosophy* (Winter 2016): https://plato.stanford.edu/archives/win2016/entries/naturalism/.

[25] Barbara Forrest, "Methodological Naturalism and Philosophical Naturalism: Clarifying the Connection," *Philo* 3.2 (2000): 7–29.

[26] For recent discussions of Mesopotamian empiricism, see Jan Dietrich's article in this volume and Marc Van de Mieroop, *Philosophy before the Greeks: The Pursuit of Truth in Ancient Babylonia* (Princeton: Princeton University Press, 2015), 10.

[27] Van de Mieroop, *Philosophy before the Greeks*, 88.

I would even suggest that the attention to animal sensory experience is indeed analogous to the Romantic Pastoral tradition from the late eighteenth century in Western Europe, itself a movement of landscape representation spurred by scientific naturalism. Pastoral landscape paintings of this modern period evoked an experience of sensing nature in all of its synaesthetic glory, but also an experience of transcendence and contemplation of divine presence. European artists represented nature either as "a comforting source of physical and spiritual sustenance" or as a sublime force of uncontrolled activity.[28]

I suggest that the images of sentient animals reacting to their natural habitats brought the audience more into the scene to create a *déja-vu*-like "as if you were here" feeling for the viewer, perhaps even due to the brain's anatomy. Davide Nadali has argued this for other scenes in Neo-Assyrian art, when he concludes "through movement we perceive the world and we are thus perceived as being in the world ... *moveo ergo sum*."[29] For the human brain contains mirror neurons that allow the brain to see and experience again what was felt in the past.[30] The brain also has the ability to leave little morsels of sensory perception with which humans can bring back a memory. In bringing back a specific place experienced during a moment in the past, the brain allows that moment to become timeless and eternalized for the sensing human. When an individual was surrounded in the Neo-Assyrian palace rooms by narrative reliefs with repetitive landscape elements, the punctuated little vignettes and details of animal behavior might also have served as wayfinding spots, sensorially aiding to bring the memory of the past outdoor events to the present in the interior of the palace. Cognitive scientists have suggested that the brain's hippocampus region serves as an internal human

---

[28] Lauren Rabb, "Nineteenth Century Landscape—The Pastoral, the Picturesque and the Sublime," University of Arizona Museum of Art, http://www.artmuseum.arizona.edu/events/event/19th-century-landscape-the-pastoral-the-picturesque-and-the-sublime. See also John Hunt, ed., *The Pastoral Landscape: Studies in the History of Art* (New Haven: National Gallery of Art, Yale University Press, 1999).

[29] Davide Nadali, "*Moveo ergo sum*, Living in the Space around Us: Distance Perspective and Reciprocity," in *Corps, image et perception de l'espace de la Mésopotamia au monde classique*, ed. Nicolas Gillman and Ann Shafer (Paris: L'Harmattan, 2014), 33–55 (45); Nadali, "Interpretations and Translations, Performativity and Embodied Simulation: Reflections on Assyrian Images," in *Leggo! Studies Presented to Frederick Mario Fales on the Occasion of His Sixty-Fifth Birthday*, ed. Giovanni B. Lanfranchi, Daniele Morandi Bonacossi, Cinzia Pappi, and Simonetta Ponchia (Wiesbaden: Harrasowitz Verlag, 2012), 583–95.

[30] See Cory D. Crawford, "Relating Image and Word in Ancient Mesopotamia," in *Critical Approaches to Ancient Near Eastern Art*, ed. Brian A. Brown and Marian Feldman (Berlin: de Gruyter, 2014), 241–64 (249); Nadali, *Interpretations and Translations*, 591; Harry Francis Mallgrave, *Architecture and Embodiment: Implications of the New Sciences and Humanities for Design* (London: Routledge, 2013), 161–64.

Global Positioning System (GPS), capturing sensory moments to bring back the actual experience of being in a unique place and space.[31] This brain anatomy allows that the images on the walls surrounding the viewer helped his or her sensing body to "re-experience the event" in more than visual ways (for example, using the sense of proprioception).[32] In turn this feeling experience could become transcendental or awe-inspiring when encountering the animals in the art. This re-experience was engaged not just due to the choice of animals and placement of scenes within the larger narratives, but also in the way in which the artists depicted the sensing experiences and behaviors of animals as if in nature outside.

Many animals from the reliefs seem stock and static: heavily caparisoned horses pulling chariots, lions frozen in *rigor mortis*-like states of dying, cartoon-like exotic animals, or space-filling creatures in rivers or seas. Some, however, also show movement and reaction, especially in relation to their specific landscapes and surroundings. Even the stationary horses sometimes buck at their handlers by opening their mouths and raising their hooves as their grooms reach up to control or soothe them (fig. 8).

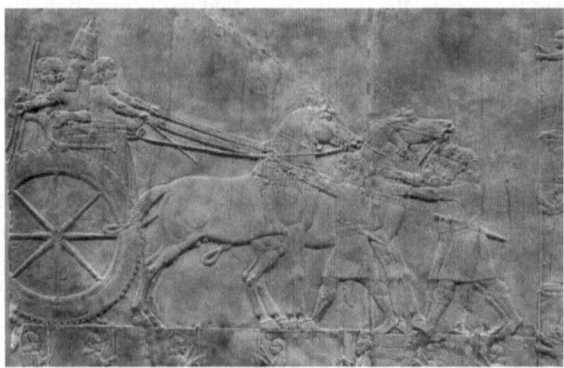

Fig. 8. Horses bucking during muster. Palace of Ashurbanipal, Nineveh. BM 124858-9. Courtesy of Trustees of the British Museum.

Like a lion or an antelope in Ashurbanipal's North Palace at Nineveh, one of the monkeys in the famous tribute scene from Ashurnasirpal II's palace at Nimrud turns his head back, apparently having sensed something behind him, perhaps in apprehension or perhaps exhibiting his natural curiosity (fig. 9). A similar you-are-here moment filled with sentient beings occurs when the wild onager turns his

---

[31] Mirror neurons and the idea of wayfinding receptors in the brain have been studied by psychologists and neurologists since the 1990s; see E. Bruce Goldstein and James R. Brockmole, *Sensation and Perception*, 10th ed. (Boston: Cengage Learning, 2017), 155–60.

[32] Nadali, *Interpretations and Translations*.

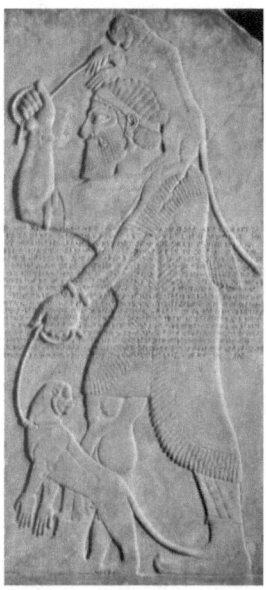

Fig. 9. Tributary carrying monkey to king. Palace of Ashurnasirpal II, Nimrud. BM 124562. Courtesy of Trustees of the British Museum.

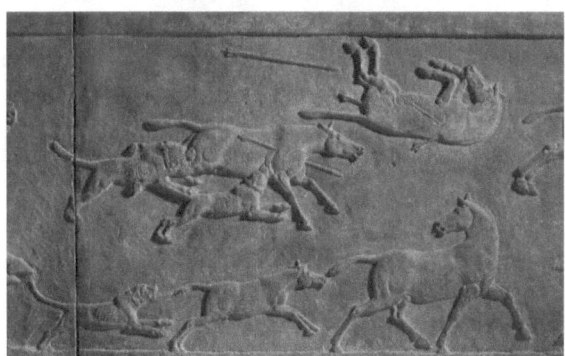

Fig. 10. Hunt of wild onager. Palace of Ashurbanipal, Nineveh. BM 124867-75. Courtesy of Trustees of the British Museum.

head back to watch his herd-mates captured in the hunt (fig. 10). While all other animals face forward, running away from the imminent danger, the Assyrian artists have shown this one turning back, and again, the open mouth and wide eyes as well as craned neck capture a living, breathing, sensing animal in a behavior observed in the wild (which is ironic, as this scene clearly takes place in a man-made game park).[33] The singular animal with head turned emerges as a trope here—one that nevertheless draws the viewer's attention and separates itself from the forward motion of the narrative.[34] For the native Assyrian courtiers who might have passed these reliefs in the palace routinely, the pictorial moment also could have resonated with their knowledge of royal inscriptions. The fleeing-in-the-face-of-fear corresponds with the use of the adverb *kīma* ("like") in animal metaphors found frequently in royal inscriptions. For example, Sennacherib described his enemies "who were weary and fled like deer" in the face of his onslaught.[35]

Returning to Ashurbanipal's dogs, the bared teeth and wrinkled snouts of Ashurbanipal's dogs certainly associate their ferocity with the upcoming royal hunt as they march down a corridor at Nineveh (see fig. 4). But there are other dogs from Ashurbanipal's reliefs with their mouths closed, not bearing their teeth. One dog—and I think the placement of his snout is purposeful—sniffs the hindquarters of the other in the typical greeting behavior of dogs. The dogs are recognized here as sentient beings, and the viewer experiences the dogs as living and acting as animals observed naturally. That Mesopotamians noticed the behavior of dogs is apparent from a Sumerian proverb, where a father warns his perverse son not to ignore humanity "like a dog with his head on the ground sniffing" or "like a dog licking his member with his tongue."[36] Even in watery scenes, occasionally the natural behaviors of animals can be picked out, as in the famous siege of a Phoenician city from Sargon's Palace at Khorsabad, which shows a crab and a fish locked in mortal combat (fig. 11). This vignette, unique among the many staid creatures floating around it that do not interact, shows animal behavior in the wild, but it might have been jarring to an ancient viewer carefully perusing the reliefs who was used to seeing repeated images of single animals isolated amongst the wavy lines in static, inanimate states. The actively sensing animals are the wayfinding spots in the mental GPS. At that moment of reception, what other levels

---

[33] Elnathan Weissert, "Royal Hunt and Royal Triumph in a Prism Fragment of Ashurbanipal," in *Assyria 1995: Proceedings of the Tenth Anniversary of the Neo-Assyrian Text Corpus*, ed. S. Parpola and R. M. Whiting (Helsinki: The Neo-Assyrian Text Corpus Project, 1997), 339–58.

[34] For discussion of narratives and time in Assyrian art, see Chiko Watanabe, "Style of Pictorial Narratives in Assurbanipal's Reliefs," in Brown and Feldman, *Critical Approaches to Ancient Near Eastern Art*, 345–70.

[35] Sennacherib 1.35 (RINAP 3.1:34).

[36] Samuel Noah Kramer, "A Father and His Perverse Son: The First Example of Juvenile Delinquency in Recorded History," *Crime and Delinquency* 3 (1957): 169–73; and Åke W. Sjøberg, "Der Vater und sein missratener Sohn," *JCS* 25 (1973): 105–69, esp. 119. I thank Nicla de Zorzi (see also in this volume) for these references, whose work on dogs will appear as "Of Raving Dogs and Promiscuous Pigs: Mesopotamian Animal Omens in Context," in *Magikon zoon: Animal et magie / The Animal Magic*, ed. Korshi Dosoo and Jean-Charles Coulon (Turnhout: Brepols, forthcoming).

of meaning of the contest between the two sea creatures were pondered by an ancient viewer informed by his or her own sensory experiences and ideas about the world?

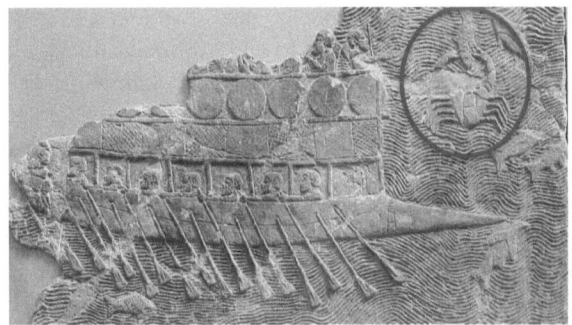

Fig. 11. Crab and fish from water scene. Palace of Sennacherib, Nineveh. BM 124772. Courtesy of Trustees of the British Museum.

I suggest that these sensing animal details and vignettes, especially those associated with other landscape elements such as trees, gardens, water, and even mountains, were meant to be transcendent. By transcendent I mean the little moments that suspend the narrative—they are atemporal, timeless—and in so doing they excavate a moment, retrieved from deep in the brain's memory, that allows the individual to integrate the physical, spiritual, cognitive, and sensorial forms of existence and leads to contemplation of one's place in the universe. My argument here is influenced by the work on the Assyrian intellect of Mehmet-Ali Ataç. Ataç takes the symbolic and religious elements of the natural scenes of animals within landscapes into the *cognitive* realm, suggesting that the detailed animal anatomy in Neo-Assyrian art relates to the Assyrian ordering of the world, or ontology. He also argues that the idyllic Garden Scene of Ashurbanipal was a complex puzzle of concepts, signaling to Assyrian courtly scholars the idea of pastoral transcendence in life and death.[37] Javier Alvarez-Mon further develops the function of the natural world as transcendent in an article on landscapes in ancient Near Eastern art, with a focus on Iran. He suggests that both the geographic and topographic elements surrounding the Elamite rock relief at Kurangun, which deliberately overlooked an Abzu-like natural lustral basin, contributed to the sense that it was a place of religious ritual and numinosity. This *feeling* experience, in addition to

---

[37] Mehmet-Ali Ataç, *The Mythology of Kingship in Neo-Assyrian Art* (Cambridge: Cambridge University Press, 2010). Compare also the liminal capabilities of landscapes of pastoral scenes in Roman painting, as discussed in Caitlín E. Barrett, "Recontextualizing Nilotic Scenes: Interactive Landscapes in the Garden of the Casa dell'Efebo, Pompeii," *AJA* 121.2 (2017): 293–332.

sensuous or emotional, could also have been a transcendent religious experience, Alvarez-Mon argues.[38]

In addition, there is a good deal of literary and other textual evidence to support the idea that a landscape full of vegetation and animals behaving naturally was a space for liminal and transcendent experiences. In the Sumerian myth of Enki and Ninhursag, as Anne-Caroline Rendu Liosel has noted, a sacred garden provided the setting for Enki's insemination of the earth with life thus acting as an ambiguous and liminal space where the human and the divine met.[39] According to ritual texts, as part of the Akītu (New Year's Festival) celebrations in both Assyria and Babylonia, the gods Nabu and Marduk accompanied by their divine consorts Tašmetum and Nanāya, enjoy marriage, sex, leisure, and exercise (Nabu "stretches his legs") in fertile gardens adjoining their festival houses.[40] And in Neo-Assyrian royal inscriptions, which deliberately invoke these divine landscapes for ideological purposes, the kings describe their gardens with fruits, flowers and animals reproducing in abundance as sites of "wonder," "joy," and "delight" (for example on the Banquet Stele of Ashurnasirpal II).

My ascription of transcendental meaning to animal images fits with Irene J. Winter's work on Mesopotamian aesthetics, where she argues that "the primary role of the aesthetic was to provide a conduit for encountering the divine."[41] I suggest that these vignettes allow the audience in the palaces to notice, observe, remember, and *exclaim* at the universe given to them by the gods. This also relates to the experiences of liminality, wonder, awe, or even majesty that art inspires.

---

[38] Javier Alvarez-Mon, "Aesthetics of the Natural Environment in the Arts of the Ancient Near East: The Elamite Rock-Cut Sanctuary of Kurangun," in Brown and Feldman, *Critical Approaches to Ancient Near Eastern Art*, 742–71.

[39] Beate Pongratz-Leisten, *Religion and Ideology in Assyria*, Studies in Ancient Near Eastern Records 4 (Berlin: de Gruyter, 1994); Anne-Caroline Rendu Loisel, "Heurs et malheurs du jardinière dans la littérature Sumérienne," in *Mondes clos cultures et jardins*, ed. Daniel Barbu, Philippe Borgeaud, Mélanie Lozat, and Youri Volokhine (Paris: Infolio, 2013), 70.

[40] Pongratz-Leisten, *Religion and Ideology in Assyria*; Pongratz-Leisten, "Sacred Marriage and the Transfer of Divine Knowledge: Alliances between Gods and the King in Ancient Mesopotamia," in *Sacred Marriages: The Divine-Human Sexual Metaphor from Sumer to Early Christianity*, ed. Martti Nissinen and Risto Uro (Winona Lake, IN: Eisenbrauns, 2008), 65; Steven W. Cole and Peter Machinist, eds., *Letters from Assyrian and Babylonian Priests to Kings Esarhaddon and Assurbanipal*, SAA 13 (Helsinki: Helsinki University Press, 1998), 78; Karen Radner, "How Did the Neo-Assyrian Kings See Their Land and Resources?," in *Rainfall and Agriculture in Northern Mesopotamia: Proceedings of the Third MOS Symposium (Leiden, May 21–22, 1990)*, ed. R. M. Jas (Leiden: Nederlands Instituut voor het Nabije Oosten, 2000), 233–46; Ataç, *Mythology of Kingship in Neo-Assyrian Art*.

[41] Irene J. Winter, "Aesthetics in Ancient Mesopotamian Art," in *Civilizations of the Ancient Near East*, ed. Jack M. Sasson (New York: Scribner's Sons, 1995), 2573.

Ann Shafer argues that Neo-Assyrian landscape images might have invoked "alternative perceptions, temporalities and phenomenal levels [of reception]."[42] Marian Feldman has suggested that for Assyrians, foreign portable works, such as Phoenician metal bowls or ivory objects, inspired a sense of emotional or sensory enchantment in the viewers, allowing an "unstable, even mystical experience."[43] Similarly, the Neo-Assyrian reliefs and the images on them are at once mundane and lived daily through the senses. At the same time the tiny differences in details carved by the artists were synaesthetically and perhaps transcendentally awe-inspiring.

In all of this death and action, life flourishes or is extinguished at the hands of the gods and kings. The depiction and reception of the sentient experiences of animals in relief art was potentially transcendent and aided by the anatomy and possibility of the human brain. In those moments of transcendent naturalism, the Assyrians were observing the ubiquitously experienced and unavoidably present cycle of life and death that the gods imparted to mortal beings. But also, and perhaps more importantly, they experienced the transcendental potential—evocative moments—of touching, seeing, smelling, feeling themselves in the midst of it all, or to borrow Oppenheim's words, as an essential part of the integrated whole.

BIBLIOGRAPHY

Albenda, Pauline "Landscape Bas-Reliefs in the Bīt-Hilani of Ashurbanipal." *BASOR* 224 (1976–1977): 49–72.

———. "Lions on Assyrian Wall Reliefs." *JANES* 6 (1974): 1–27

Alvarez-Mon, Javier. "Aesthetics of the Natural Environment in the Arts of the Ancient Near East: The Elamite Rock-Cut Sanctuary of Kurangun." Pages 742–71 in *Critical Approaches to Ancient Near Eastern Art*. Edited by Brian A. Brown and Marian Feldman. Berlin: de Gruyter, 2014.

Ataç, Mehmet-Ali. "'Imaginal' Landscapes in Assyrian Imperial Monuments." Pages 383–423 in *Experiencing Power, Generating Authority: Cosmos, Politics and the Ideology of Kingship in Ancient Egypt and Mesopotamia*. Edited by Jane A. Hill, Philip Jones, and Antonio J. Morales. Philadelphia: University of Pennsylvania Press, 2013.

———. *The Mythology of Kingship in Neo-Assyrian Art*. Cambridge: Cambridge University Press, 2010.

Bahrani, Zainab. *The Graven Image: Representation in Babylonia and Assyria*. Philadelphia: University of Pennsylvania Press, 2003.

———. *Women of Babylon: Gender and Representation in Mesopotamia*. London: Routledge, 2001.

---

[42] Ann Shafer, "The Assyrian Landscape as Ritual," in Brown and Feldman, *Critical Approaches to Ancient Near Eastern Art*, 729.

[43] Marian Feldman, *Communities of Style: Portable Luxury Arts, Identity and Collective Memory in the Iron Age Levant* (Chicago: University of Chicago Press, 2014), 128–30.

Barnett, Richard David. *Sculptures from the North Palace of Assurbanipal at Nineveh.* London: British Museum Press, 1976.

Barrett, Caitlín E. "Recontextualizing Nilotic Scenes: Interactive Landscapes in the Garden of the Casa dell'Efebo, Pompeii." *AJA* 121.2 (2017): 293–332.

Breniquet, Catherine. "Animals in Mesopotamian Art." Pages 145–68 in *A History of Animals in the Ancient Near East.* Edited by Billie Jean Collins. HdO 64. Leiden: Brill, 2002.

Cole, Steven W., and Peter Machinist, eds. *Letters from Assyrian and Babylonian Priests to Kings Esarhaddon and Assurbanipal.* SAA 13. Helsinki: Helsinki University Press, 1998.

Collins, Paul. "Trees and Gender in Neo-Assyrian Art." *Iraq* 68 (2006): 99–107.

Crawford, Cory D. "Relating Image and Word in Ancient Mesopotamia." Pages 241–64 in *Critical Approaches to Ancient Near Eastern Art.* Edited by Brian A. Brown and Marian Feldman. Berlin: de Gruyter, 2014.

Deller, Karlheinz. "Assurbanipal in der Gartenlaube," *Baghdader Mitteilungen* 18 (1987): 229–38.

De Zorzi, Nicla. "Of Raving Dogs and Promiscuous Pigs: Mesopotamian Animal Omens in Context." In *Magikon zoon: Animal et magie / The Animal Magic.* Edited by Korshi Dosoo and Jean-Charles Coulon. Turnhout: Brepols, forthcoming.

Evans, Jean. *The Lives of Sumerian Sculpture.* Cambridge: Cambridge University Press, 2014.

Feldman, Marian. *Communities of Style: Portable Luxury Arts, Identity and Collective Memory in the Iron Age Levant.* Chicago: University of Chicago Press, 2014.

Forrest, Barbara. "Methodological Naturalism and Philosophical Naturalism: Clarifying the Connection." *Philo* 3.2 (2000): 7–29.

Goldstein, E. Bruce, and James R. Brockmole. *Sensation and Perception.* 10th ed. Boston: Cengage Learning, 2017.

Graff, Sarah B. "The Head of Humbaba." *AR* 14 (2013): 129–44.

Guinan, Ann. "A Severed Head Laughed: Stories of Divinatory Interpretation." Pages 13–40 in *Magic and Divination in the Ancient World.* Edited by Leda Ciraolo and Jonathan Seidel. Ancient Magic and Divination 2. Groningen: Styx, 2002.

Hamilakis, Yannis. *Archaeology and the Senses: Human Experience, Memory and Affect.* Cambridge: Cambridge University Press, 2013.

Harmanşah, Ömür. *Of Rocks and Water: Towards an Archaeology of Place.* Joukowsky Institute Publications 5. Oxford: Oxbow, 2014.

———. "'Source of the Tigris': Event, Place and Performance in the Assyrian Landscapes of the Early Iron Age." *Archaeological Dialogues* 14 (2007): 179–204.

Hunt, John, ed. *The Pastoral Landscape: Studies in the History of Art.* New Haven: National Gallery of Art, Yale University Press, 1999.

Kramer, Samuel Noah. "A Father and His Perverse Son: The First Example of Juvenile Delinquency in Recorded History." *Crime and Delinquency* 3 (1957): 169–73.

Mallgrave, Harry Francis. *Architecture and Embodiment: Implications of the New Sciences and Humanities for Design.* London: Routledge, 2013.

Marcus, Michelle I. "Geography as Visual Ideology: Landscape, Knowledge and Power in Neo-Assyrian Art." Pages 193–202 in *Neo-Assyrian Geography.* Edited by M. Liverani. Quaderni di Geografia Storica 5. Rome: Herder, 1995.

Nadali, Davide. "Interpretations and Translations, Performativity and Embodied Simulation: Reflections on Assyrian Images." Pages 583–95 in *Leggo! Studies Presented to Frederick Mario Fales on the Occasion of His Sixty-Fifth Birthday*. Edited by Giovanni B. Lanfranchi, Daniele Morandi Bonacossi, Cinzia Pappi, and Simonetta Ponchia. Wiesbaden: Harrassowitz Verlag, 2012.

———. "*Moveo ergo sum*, Living in the Space around Us: Distance Perspective and Reciprocity." Pages 33–55 in *Corps, image et perception de l'espace de la Mésopotamia au monde classique*. Edited by Nicolas Gillman and Ann Shafer. Paris: L'Harmattan, 2014.

———. "Neo-Assyrian State Seals: An Allegory of Power." *SAAB* XVIII (2009–2010): 215–44.

Oppenheim, A. Leo. "Man and Nature in Mesopotamian Civilization." Pages 634–66 in *The Dictionary of Scientific Biography* 15. New York: Scribner's Sons, 2008.

Papineau, David. "Naturalism." In *The Stanford Encyclopedia of Philosophy* (Winter 2016): https://plato.stanford.edu/archives/win2016/entries/naturalism/

Pongratz-Leisten, Beate. "Melammu." In *The Encyclopedia of Ancient History*. Malden, MA: Blackwell, 2012. doi:10.1002/9781444338386.wbeah24143.

———. *Religion and Ideology in Assyria*. Studies in Ancient Near Eastern Records 4. Berlin: de Gruyter, 1994.

———. "Sacred Marriage and the Transfer of Divine Knowledge: Alliances between Gods and the King in Ancient Mesopotamia." Pages 43–73 in *Sacred Marriages: The Divine-Human Sexual Metaphor from Sumer to Early Christianity*. Edited by Martti Nissinen and Risto Uro. Winona Lake, IN: Eisenbrauns, 2008.

Rabb, Lauren. "Nineteenth Century Landscape—The Pastoral, the Picturesque and the Sublime." University of Arizona Museum of Art. http://www.artmuseum.arizona.edu/events/event/19th-century-landscape-the-pastoral-the-picturesque-and-the-sublime.

Radner, Karen. "How Did the Neo-Assyrian Kings See Their Land and Resources?" Pages 233–46 in *Rainfall and Agriculture in Northern Mesopotamia: Proceedings of the Third MOS Symposium (Leiden, May 21–22, 1990)*. Edited by R. M. Jas. Leiden: Nederlands Instituut voor het Nabije Oosten, 2000.

Reade, Julian E. "The Assyrians as Collectors: From Accumulation to Synthesis." Pages 255–66 in *From the Upper Sea to the Lower Sea: Studies on the History of Assyrian and Babylonia in Honour of A. K. Grayson*. Edited by Grant Frame. Leiden: Nederlands Instituut voor het Nabije Oosten, 2004.

———. "Ideology and Propaganda in Assyrian Art." Pages 329–43 in *Power and Propaganda*. Edited by Mogens Trolle Larsen. Copenhagen: Akademisk Forlag, 1979.

Rendu Loisel, Anne-Caroline. "Heurs et malheurs du jardinière dans la littérature Sumérienne." Pages 67–84 in *Mondes clos cultures et jardins*. Edited by Daniel Barbu, Philippe Borgeaud, Mélanie Lozat, and Youri Volokhine. Paris: Infolio, 2013.

———. "When Gods Speak to Men: Reading House, Street and Divination from Sound in Ancient Mesopotamia (First Millennium BC)." *JNES* 75.2 (2016): 291–309.

Russell, John M. *Sennacherib's Palace without Rival at Nineveh*. Chicago: University of Chicago Press, 1991.

Shafer, Ann. "The Assyrian Landscape as Ritual." Pages 713–39 in *Critical Approaches to Ancient Near Eastern Art*. Edited by Brian A. Brown and Marian Feldman. Boston: de Gruyter, 2014.

———. "Assyrian Royal Monuments on the Periphery: Ritual and the Making of Imperial Space." Pages 133–59 in *Ancient Near Eastern Art in Context: Studies in Honor of Irene J. Winter by Her Students*. Edited by J. Cheng and M. Feldman. Leiden: Brill, 2007.

Sjøberg, Åke W. "Der Vater und sein missratener Sohn." *JCS* 25 (1973): 105–69.

Strawn, Brent A. *What Is Stronger Than a Lion? Leonine Image and Metaphor in the Hebrew Bible and the Ancient Near East*. OBO 212. Fribourg: Academic Press, 2005

Thomason, Allison. *Luxury and Legitimation: Royal Collecting in Ancient Mesopotamia*. Aldershot: Ashgate; London: Routledge, 2005.

———. "Representations of the North Syrian Landscape in Neo-Assyrian Art." *BASOR* 323 (2001): 63–96.

———. "The Sense-Scapes of Neo-Assyrian Capital Cities: Royal Authority and Bodily Experience." *Cambridge Archaeological Journal* 26.2 (2016): 243–64.

Van de Mieroop, Marc. *Philosophy before the Greeks: The Pursuit of Truth in Ancient Babylonia*. Princeton: Princeton University Press, 2015.

Watanabe, Chiko. *Animal Symbolism in Mesopotamia: A Contextual Approach*. Vienna: Institut für Orientalistik der Universität Wien, 2002.

———. "Style of Pictorial Narratives in Assurbanipal's Reliefs." Pages 345–70 in *Critical Approaches to Ancient Near Eastern Art*. Edited by Brian A. Brown and Marian Feldman. Berlin: de Gruyter, 2014.

Weissert, Elnathan. "Royal Hunt and Royal Triumph in a Prism Fragment of Ashurbanipal." Pages 339–58 in *Assyria 1995: Proceedings of the Tenth Anniversary of the Neo-Assyrian Text Corpus*. Edited by S. Parpola and R. M. Whiting. Helsinki: The Neo-Assyrian Text Corpus Project, 1997.

Winter, Irene J. "Aesthetics in Ancient Mesopotamian Art." Pages 2569–80 in *Civilizations of the Ancient Near East*. Edited by Jack M. Sasson. New York: Scribner's Sons, 1995.

———. "Radiance as an Aesthetic Value in the Art of Mesopotamia, with Some Indian Parallels." Pages 123–32 in *Art, the Integral Vision: A Volume in Felicitation of Kapila Vatsyayan*. Edited by Baidyanath M. Saraswati, S. C. Malik, and Madhu Khanna. New Delhi: Printworld, 1994.

———. "Royal Rhetoric and the Development of Historical Narrative in Neo-Assyrian Reliefs." *Studies in Visual Communication* 7 (1981): 2–38.

———. "Tree(s) on the Mountain: Landscape and Territory on the Victory Stele of Naram-Sin of Agade." Pages 63–72 in *Landscapes: Territories, Frontiers and Horizons in the Ancient Near East*. Edited by Lucio Milano, Stefano de Marino, Frederick Mario Fales, and Giovanni B. Lanfranchi. HANE/M 3.1. Padua: Sargon, 2000.

ANCIENT EGYPT

SOUND STUDIES AND VISUAL STUDIES APPLIED TO ANCIENT EGYPTIAN SOURCES

Dorothée Elwart and Sibylle Emerit

INTRODUCTION

The aim of this paper is to show how the approaches developed by sound studies and visual studies may renew our understanding of the sources from ancient Egypt. The fields covered by sound studies, on one hand, and visual studies, on the other, are not the same since the former concerns the sense of hearing and the latter the sense of sight, but their approaches both deal with cultural and social identity. Since perception and cognition mechanisms are an integral part of sound studies and visual studies, the images, sounds, objects, and also architecture should be studied on the basis of their role and function. Visual and aural perceptions are by no means trivial; they have an emotional impact that can condition beliefs. Each culture has a policy and an economy of visual perception and sound designed to lead to specific emotions. This was also the case in the ancient Egyptian world.

Starting from a general overview of the theoretical and methodological frameworks of sound studies and visual studies, this paper gives several examples taken from the ancient Egyptian sources to illustrate the relevance of this approach. Musical instruments, as sound and iconic objects, provide a good example of how images and sounds deserve to be apprehended as a whole, but also as driving forces used for religion purpose. More generally, a sensory reading of ancient Egyptian rites leads us to reexamine space in temples, by taking into account iconographic and textual material relating to music, dance, and joy. As discussed below, the temple of Dendara is a case study particularly interesting for the combination of sound studies and visual studies within a religious environment.

Theoretical and Methodological Frameworks

From Music to Sound Studies

The concept of music itself, used by three renowned specialists of pharaonic music—Victor Loret (1859–1946), Curt Sachs (1881–1958), and Hans Hickmann (1908–1968)—is inappropriate as it leads researchers to apply occidental classification to ancient Egyptian material. In most societies studied by ethnomusicologists, there is no equivalent term for the word *music*. Music is not named as such and is not dissociated from dance and singing. In other words, music is experienced across body sensations. Similarly, there is no generic term for music in ancient Egyptian, nor for dancing. Only one word, *kheru* (*ḫrw*), refers to all forms of sound manifestations, whether they are noisy or musical, related to dance or emotion.[1] This broad meaning of *kheru* opens new perspectives in analyzing ancient Egyptian sources.

The work being currently carried out by researchers in ethnomusicology and anthropology of music invites us to bring down the artificial barriers between disciplinary fields and objects of study in order to perform analysis on a broader scale.[2] Renewing our knowledge of ancient Egyptian music requires us to take sound as a whole as an object to be studied not only in relation to musical manifestations, but also in relation to other expressions, within the general framework of the sensory studies. On this basis, the three major epithets of the goddess Hathor, which define her as mistress of "music" (*nbt ḥst*), "dance" (*nbt ibȝ*), and "joy" (*nbt ȝwt-ib*), perfectly illustrate the importance of having a multisensorial approach to ancient Egyptian sources. The semantic field of sound has a lot of items with links to dance and emotions in ancient Egyptian. A lexicographical analysis from an emic perspective is the necessary first stage to go through to apply a sound studies approach on these sources. Visual studies are also involved because images are an essential element of the hieroglyphic pictorial writing system.

A lexicographical approach can help to avoid, as much as possible, confusion with contemporary categories. The words will indeed reveal the way in which sounds were perceived and constructed, whether through a range of expressions developed by the speakers themselves, through the interpretive

---

[1] The results of the lexicographical analysis of the word *kheru* have been presented by Sibylle Emerit during the international round-table *De la cacophonie à la musique: La perception du son dans les sociétés antiques*, held at l'École française d'Athènes in 2014 and organized by Sibylle Emerit, Sylvain Perrot, and Alexandre Vincent. The proceedings will be published by the Institut français d'archéologie orientale (IFAO).

[2] Nathalie Fernando and Jean-Jacques Nattiez, eds., *Ethnomusicologie et anthropologie de la musique: Une question de perspective*, Anthropologie et sociétés 38 (2014).

imagery applied to them, or through the way in which they categorize different aural phenomena. If it might initially appear simple to identify the vocabulary of sound, one soon realizes that it is not so easy to grasp the nuances. Many words and expressions that describe enjoyment or pain seem to have a musical connotation, as the word *nhm* (*nhm*), which means "shout" or "shouting with joy."[3] Indeed, this word is written during the Ptolemaic period with the sign of a woman playing tambourine. It is perhaps because the heart beats more intensively when someone feels an emotion.

The sources concerning sounds have been rarely examined from an anthropological perspective before the research programme named Soundscapes and Urban Spaces in the Ancient Mediterranean.[4] One of the goals of this research programme is to develop a dialogue between specialists of different cultures of antiquity around a common theme, that of sound perception, its production, and its use in ancient societies.[5] The historicity of aural perception is a given that is no longer contested. Sound is an object of culture, and it is recognized that each group of individuals has a certain relationship with sound that distinguishes it from other groups. In this sense, sound is an object of historical study.

In order to clearly draw a parallel between the two fields of research (sound and visual), the phrase *sound studies* has been privileged over *soundscape studies* in the title of this paper. In fact, there is a distinction between sound studies and soundscape studies. Sound studies are devoted to the sound in itself, in its acoustic and technical dimension, while soundscape studies take into account the context of transmission and reception of the sound message by an individual or a society inside an acoustic environment.[6] However, since the publication of

---

[3] *Wb* 2:285.7–18.

[4] This research programme has been established in 2012 between the three French Schools Abroad, namely, the IFAO, the École française d'Athènes, and the École française de Rome.

[5] See the first volume of this research programme, Sibylle Emerit, Sylvain Perrot, and Alexandre Vincent, eds., *Le paysage sonore de l'Antiquité: Méthodologie, historiographie et perspectives, Actes de la journée d'études tenue à l'École française de Rome, le 7 janvier 2013*, RAPH 40 (Le Caire: IFAO, 2015). The included article of Sibylle Emerit, "Autour de l'ouïe, de la voix et des sons: Approche anthropologique des 'paysages sonores' de l'Égypte ancienne," 115–54, gives the bibliography related to this subject in Egyptology and suggests future research for taking advantage of the ancient Egyptian sources. Two recent publications have to be added: Alexandra von Lieven, "Sounds of Power: The Concept of Sound in Ancient Egyptian Religion," in *Religion für die Sinne / Religion for the Senses*, ed. Philipp Reichling and Meret Strothmann, Artificium 58 (Oberhausen: Athena, 2016), 25–35; and Erika Meyer-Dietrich, *Auditive Räume des alten Ägypten: Die Umgestaltung einer Hörkultur in der Amarnazeit*, CHANE 92 (Leiden: Brill, 2018).

[6] Alexandre Vincent, "Paysage sonore et sciences sociales: Sonorités, sens, histoire," in Emerit, Perrot, and Vincent, *Le paysage sonore de l'Antiquité*, 18–19.

the book of Jonathan Sterne in 2003, a major evolution has occurred in the way sound studies tackle their research questions.[7] The author invites scholars to study historical, political, and philosophical events also from the point of view of the sound and, by proceeding so, to come closer to the research problems of cultural studies. In both cases, the aim of the sound studies and soundscape studies is to situate the sound inside a cultural context to understand its different uses within a society: music, sounds, and noises produced by a group are all elements that constitute its sound identity and reveal the way it functions.

From Art History to Visual Studies

The book of Daniel Dubuisson and Sophie Raux explores the issues covered by visual studies.[8] This field of research, born in 1995, is committed to studying all types of image used by a cultural group.[9] In that respect, this approach has to be distinguished from art history, which studies only masterpieces of visual artifacts. However, the border between these two subjects is not rigid, and the scope of the visual studies is wider: it concerns images in the broadest sense of the term, which includes visual artifacts, but also all visual signs such as clothes, furniture, writings, ornaments, effigies, symbols, tattoos, and urban settings (monuments and architectural elements).[10] In fact, images, symbols, and buildings create visual universes. They are social and cultural creations through which a society shows itself. Any human culture or group thus possesses a visual identity based on a codified repertoire of signs immediately recognizable and interpretable by their members. Unlike art history, visual studies do not carry out a distinction between high and low art.

In the field of Egyptology, many works have focused on the semiology of the image, as well as on its performativity. With regard to visual studies, three recent publications have to be mentioned. In his monograph, Kai Widmaier invites Egyptologists to follow the path of visual studies.[11] According to this author, the methods of art history used to analyze ancient Egyptian images tend to apply a Western conception of art: "Images can, therefore, be seen and understood in completely different ways in which these images were perceived by

---

[7] Jonathan Sterne, *The Audible Past: Cultural Origins of Sound Reproduction* (Durham, NC: Duke University Press, 2003).

[8] Daniel Dubuisson and Sophie Raux, eds., *À perte de vue: Les nouveaux paradigmes du visuel* (Dijon: Les presses du réel, 2015).

[9] Daniel Dubuisson and Sophie Raux, "Entre l'histoire de l'art et les Visual Studies: Mythe, science et idéologie," *Histoire de l'Art* 70 (2012): 99.

[10] Dubuisson and Raux, *À perte de vue*, 8.

[11] Kai Widmaier, *Bilderwelten: Ägyptische Bilder und ägyptologische Kunst: Vorarbeiten für eine bildwissenschaftliche Ägyptologie*, PAe 35 (Leiden: Brill, 2017).

those who created them."¹² To be able to understand the way that an image was perceived by the observer, the context where it has been created must be taken into account. Ludwig D. Morenz also suggests various approaches to interpret pharaonic images in a perspective of visual anthropology.¹³ Morenz defines three main areas in which the production and reception of images play a decisive role in ancient Egypt: the manner to comprehend the death, the relations with the world of the gods, and the way to stage the power.¹⁴ For Morenz, in all these areas, image is used to make visible the invisible. He also reminds us that several iconographic themes had been recurrent during three millennia in order to impose the power of monarchy. These images were a strong cultural referent and contributed to build a specific visual universe. In his article, Jan Assmann reconsiders the idea of permanence, which seems to be a fundamental feature of the pharaonic society: images or monuments must be sustainable over time.¹⁵ This is even underlined by the root of the Egyptian word *mnw* ("monument"), which is *mnj* ("enduring"). For instance, an Egyptian temple has a monumental function that imposes itself visually on the faithful and marks in the landscape a border with the sacred. Assmann also emphasizes the performative power of the image, particularly in rituals context (worship or execration), when a short-lived image is created in order to make a divine entity to appear into a sensitive form. This "iconic action" depends on the religious beliefs from which symbolic objects are deriving. To do so, a spatiotemporal framework is necessary to give all the power to the performative action. At the end, the image must be destroyed or hidden for the efficacy of the ritual. Beside this iconic action, it can be assumed that the performativity of words, sound, music, and also silence played a role in the rituals. Did the ancient Egyptians seek to combine the two senses to obtain a ritual efficacy?

MUSICAL INSTRUMENTS AS AUDIO AND VISUAL VECTORS

The Visual Dimension of Bells

Musical instruments give an excellent illustration on the way sound studies and visual studies may converge. For instance, the iconography of the harps, depicted on the musical scenes of private tombs, shows that this type of musical

---

¹² Widmaier, *Bilderwelten*, XL.

¹³ Ludwig D. Morenz, *Anfänge der ägyptischen Kunst: Eine problemgeschichtliche Einführung in ägyptologische Bild-Anthropologie*, OBO 264 (Fribourg: Presses Universitaires, 2014).

¹⁴ Morenz, *Anfänge der ägyptischen Kunst*, 4.

¹⁵ Jan Assmann, "Le pouvoir des images: De la performativité des images en Égypte ancienne," in *Penser l'image II: Anthropologies du visuel*, ed. Emmanuel Alloa (Dijon: Les presses du réel, 2015), 173–206.

instrument was richly decorated since the Old Kingdom, but only a few artifacts still preserve a painting on their sound-box.[16] Apparently, this kind of object was made to produce a sound and have a visual impact. Similarly, bells and sistra are often richly ornamented, soliciting two senses at the same time. These idiophones were used for ritual purposes, and their iconography refers clearly to the world of the gods. Unfortunately, the corpus of decorated bells is poorly dated (from late period to Roman period), the provenance mostly unrecorded and the contexts of discoveries (tomb?, temple?, house?) rarely known.[17] For instance, the British Museum preserves two small egg-shaped bells in the form of Bes, one made in blue-gaze faience (BM EA66619), the other in bronze (BM EA6374).[18] Their provenance is unrecorded. The first one is said to be from the Ptolemaic period, the second one from the Roman period. Whereas the back is damaged on one, the other is decorated with a bovine head (?) and two lizards. Several decorated bells can also be found at the Cairo Museum, the Petrie Museum (London), the Museum of Fine Arts (Boston), the Metropolitan Museum of Art (New York), the Louvre Museum (Paris), and the Neues Museum (Ägyptisches Museum und Papyrussammlung, Berlin).[19] Their comparison gives an idea of the most recurrent iconography. The face of Bes appears alone regularly[20] or with other patterns like animal heads (jackal [Anubis?], ram [Amon?], bovine [Hathor?], lioness [Sekhmet?]), a dwarf, an udjat-eye, or a lizard).[21] Occasionally,

---

[16] Mohamed Abdel Rahiem, "Decoration of Ancient Egyptian Harps," in *Laut und Leise: Der Gebrauch von Stimme und Klang in historischen Kulturen*, ed. Erika Meyer-Dietrich, Mainzer Historische Kulturwissenschaften 7 (Bielefeld: Transcript, 2011), 89–120.

[17] See Hans Hickmann, *Instruments de musique*, Catalogue général des antiquités égyptiennes du Musée du Caire (Le Caire: IFAO, 1949), CG 69298: 49, pl. XXVI C (Tanis); CG 69299: 49, pl. XXVI A, B, (Qaou el-Kebir); CG 69603: 65, pl. XXIII B (Saqqara).

[18] Robert D. Anderson, *Musical Instruments*, Catalogue of Egyptian Antiquities in the British Museum 3 (London: British Museum Publications, 1976), 38 no. 47, fig. 66 (BM EA66619); 32 no. 33, fig. 48 (BM EA6374).

[19] For some references, see Dominique Bénazeth and Alain Delattre, "Cloches et clochettes dans l'Égypte chrétienne," in *Études coptes XIV*, ed. Anne Boud'hors et Catherine Louis, Cahiers de la Bibliothèque Copte 21 (Paris: de Boccard, 2016), 258 no. 75.

[20] For instance: Cairo CG 69276 (Hickmann, *Instruments de musique*, 42 pl. XXIII A); Museum of Fine Arts Boston 03.1666 ("Bell with the Face of the God Bes," mfa Boston, http://www.mfa.org/collections/object/bell-with-the-face-of-the-god-bes-130475); Petrie Museum UC33266, UC37492 (William Matthew Flinders Petrie, *Amulets Illustrated by the Egyptian Collection in University College* [London: Constable, 1914], 28 pl. XLIX 124 c).

[21] For instance: Cairo CG 68298a (Hickmann, *Instruments de musique*, 49 pl. XXVI C); BM EA17094, BM EA38160, BM EA6376, BM EA6378, BM EA67105 (Anderson, *Musical Instruments*, no. 36: 33, figs. 51–52; no. 37: 34, figs. 53–54; no. 34: 33, fig. 49;

the headdress of the god Bes, or Bes himself, serves as a handle;[22] on a bell held in the Cairo Museum, Bes is shaped twice, back-to-back, with a circular rim between the legs. The sense of touch is probably also invoked when grasping the instrument, but a hole is always present at the back of the headdress or at the top of the bell to allow its hanging. Further investigations would be required to explain the association between Bes and the other symbols and to get a better understanding of this type of musical instrument.

However, the apotropaic function of these objects is not in doubt. Since the New Kingdom, Bes is known as a powerful apotropaic deity who protects birth, childhood, and by extension, the rebirth of the deceased.[23] He repels evil spirits by his ugliness and by playing all sorts of musical instruments such as the harp, lute, oboe, or tambourine. Highly worshipped in Egypt during the Ptolemaic and Roman periods, it is not surprising to find his face on bells, even if we do not know for what kind of ceremonies the sound of these bronze instruments was used. A funerary overtone has to be considered that bells with heads of mythological animals were found in the cemetery of Naukratis at the end of the nineteenth century.[24] Furthermore, the head of jackal symbolizes certainly Anubis, which is a crucial god in funerary rites of passage. The fact that some bells are made in blue-glazed faience and are similar to amulets could confirm this funeral function. Bell-shaped amulets were used for the protection of the de-

---

no. 35: 33, fig. 50; no. 38: 34–35, figs. 55–56); The Metropolitan Museum of Art 1985.73 ("Bell in the Form of Bes," the MET, https://metmuseum.org/art/collection/search/551369).

[22] On the bell CG 69295, Bes is shaped twice back-to-back (Hickmann, *Instruments de musique*, 48 pl. XXVII c).

[23] James F. Romano, *The Bes-Image in Pharaonic Egypt* (Ann Arbor, MI: University Microfilms International, 1989); Marteen Raven, "Women's Bed from Deir el-Medina," in *The Workman's Progress Studies in the Village of Deir al-Medina and Other Documents from Western Thebes in Honour of Rob Demarée*, ed. Rob Demarée, Ben J. J. Haring, and Olaf Ernst Kaper (Leiden: Nederlands Instituut voor het Nabije Oosten; Leuven: Peeters, 2014), 191–204; Benjamin Hinson, "Dead Ringers: The Mortuary Use of Bells in Late Pharaonic Egypt," in *A True Scribe of Abydos: Essays on First Millenium Egypt in Honour of Anthony Leahy*, ed. Claus Jurman, Bettina Bader, David Aston, OLA 265 (Leuven: Peeters, 2017), 187–88.

[24] Museum of Fine Arts Boston 88.751, 88.752 ("Bell," mfa Boston, http://www.mfa.org/collections/object/bell-131441; and "Bell," mfa Boston, http://www.mfa.org/collections/object/bell-131442); see Aurélia Masson, "Bronze Votive Offerings," in *Naukratis: Greeks in Egypt*, ed. Alexandra Villing et al. (London: British Museum, 2016), 12–13, http://www.britishmuseum.org/research/online_research_catalogues/ng/naukratis_greeks_in_egypt/material_culture_of_naukratis/bronze_offerings.aspx. For others references, see Hinson, "Dead Ringers," 187.

ceased: four of them, without any decoration, were found in a roman grab at Tounah el Gebel with other kinds of amulets.²⁵

The Visual and Audio Dimensions of Sistra

In contrast to bells, interpreting sistra is easier because textual and iconographic sources accompany the archaeological objects. As sistra produce sounds (idiophones) and take the shape of Hathor²⁶ (her fontal face), they should be understood as vectors of audio-visual emotions. They often appear in ritual scenes depicted on the walls of the temples during the Greco-Roman period, acting as an instrument of Hathor appeasement (see below "Ritual Efficacy of Sistra").

Usually two types of sistra are defined according to the nature of the upper-part fixed above the handle: an arch fitted with crossbars and loose metal rings (the so-called arched-sistrum), or an element taking the shape of a *bekhen*-door, a monumental door with scrolls on each side, often represented with an uraeus (the female cobra) standing in it (the so-called *bekhen*-sistrum).²⁷

bekhen-door   *bekhen*-door with scrolls

While *bekhen*-sistra were more frequently made of faience,²⁸ arched-sistra have been almost exclusively made of bronze.²⁹ This double typology is reflected in the ancient Egyptian hieroglyphic script, where the two sistra have their own sign:

---

²⁵ Dieter Kessler and Patrick Brose, *Ägyptens letzte Pyramide: Das Grab des Seuta(s) in Tuna el-Gebel* (Vaterstetten: Verlag Patrick Brose, 2008), 40 pl. 41 and 46. Hinson's theory, which considers that bells were mainly deposited in children's tombs, seems too much reductive ("Dead Ringers," 179–201).

²⁶ Sistra are two of the sacred objects devoted to the goddess Hathor, see François Daumas, "Les objets sacrés d'Hathor au temple de Dendara," *Bulletin de la société française d'égyptologie* 57 (1970): 7–18.

²⁷ The Egyptological literature has erroneously given that sistrum the name of naos-sistrum. See, for instance, Marleen Reynders, "Sšš.t and sḫm: Names and Types of the Egyptian Sistrum," in *Egyptian Religion: The Last Thousand Years, Studies Dedicated to the Memory of Jan Quaegebeur*, ed. Willy Clarysse, Antoon Schoors and Harco Willems, 2 parts, OLA 85 (Leuven: Peeters, 1998), 1013–26. But the monument involved here cannot be referred to as a naos as it is clearly a doorway.

²⁸ The ancient Egyptian faience is a quartz glazed with a blue-green color obtained from copper oxide. See, for instance, Louvre E 8063, N 5038, E 5654, E 10244, E 3668, AF 2937, E 4432 and N 3802 (Christiane Ziegler, *Catalogue des instruments de musique égyptiens* [Paris: Éditions de la réunion des musées nationaux, 1979], 40 IDM 22; 45 IDM 34–37; 46 IDM 38–40); BM EA6359, BM EA38173 (Anderson, *Musical Instru-*

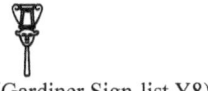

bekhen-sistrum (Gardiner Sign-list Y8)   arched-sistrum (Gardiner Sign-list Y18)

Two Egyptian words are used to designate the two types of sistra in the hieroglyphics texts, especially those from the Greco-Roman period: *sesheshet* (*sššt*) and *sekhem* (*sḫm*). Used as classifiers,[30] the signs previously mentioned show that that *sšš(t)* designates the *bekhen*-sistrum and *sḫm* the arched-sistrum:

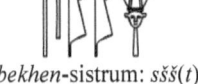 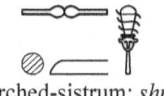

bekhen-sistrum: *sšš(t)*   arched-sistrum: *sḫm*

However, if there are two types of object as well as two distinct terms, the function is identical for the two sistra, as they both bear and act as audio and visual vectors, in a kind of cross, complementary approach:

	Reading	Function
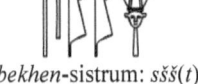	*sššt* →	1—**sound**: onomatopoeia "*sesheshet*"
	+ *bekhen*-*sistrum* as classifier →	2—**image**: *bekhen*-door with lateral volutes and frontal Hathor's head specific to the object
	sḫm →	1—**image**: *sekhem*, lit. "divine image"
	+ *arched*-*sistrum* as classifier →	2—**sound**: jangles produced by the crossbars and rings within the arch.

---

ments, 53 no. 70, fig. 94; 55 no. 73, fig. 97); Cairo CG 69321, CG 69322, CG 69325 (Hickmann, *Instruments de musique*, 83–84 pl. LII, C and D; 84 pl. LV, A and B; 85 pl. LIX, A and B). A better photo of CG 69325 has been published by Dorothée Elwart, "Sistren als Klang des Hathorkultes," in *Laut und Leise: Der Gebrauch von Stimme und Klang in historischen Kulturen*, ed. Erika Meyer-Dietrich, Mainzer Historische Kulturwissenschaften 7 (Bielefeld: Transcript, 2011), 39.

[29] Some bronze arched-sistra are richly decorated; see, for example, Louvre E 8076 (Ziegler, *Catalogue des instruments*, 58 IDM 76), E 11158 (ibid., 60 IDM 78), E 11201 (Christiane Ziegler, "Le sistre d'Henouttaouy," *Revue du Louvre* 1 [1977]: 1–4), and N 4272 (Ziegler, *Catalogue des instruments de musique égyptiens*, 56 IDM 67); BM EA36310, BM EA38172 (Anderson, *Musical Instruments*, 41 no. 51, figs. 70–71 and no. 52, figs. 72–73), Cairo CG 69316 (Hickmann, *Instruments de musique*, 80–81 pl. XLV, XLVI, A, B, C).

[30] A classifier is a hieroglyph placed at the end of a word, in order to specify its meaning.

As for the *bekhen*-sistrum, the Egyptian word $sšš(t)$[31] (*seshesh*) used to designate it is clearly onomatopoetic and evokes the sound that the object itself produces when shacked. The *bekhen* feature exhibiting the frontal head is a clear image of the goddess herself. The whole columns inside the pronaos of the temple of Dendara (fig. 1) precisely represent Hathor with her frontal head crowned by the *bekhen*-door and are as many monumental images of the main goddess of the temple.

As for the arched-sistrum, the relationship is reversed as the notion of image is taken on by the ancient Egyptian word $sḫm$[32] (*sekhem*), which designates simultaneously "figure," "representation," or "divine statue," whereas the sound related aspect of the sistrum is to be found in the arch fitted with the crossbars and loose metal rings. Shaking the sistra rattles the crossbars and the rings together.

This means that, whatever its type or its name, a sistrum adds the notions of sound and image.[33] In a general way, sistra are to be thus understood as vectors of audio and visual emotions.

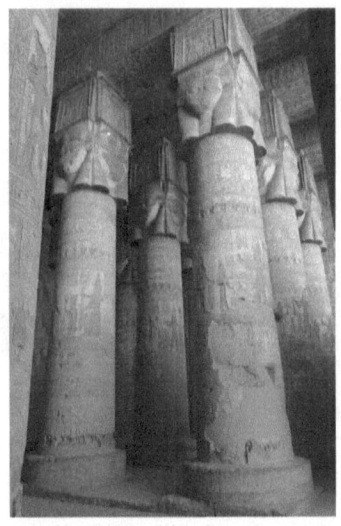

Fig. 1. Hathoric columns, Pronaos of Hathor temple, Dendara
© Sibylle Emerit (IFAO, CNRS UMR 5189)

---

[31] *Wb* 3:486.19.

[32] *Wb* 4:251.18.

[33] For more details, see Dorothée Elwart, "Le sistre, le son et l'image," in *Offrandes, rites et rituels dans les temples d'époques ptolémaïque et romaine: Actes de la journée d'études de l'équipe EPHE (EA 4519) "Égypte ancienne; Archéologie, langue, religion,"* Paris, 27 juin 2013, ed. Christiane Zivie-Coche, Cahiers Égypte nilotique et méditerranéenne 10 (Montpellier: Université Paul Valéry, 2015), 109–21.

Ritual Efficacy of Sistra

The scenes decorating Egyptian temples, especially during the Greco-Roman period, show quite frequently the pharaoh holding two sistra (fig. 2) with the aim, the texts say, to appease the goddess facing him, in most cases Hathor.[34] In Ptolemaic studies, these scenes are, in a generic way, referred to as "offering scenes," but it would be useful to bear in mind that this appellation is especially misleading for the scenes where sistra are involved. According to the texts, the sistra are not objects offered as such, but they are the tool, the vector by which the rite of appeasement is performed through sound and image. In other words, sistra are, as vector of audio-visual emotions, a key instrument of Hathor appeasement.

The actions in question in these scenes are a reference to the myth of the Distant Goddess[35] and are ritual instantiations of the appeasement achieved by

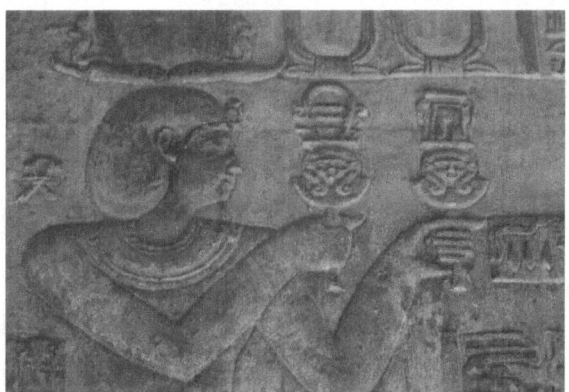

Fig. 2. Pharaoh holding two sistra, chapel Hut-sechechet of Hathor Temple, Dendara
© Dorothée Elwart (LabEx Hastec, EPHE-PSL)

---

[34] See Dorothée Elwart, *Apaiser Hathor: Le rite de présentation des sistres à Dendara* (PhD diss., École Pratique des Hautes Études; Universität zu Köln, 2013).

[35] The myth of the Distant Goddess is known by many Late period sources, written in hieroglyphs (temple texts) or in demotic (cursive writing used especially for organically supports such as ostraca and papyri). At the beginning of the twentieth century, Hermann Junker and Wilhelm Spiegelberg were entering the studies about the myth. Hermann Junker, *Der Auszug der Hathor-Tefnut aus Nubien* (Berlin: Preussische Akademie der Wissenschaften, 1911); Wilhelm Spiegelberg, *Der ägyptische Mythus vom Sonnenauge (der Papyrus der Tierfabeln—"Kufi"): Nach dem Leidener demotischen Papyrus I 384* (Strassburg: Strassburger Druckerei und Verlagsanstalt, 1917). So many researchers have since worked on the texts relating to the myth of the Distant Goddess that it would be impossible to quote here all of them. For the orgiastic feasts linked to this myth, see the recent bibliography quoted in Joachim Friedrich Quack and Kim Ryholt, *Demotic Literary Texts from Tebtunis and Beyond: The Carlsberg Papyri* 11, CNI Publications 36 (Copenhagen: Museum Tusculanum Press, 2019), 145, n.6.

the gods Shu and Thot in order to put an end to the carnage and devastation done by the goddess when she was exiled in Nubia as a fierce lioness. The appeasement rituals aim at changing the goddess's behavior and state by converting her anger into joy.

In the texts, the emotions felt by the goddess are expressed through a very rich lexicon. For the concept of anger, the terms reflect a wide range of grades of intensity. The more violent angers are expressed by words as *neshen* (*nšn*) and *denden* (*dndn*)[36]:

neshen (nšn) denden (dndn)

These lexemes are bounded to the violent and damaging god Seth by their classifiers: the slaughtered Sethian animal for the former, the oryx head for the latter.

Sethian animal oryx head

If both *neshen* (*nšn*) and *denden* (*dndn*) designate some violent angers, the *neshen*-fury only, by its presence in temporal clauses such as "at the time of the *neshen*-fury" or "after her *neshen*-fury," which expresses the tipping-point of the rite, is to be understood as the primary anger of the lioness goddess and has to be destroyed in priority.

Sounds and image of the sistra are thus ritually acting through the pharaoh's hands in order to neutralize the angers of Hathor, the *neshen*-fury, in the first place (see below for how the terms of anger have been spread at some specific places in the temple according to their nature and intensity).

THE TEMPLE OF DENDARA FROM THE PERSPECTIVE OF SOUND STUDIES AND VISUAL STUDIES

Musicians inside a Religious Space

Spaces should be experienced "not only by seeing but also by listening."[37] The book of Barry Blesser and Linda-Ruth Salter is an invitation to study monuments from a sonic point of view. Usually an architecture is considered only

---

[36] *Wb* 2:341.1; *Wb* 5:471.1–19.

[37] Barry Blesser and Linda-Ruth Salter, *Spaces Speak, Are You Listening? Experiencing Aural Architecture* (Cambridge, MA: MIT Press, 2007), quotation taken from abstract.

from the visual aspect of its structure, rarely from its acoustic sensation. The Egyptian temple has never actually been studied from that perspective.

The temple of Dendara is a major place to conduct a study on the senses, because the temple is dedicated to Hathor, the goddess of music, who was worshipped with musical instruments: harps, tambourines, and sistra. An architectural analysis of the monument has shown the role of light in its conception.[38] The place of sound and visual perception across the architecture of the monument and their respective influence on rites, processions, and festivals has never been addressed, at least until recently. Indeed, Barbara Richter shows, in her doctorate thesis, the relationship between texts and iconography within a unified architectural space, the *pr-wr* sanctuary of the temple of Hathor at Dendara, which is the main cult chamber of the naos.[39] Her study is devoted solely to this room in order to analyze in detail how the aural and visual scribal techniques are used to reveal different aspects of the cult of the goddess. The aim of these techniques is to create a network of interrelationships between texts (which included the aural and visual dimensions of the hieroglyphics), iconography (ritual scenes and other pictorial decorations depicted on the walls), and their respective location inside a three-dimensional space. This kind of analysis gives a better understanding of the rituals and their meanings because the translation of the texts is taking into consideration the context. One must look at the temple and the temenos levels to see how the sense of hearing and the sense of sight were used inside a sacred space.

The religious space of Dendara includes several buildings that do not have the same functions or the same relations to sound. The decoration of the rooms, but also those of the two *mammisi* (place of birth) and of the Osirian chapels situated on the roof of the main temple, allow one to observe musicians at work in certain spaces, as well as dancers, while the texts inform us about how the senses were solicited for the cult of the goddess Hathor. Beside the sistra often held by the king (who is the supreme priest), the goddess herself (Hathor or the seven Hathor) is also shown playing sistra or tambourines on the lintel of the outer entrance of several rooms or on the jamb of the door; in other words, this iconography is located in spaces of "passage."[40] On the inner lintel of the *per-wer* sanctuary and of the barque sanctuary,[41] the goddess Meret plays the harp

---

[38] Pierre Zignani, *Le temple d'Hathor à Dendara: Relevés et étude architecturale*, Bibliothèque d'Étude 146 (Le Caire: IFAO, 2010).

[39] Barbara Richter, *The Theology of Hathor of Dendara: Aural and Visual Scribal Techniques in the Per-Wer Sanctuary*, Wilbour Studies 4 (Atlanta: Lockwood, 2016).

[40] See, for instance, Émile Chassinat, *Le temple de Dendara*, vol. 4 (Le Caire: IFAO, 1935), pl. CCCIV.

[41] Émile Chassinat, *Le temple de Dendara*, vol. 1 (Le Caire: IFAO, 1934), pl. XLVIII–L; Chassinat, *Le temple de Dendara*, vol. 3 (Le Caire: IFAO, 1935), pl. CLXXX (left), CLXXXI.

just in front of the place where the statue and the barque of the goddess was daily worshipped, which seems to prove that the sound was permitted in the most sacred area of the temple. In theory, the naos was accessible only to priests. This raises the issue of who played the role of the goddesses making music during cult activities.

Only scenes present in the pronaos of the temple show a procession with musicians, who are not divine (fig. 3).[42] They are carved on the base of the columns that border the central path of the pronaos, which is the huge room that precedes the naos. All the musicians are facing the interior of the temple in order to welcome the goddess when she is going out from the naos for religious festivals. The intention of this decoration is to make effective their presence. Deities and human beings play together, side by side, which indicates that this room was an open space to the public, unlike the naos.[43]

In all these examples, it is obvious that the iconography of the temple of Dendara reveals a visual and sound staging of music within the architecture itself. The same observation can be done with the scenes of presenting the sistra.

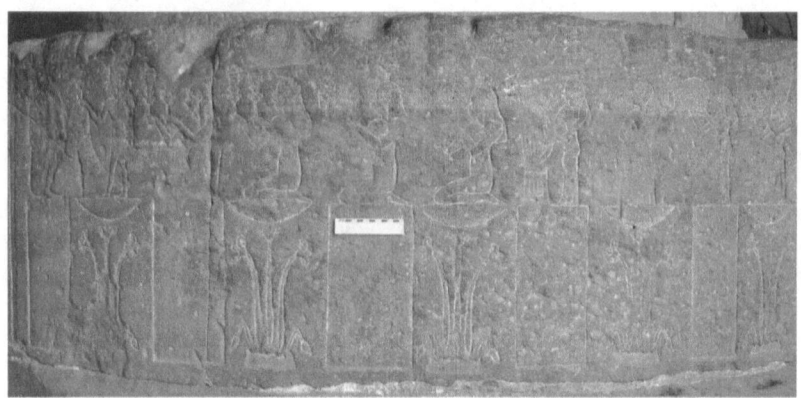

Fig. 3. Musicians procession, Pronaos of Hathor temple, Dendara
© Sibylle Emerit (IFAO, CNRS UMR 5189)

---

[42] Sylvie Cauville, *Le temple de Dendara*, vol. 13 (book unpublished, but the author gave the access for a while at the following address: http://www.dendara.net), pl. 117.

[43] The procession of the musicians of the pronaos is to be published in Sibylle Emerit, "Musiciens et processions dans le temple d'Hathor à Dendara: Iconographie et espace rituel," in *Représenter la musique dans l'Antiquité*, Musique-Images-Instruments 18 (forthcoming).

Specific Places for Sounds and Images of Sistra

In Dendara, it appears that the appeasement ritual with sistra contained a progression from sound to image. Evidence of this can be found in the ritual scenes and their texts, in connection with their position within the temple. When represented alone, the *bekhen*-sistrum is used to produce a *seshesh* (*sšš*) sound intended to annihilate the *neshen*-fury, namely, the primary fury, of the goddess while she is still in Nubia. This first part of the rite is located on the external walls of the Hathor temple, or on the doors of the site of Dendara, that is to say, places where people can come and go and where the procession accompanying the return of the Distant Goddess could obviously take place, before she entered her temple again.[44] According to the texts, the final step to the appeasement ritual is done by the arched-sistrum alone, which is raised (*s'ḥ'*) at the appearance (*ḫ'w*) of the goddess, before her union with the Sun. The rite of raising up the arched-sistrum takes place mainly in the well named "room of apparitions" or in the crypts of the Hathor temple, which are closed or subterranean rooms.[45] The arched-sistrum thus symbolizes the settling of the appeased goddess in her temple. The temporal progress of the rite, which is expressed by the use of the sounds (*seshesh*) and then of the image (*sekhem*) of the sistra, is moreover reflected in the locations of the scenes in the temple.

Still in Dendara, occurrences of the presentation of the two sistra (*ir sššt sḫm*), which involve both sound and image at the same time, are usually arranged in a symmetrical manner. Scenes are located, for example, on both sides of the external wall of the main sanctuary, while some others take place symmetrically on door lintels or jambs on the main axis of the temple, that is, on the passage way to the main sanctuary.[46]

Another example of the spatial progression of the ritual is given by the previously mentioned terms related to anger: the *neshen*-fury and the *denden*-rage. Texts say that the first one has to be pushed back, sent away (*sb nšn*) while the latter has to be expelled, driven off (*rwj dndn*). When mentions of these two expressions are spotted within the temple, they occupy two distinct spaces. The

---

[44] For an example on the wall, see Sylvie Cauville, *Le temple de Dendara*, vol. 12 (Le Caire: IFAO, 2007), Tableau XIII, 120–21, pl. 73. For an example on the door, see the Isis door in Cauville, *Le temple de Dendara: La Porte d'Isis* (Le Caire: IFAO, 1999), Tableau no. 24, 33, 3–12, pls. 4, 5, 41.

[45] For an example from the "room of apparitions," see François Daumas, *Le temple de Dendara*, vol. 9 (Le Caire: IFAO, 1987), Tableau IV, 66–67, pl. DCCCXXX. For an example in the crypts, see Émile Chassinat, *Le temple de Dendara*, vol. 5 (Le Caire: IFAO, 1952), Tableau I, 61–62, pl. CCCLVIII and CCCLXVI.

[46] For an example from the external wall, see Chassinat, *Le temple de Dendara*, 1:100–101, pl. LXXV and 132–33, pl. LXXIX. For an example of lintels, see Daumas, *Le temple de Dendara*, 9:3 and 4, pl. DCCCXII. For an example of jambs, see Chassinat, *Le temple de Dendara*, 4:52–53 and 55, pl. CCLXXII.

sb nšn action is clearly located at the temple entrance, at the pronaos, and on the external walls of both, pronaos and naos, whereas the *rwj dndn* action appears more specifically inside the temple. We therefore have a progress of the appeasement, from the entrance toward the back of the temple. The primary anger (*neshen*) would be annihilated first, when entering the temple and in its first room (the pronaos). Then the appeasement would be carried on by addressing the *denden*-anger, which is less offensive than the *neshen* one, in the rooms inside the temple.

The appeasement of Hathor by means of sound and image conveyed by the sistra is thus spatially expressed in the temple of Dendara by following the main axis and by a repartition between the surroundings and first rooms, on the one hand, and the internal chapels and crypts, on the other.

Conclusion

The role of the senses in ancient Egyptian rituals can be enlightened by employing the theoretical and methodological frameworks of sound studies and visual studies.

The various examples presented in this article show how the joint use of sound and image contribute to ritual efficiency, at the level of both the instrument and of the temple. A musical instrument is used both as a sound producer and as a religious image, capable of inducing a change of state. This change of state—which fluctuates in intensity—follows a path inside and outside the temple, which is determined by the course of the ritual.

Ancient Egyptians did recognize the efficiency of combining visual and aural sensitivity inside a ritual space in order to create religious experience. As Blesser and Salter notes, "visual and aural sensitivity often align and reinforce each other. For example, the visual vastness of a cathedral communicates through the eyes, while its enveloping reverberation communicates trough the ears. For those with ardent religious beliefs, both senses create a feeling of being in the earthly home of their deity."[47] This specific example invites us to examine the Egyptian temple as aural and visual architecture.

The site of Dendara constitutes an exceptional case study with which to explore the idea of the sensorial experience of the divine within a sacred place. The examples put forward in the article demonstrate that the choice in the words and in the images, as well as their location in the temple, are not a matter of chance. On the contrary, words and images are choreographed in a three-dimensional space, which is also the space lived and experienced by the actors of the cult. When considering the architectural context, as well as the location of texts and images, an aural and visual topography takes shape. This topography

---

[47] Blesser and Salter, *Spaces Speak*, 3.

helps us to comprehend the sensory dimensions of ancient Egyptian cultic practices. Nowadays, ethnomusicologists and acoustic experts work together to understanding how a religious space induces sensory experiences of the audience and performers of rites.[48] The way a temple is built, sounds, is engraved with texts and images, and is filled up with objects leads the people to feel the space and to see it as a visual and aural landmark. In this context, an interesting question would be whether the way a building sounds has an influence on the way a rite is performed and experienced by a priest. One could also address the question of aural borders inside a sacred space, where some zones are dedicated to silence and others to collective exultation.

This multisensorial approach to religion through the senses of hearing and sight seems to be particularly suitable to ancient Egypt as two deities, namely, Ir ("The-One-Who-Sees") and Sedjem ("The-One-Who-Hears"), embody those two senses. Instructions related to sound are also attested in the so-called Recommendations to the Priests, as well as in some taboos in the cult of Osiris, which specifically concern music.[49]

More generally, the new research avenues opened by multisensory studies will provide the framework for a finer understanding of ancient Egyptian rituals and how the religious space was felt through senses. Finally, it seems clear that an anthropological approach, encompassing senses and emotions, has a key role to play in the study of ancient Egyptian music and rituals as it can renew our understanding of them.

LINKS TO THE BRITISH MUSEUM COLLECTION ONLINE TO SEE EXAMPLES OF BELLS AND SISTRA

BM EA66619 (see note 18): "Bell, Modell," The British Museum, http://www.britishmuseum.org/research/collection_online/collection_object_details.aspx?assetId=54511001&objectId=152068&partId=1.

BM EA6374 (see note 18): "Bell," The British Museum, http://www.britishmuseum.org/research/collection_online/collection_object_details.aspx?assetId=415398001&objectId=176365&partId=1.

BM EA38160 (see note 21): "Bell," The British Museum, http://www.britishmuseum.org/research/collection_online/collection_object_details.aspx?assetId=988834001&objectId=166687&partId=1.

---

[48] Workshop organized by Christine Guillebaud, Frédéric Keck, and Catherine Lavandier: "Worship Sound Spaces. Sound Perception of Places of Worship (of Different Religions) via a Multidisciplinary Anthropological and Acoustic Approach," musée du Quai Branly, 3–4 November 2015 (Paris). For more information see Milson, http://milson.fr/.

[49] Emerit, "Autour de l'ouïe," 133–34.

BM EA38173 (see note 28): "Sistrum," The British Museum, http://www.britishmuseum.org/research/collection_online/collection_object_details. aspx?assetId=312946001&objectId=166674&partId=1.

BM EA38172 (see note 29): "Sistrum/Core," The British Museum, http://www.britishmuseum.org/research/collection_online/collection_object_details. aspx?assetId=1444437001&objectId=166675&partId=1

BIBLIOGRAPHY

Anderson, Robert D. *Musical Instruments*. Catalogue of Egyptian Antiquities in the British Museum 3. London: British Museum Publications, 1976.

Assmann, Jan. "Le pouvoir des images: De la performativité des images en Égypte ancienne." Pages 173–206 in *Penser l'image II: Anthropologies du visuel*. Edited by Emmanuel Alloa. Dijon: Les presses du réel, 2015.

Bénazeth, Dominique, and Alain Delattre. "Cloches et clochettes dans l'Égypte chrétienne." Pages 251–80 in *Études coptes XIV*. Edited by Anne Boud'hors et Catherine Louis. Cahiers de la Bibliothèque Copte 21. Paris: de Boccard, 2016.

Blesser, Barry, and Linda-Ruth Salter. *Spaces Speak, Are You Listening? Experiencing Aural Architecture*. Cambridge, MA: MIT Press, 2007.

Cauville, Sylvie. *Le temple de Dendara*. Vol. 12. Le Caire: IFAO, 2007.

———. *Le temple de Dendara*. Vol. 13. Unpublished manuscript.

———. *Le temple de Dendara: La Porte d'Isis*. Le Caire: IFAO, 1999.

Chassinat, Émile. *Le temple de Dendara*. Vol. 1. Le Caire: IFAO, 1934.

———. *Le temple de Dendara*. Vol. 3. Le Caire: IFAO, 1935.

———. *Le temple de Dendara*. Vol. 4. Le Caire: IFAO, 1935.

———. *Le temple de Dendara*. Vol. 5. Le Caire: IFAO, 1952.

Daumas, François. *Le temple de Dendara*. Vol. 9. Le Caire: IFAO, 1987.

———. "Les objets sacrés d'Hathor au temple de Dendara." *Bulletin de la société française d'égyptologie* 57 (1970): 7–18.

Dubuisson, Daniel, and Sophie Raux, eds. *À perte de vue: Les nouveaux paradigmes du visuel*. Dijon: Les presses du réel, 2015.

———. "Entre l'histoire de l'art et les Visual Studies: Mythe, science et idéologie." *Histoire de l'Art* 70 (2012): 95–103.

Elwart, Dorothée. *Apaiser Hathor: Le rite de présentation des sistres à Dendara*. PhD diss., École Pratique des Hautes Études; Universität zu Köln, 2013.

———. "Le sistre, le son et l'image." Pages 109–21 in *Offrandes, rites et rituels dans les temples d'époques ptolémaïque et romaine: Actes de la journée d'études de l'équipe EPHE (EA 4519) "Égypte ancienne; Archéologie, langue, religion," Paris, 27 juin 2013*. Edited by Christiane Zivie-Coche. Cahiers Égypte nilotique et méditerranéenne 10. Montpellier: Université Paul Valéry, 2015.

———. "Sistren als Klang des Hathorkultes." Pages 37–60 in *Laut und Leise: Der Gebrauch von Stimme und Klang in historischen Kulturen*. Edited by Erika Meyer-Dietrich, Mainzer Historische Kulturwissenschaften 7. Bielefeld: Transcript, 2011.

Emerit, Sibylle. "Autour de l'ouïe, de la voix et des sons: Approche anthropologique des 'paysages sonores' de l'Égypte ancienne." Pages 115–54 in *Le paysage sonore de l'Antiquité: Méthodologie, historiographie et perspectives, Actes de la journée d'études tenue à l'École française de Rome, le 7 janvier 2013*. Edited by Sibylle Emerit, Sylvain Perrot, and Alexandre Vincent. RAPH 40. Le Caire: IFAO, 2015.

———. "Musiciens et processions dans le temple d'Hathor à Dendara: Iconographie et espace rituel." In *Représenter la musique dans l'Antiquité*. Musique-Images-Instruments 18. Forthcoming.

Emerit, Sibylle, Sylvain Perrot, and Alexandre Vincent, eds. *Le paysage sonore de l'Antiquité: Méthodologie, historiographie et perspectives, Actes de la journée d'études tenue à l'École française de Rome, le 7 janvier 2013*. RAPH 40. Le Caire: IFAO, 2015.

Fernando, Nathalie, and Jean-Jacques Nattiez, eds. *Ethnomusicologie et anthropologie de la musique: Une question de perspective*. Anthropologie et sociétés 38 (2014).

Hickmann, Hans. *Instruments de musique*. Catalogue général des antiquités égyptiennes du Musée du Caire. Le Caire: IFAO, 1949.

Hinson, Benjamin. "Dead Ringers: The Mortuary Use of Bells in Late Pharaonic Egypt." Pages 179–201 in *A True Scribe of Abydos: Essays on First Millenium Egypt in Honour of Anthony Leahy*. Edited by Claus Jurman, Bettina Bader, David Aston. OLA 265. Leuven: Peeters, 2017.

Junker, Hermann. *Der Auszug der Hathor-Tefnut aus Nubien*. Berlin: Preussische Akademie der Wissenschaften, 1911.

Kessler, Dieter, and Patrick Brose. *Ägyptens letzte Pyramide: Das Grab des Seuta(s) in Tuna el-Gebel*. Vaterstetten: Verlag Patrick Brose, 2008.

Masson, Aurélia. "Bronze Votive Offerings." Pages 12–13 in *Naukratis: Greeks in Egypt*. Edited by Alexandra Villing et al. London: British Museum, 2016.

Meyer-Dietrich, Erika. *Auditive Räume des alten Ägypten: Die Umgestaltung einer Hörkultur in der Amarnazeit*. CHANE 92. Leiden: Brill, 2018.

Morenz, Ludwig D. *Anfänge der ägyptischen Kunst: Eine problemgeschichtliche Einführung in ägyptologische Bild-Anthropologie*. OBO 264. Fribourg: Presses Universitaires, 2014.

Petrie, William Matthew Flinders. *Amulets Illustrated by the Egyptian Collection in University College*. London: Constable, 1914.

Quack, Joachim Friedrich, and Kim Ryholt. *Demotic Literary Texts from Tebtunis and Beyond: The Carlsberg Papyri 11*. CNI Publication 36. Copenhagen: Museum Tusculanum Press, 2019.

Rahiem, Mohamed Abdel. "Decoration of Ancient Egyptian Harps." Pages 89–120 in *Laut und Leise: Der Gebrauch von Stimme und Klang in historischen Kulturen*. Edited by Erika Meyer-Dietrich, Mainzer Historische Kulturwissenschaften 7. Bielefeld: Transcript, 2011.

Raven, Marteen. "Women's Bed from Deir el-Medina." Pages 191–204 in *The Workman's Progress Studies in the Village of Deir al-Medina and Other Documents from Western Thebes in Honour of Rob Demarée*. Edited by Rob Demarée, Ben J. J. Haring, and Olaf Ernst Kaper. Leiden: Nederlands Instituut voor het Nabije Oosten; Leuven: Peeters, 2014.

Reynders, Marleen. "Sšš.t and sḫm: Names and Types of the Egyptian Sistrum." Pages 1013–26 in *Egyptian Religion: The Last Thousand Years, Studies Dedicated to the*

Memory of Jan Quaegebeur. Edited by Willy Clarysse, Antoon Schoors and Harco Willems. 2 parts. OLA 85. Leuven: Peeters, 1998.

Richter, Barbara. *The Theology of Hathor of Dendara: Aural and Visual Scribal Techniques in the Per-Wer Sanctuary*. Wilbour Studies 4. Atlanta: Lockwood, 2016.

Romano, James F. *The Bes-Image in Pharaonic Egypt*. Ann Arbor, MI: University Microfilms International, 1989.

Spiegelberg, Wilhelm. *Der ägyptische Mythus vom Sonnenauge (der Papyrus der Tierfabeln—"Kufi"): Nach dem Leidener demotischen Papyrus I 384*. Strassburg: Strassburger Druckerei und Verlagsanstalt, 1917.

Sterne, Jonathan. *The Audible Past: Cultural Origins of Sound Reproduction*. Durham, NC: Duke University Press, 2003.

Vincent, Alexandre. "Paysage sonore et sciences sociales: Sonorités, sens, histoire." Pages 9–40 in *Le paysage sonore de l'Antiquité: Méthodologie, historiographie et perspectives, Actes de la journée d'études tenue à l'École française de Rome, le 7 janvier 2013*. Edited by Sibylle Emerit, Sylvain Perrot, and Alexandre Vincent. RAPH 40. Le Caire: IFAO, 2015.

von Lieven, Alexandra. "Sounds of Power: The Concept of Sound in Ancient Egyptian Religion." Pages 25–35 in *Religion für die Sinne / Religion for the Senses*, ed. Philipp Reichling and Meret Strothmann. Artificium 58. Oberhausen: Athena, 2016.

Widmaier, Kai. *Bilderwelten: Ägyptische Bilder und ägyptologische Kunst: Vorarbeiten für eine bildwissenschaftliche Ägyptologie*. PAe 35. Leiden: Brill, 2017.

Ziegler, Christiane. *Catalogue des instruments de musique égyptiens*. Paris: Éditions de la réunion des musées nationaux, 1979.

Zignani, Pierre. *Le temple d'Hathor à Dendara: Relevés et étude architecturale*. Bibliothèque d'Étude 146. Le Caire: IFAO, 2010.

FISH, FOWL, AND STENCH IN ANCIENT EGYPT

Dora Goldsmith

INTRODUCTION

The significance of the archaeology of the senses has not yet been fully recognized by Egyptologists. Some research has been done on sight[1] and hearing,[2] especially music,[3] in ancient Egyptian culture. However, no comprehensive

---

The present article contains some preliminary results of my PhD thesis entitled *The Archaeology of Smell in Ancient Egypt—A Cultural Anthropological Study Based on Written Sources* registered at the Egyptology Seminar of the Freie Universität Berlin in Berlin, Germany. My research is funded by the Ernst Ludwig Ehrlich Studienwerk. My first supervisor is Prof. Dr. Jochem Kahl, the head of the Egyptology Seminar of the Freie Universität Berlin. My second supervisor is Prof. Dr. Friederike Seyfried, the director of the Egyptian Museum and Papyrus Collection in Berlin. My PhD project is carried out within the framework of the archaeology of the senses and explores the sense of smell in ancient Egypt. Smell is a social phenomenon, a gateway of knowledge, an instrument of power, and a source of pleasure and pain; it is subject to dramatically different constructions in different societies and periods. The goal of my research is to examine the role of olfaction in all spheres of the ancient Egyptian society from the very beginning until the end of pharaonic history (3200–332 BCE) based on written evidence. Unless otherwise noted, all translations are my own.

[1] See the Eye of Horus, for example. Numerous scientific works treat the subject of the Eye of Horus from the aspect of mythology, magic, health, mathematics, and as a hieroglyphic symbol. For the latest study, see Nadine Grässler, *Konzepte des Auges im alten Ägypten*, SAK.B 20 (Hamburg: Helmut Buske, 2017).

[2] See the word *sḏm* ("to hear"), for instance. Several Egyptologists have treated the meaning of the word *sḏm*, which not only encompasses "hearing," but also "listening," "obeying" and "being attentive." For articles on hearing and sounds in ancient Egypt, see, for example, Erika Meyer-Dietrich, ed., *Laut und Leise: Der Gebrauch von Stimme und Klang in historischen Kulturen*, Mainzer Historische Kulturwissenschaften 7 (Bielefeld: transcript, 2011).

[3] See Lise Manniche, *Music and Musicians in Ancient Egypt* (London: British Museum, 1991); Sibylle Emerit, "Music and Musicians," in *UCLA Encyclopedia of Egyptology*, ed. Willeke Wendrich (Los Angeles: University of California, Department of Near

research has ever been carried out on the sense of smell,[4] touch,[5] and taste[6] in this society. Some Egyptologists mention sight as the most important sensory value in ancient Egypt.[7] In her article entitled "Foundations for an Anthropology of the Senses," Constance Classen mentions that considering sight the most significant of all senses in *all* cultures is a common mistake of European scholars and is due to the overwhelming importance of sight in European culture.[8] Classen notes that the reluctance of late twentieth century anthropologists to examine or recognize the cultural importance of smell, taste, and touch is due

---

Eastern Languages and Cultures, 2013); Emerit, "La musique pharaonique, un patrimoine plurimillénaire," in *Musiques! Échos de l'Antiquité*, ed. Sibylle Emerit et al. (Musée du Louvre-Lens, Gand: Snoeck, 2018), 48–61. Rafael Pérez Arroyo released a CD in 2004 entitled *Music in the Age of the Pyramids* with ten tracks thought to represent the music of the ancient Egyptians.

[4] The only publication to have treated smells as a whole is Lise Manniche, *Sacred Luxuries: Fragrance, Aromatherapy and Cosmetics in Ancient Egypt* (London: Opus Publishing Limited, 1999). However, this work does not treat the *role* of smell in the Egyptian culture, but mostly focuses on perfumes produced in ancient Egypt. For articles on smell, see Nathalie Beaux, "Odeur, souffle et vie," in *Mélanges offerts à Ola el-Aguizy*, ed. Faiza Haykal, Bibliothèque d'étude 164 (Cairo: Institut français d'archéologie orientale, 2015), 61–73; Alexandra von Lieven, "'Thy Fragrance Is in All My Limbs': On the Olfactory Sense in Ancient Egyptian Religion," in *Religion für die Sinne—Religion for the Senses*, ed. Phillip Reichling and Meret Strothmann, Artificium 58 (Oberhausen: ATHENA, 2016), 309–25; Robyn Price, "Sniffing out the Gods: Archaeology with the Senses," *JAEI* 17 (2018): 137–55.

[5] The closest publication on the topic is Lise Manniche, *Sexual Life in Ancient Egypt* (Zürich: Artemis, 1987).

[6] Some research has been done on the cuisine of ancient Egypt. See, for example, Ursula Verhoeven-van Elsbergen, *Grillen, Kochen, Backen im Alltag und im Ritual Altägyptens: Ein lexikographischer Beitrag* (Bruxelles: Fondation Egyptologique Reine Elisabeth, 1984). For linguistic studies on taste, see Elizabeth Steinbach-Eicke, "'Ich habe seinen Anblick geschmeckt ...': Verben der Wahrnehmung und die semantischen Beziehungen zwischen Perzeption und Kognition," in *Wissen-Wirkung Wahrnehmung: Beiträge des vierten Münchner Arbeitskreises Junge Aegyptologie*, ed. Gregor Neunert, Henrike Simon, Alexandra Verbovsek, and Kathrin Gabler, MAJA 4 (Wiesbaden: Harrassowitz, 2015), 209–25; Steinbach-Eicke, "Experiencing Is Tasting: Perception Metaphors of Taste in Ancient Egyptian," *Lingua Aegyptia* 25 (2017): 373–90.

[7] Ragnhild Bjerre Finnestad, "Enjoying the Pleasures of Sensation: Reflections on a Significant Feature of Egyptian Religion," in *Gold of Praise: Studies on Ancient Egypt in Honor of Edward F. Wente*, ed. Emily Teeter and John A. Larson, SAOC 58 (Chicago: Oriental Institute, 1999), 111–19, for example, notes that "perhaps the most important sense organ was the eye in the ancient Egyptian worship."

[8] Constance Classen, "Foundations for an Anthropology of the Senses," *International Social Science Journal* 153 (1997): 401–12.

not only to the relative marginalization of these senses in the modern West, but also to the racist tendencies of an earlier anthropology to associate the "lower" senses with the "lower" races. As sight and, to a lesser extent, hearing were deemed to be the predominant senses of "civilized" Westerners, smell, taste, and touch were assumed to predominate among "primitive" non-Westerners.

The goal of my research is to unfold the world of olfaction of the ancient Egyptians reflected by the written sources left behind, without being influenced by any modern Western sensory values and conceptions of the senses. Olfaction, as all sensory perceptions, is not only a means of apprehending physical phenomena, but also an avenue for the transmission of cultural values. Through apprehending the olfactory sensation of the ancient Egyptians, which has never been investigated before, my research topic contributes to the better understanding of the ancient Egyptian culture as a whole.

1. Fish and Fowl as the Prototype of Stench in Ancient Egypt

A general characteristic of smells in every society is that they are organized on an axis of good-bad.[9] This was no different in ancient Egypt. The hieroglyphic script and the information gained from written sources reveal that fish and birds were considered the prototype of stench in ancient Egypt. As the epitome of evil smells, fish and fowl reflect *collective* olfactory values of the ancient Egyptian society, which were culturally shaped.

Fish, Fowl, and Swamps

Multiple written sources inform us explicitly that fish, birds, and their natural environment in Egypt, the swamps of the Delta, stank.[10] The Nile Delta is found in the north of Egypt, and it is where the Egyptians went fishing and fowling.

---

[9] David E. Sutton, *Remembrance of Repasts: An Anthropology of Food and Memory* (Oxford: Berg, 2001), 88, notes that "attempts at scientific classification of smells in something equivalent to classes have led to little consensus concerning what might constitute clusters of smells and 'primary smells,' and attempted taxonomies seem forced and vague."

[10] The ancient Egyptian literary corpus also includes texts of converse nature. The literary work called The Pleasures of Fishing and Fowling, for example, praises the activity of fishing and fowling, the occupation of the fisher and fowler, and life in the swamps, far away from urban life. The Ramesside letter entitled Report on the Delta Residence states that ponds, lakes, and channels rich in various species of fish were an integral part of the city Pi-Ramesse-miamun. The scribe penning the letter describes these watery regions infested with fish as the very beauty of the urban center. In the present article, I am only focusing on written documents that regard the above as negative and evil-smelling, while acknowledging the fact that texts of converse nature also existed.

The Middle Kingdom literary work called The Dispute of a Man and His Ba makes use of the stench of fish and fowl as general olfactory values, which would be obvious to everyone.

m.k bʿḥ rn.i m.k <r sṯi> šsp sbnw m hrw rsf pt t3t
My name reeks[11] more than <the smell> of a catch of fish[12] on fishing days of burning sky. (Dispute 88–90)

m.k bʿḥ rn.i m.k r sṯi m 3p{s}<d>w r bw3t nt tri ḥr msyt
My name reeks more than the smell of marsh birds, more than a thicket of reeds full of waterfowl. (Dispute 91–93)

The text describes the area of the Nile Delta. What is meant by a "thicket of reeds" is like a wetland hammock or hydric hammock, which grows on soils that are poorly drained or that have high water tables, subject to occasional flooding. They are usually found on gentle slopes just above swamps, marshes, or wet prairies, and they tend to have a strong, unpleasant smell.

The occupation of the fisherman, who worked all day in the dangerous and evil-smelling swamps catching fish, was considered the most degrading of all professions due to the stench and danger. The Satire of Trades, a satirical teaching, states:

dd.i n.k mi wḥʿ rmw sfn.f r i3t nbt
I will speak of the fisherman also, his is the worst of all jobs. (Satire of Trades 21)

The Satire of Trades informs us that the occupation of the fowler was regarded just as lowly:

wḥʿ 3pdw sfn r-sy ḥr gmḥ iryw pt ir sw3 3pdw ẖnmw m ḥr.f ḥr.f dd.f h3nr n.i m i3dt

---

[11] The word *bʿḥ* actually means "to be detested" (*Wb* 1:450.6) and not "to stink," like *ḥnš*. However, the expression *bʿḥ rn.i* is similar in meaning to the common expression *ḥnš rn.i* ("my name stinks") known from several ancient Egyptian sources, e.g., chapter 30B of the Book of the Dead. In all sentences, where the phrase *bʿḥ rn.i* appears in The Dispute of a Man and His Ba, it is connected to bad smells. Furthermore, *bʿḥ* is classified with the fish classifier (K5), similarly to *ḥnš*, which serves to denote "stench." Thus, for *bʿḥ rn.i* "my name stinks" or "my name reeks" seems to be a perfect translation.

[12] John L. Foster and Miriam Lichtheim translated "catch of fish," while Stephen Quirke translated "dead fish." John L. Foster, *Ancient Egyptian Literature: An Anthology* (Austin: University of Texas Press, 2007), 60; Miriam Lichtheim, *The Old and Middle Kingdoms*, vol. 1 of *Ancient Egyptian Literature: A Book of Readings* (Berkeley, California: University of California Press, 1973), 166; Stephen Quirke, *Egyptian Literature 1800 BC: Questions and Readings*, Egyptology 2 (London: Golden House, 2004), 132.

The fowler is very miserable when he looks at the denizens of the sky. If marsh fowl pass by over him, then he says: "Would that I have a net!" (Satire of Trades 20)

The Dispute of a Man and His Ba contains a reference to fishermen, according to which fishermen had a terrible stench.

m.k bʿh rn.i m.k r sṯi h3mw r h3sw nw sš h3m.n.sn
My name reeks more than the smell of fishermen, more than the swamps where they fished. (Dispute 93–95)

Now let us turn to the Book of Kemit, a work compiled in the late Eleventh Dynasty, which was a compendium intended for the education of the Egyptian scribe. The second, biographical part of the book expresses the notion of the smell of home. A Theban official, writing to his superior, reports on the activities of a fellow-townsman named Au, who has been absent from home for a period of more than two years. We may guess from what follows that the occasion of the absence was a prolonged hunting and fishing expedition somewhere in the north of Egypt, probably in the swamplands of the Delta. Returning home, Au gets himself cleaned up, perfumed, and dressed in fresh garments.

snḏm ib.i pn rdit iwt 3w m3.n.i sw m hmtnwt.f rnpt wrh m ʿntyw m pwnt hnmw t3 nṯr sd m d3iw n ir.i i3dw m3.n.f hnty dd.s is 3w m3.n.k hmt.k iw mr rm.s ṯw iw rmm.s ṯw hr rmw.k m grh 3pdw.k m hrw
As for what might make me glad, it is that Au be allowed to return. When I last saw him in his third year (of training), he was anointed with the myrrh of Punt, the fragrance of the land of the god, and clothed in a kilt of my making. Only as a child he visited the palace. She said "Go Au and see your wife! How bitterly she weeps for you! How bitterly she weeps for you because of your (catching) *fish* by night and your (snaring) *fowl* by day!" (Kemit 6–8)

The principal theme of this section is homesickness in a far place. After years of being far away from home, Au returns to Thebes, to his former civilized mode of life and finds himself dressed again in linen anointed with fragrant unguents.[13] Two worlds are contrasted here, the world of a faraway land and the world of the homeland. The remote land is represented by fish, fowl, and the notion of being away from home and from one's family. Even though it is not said explicitly, the text metaphorically reveals that the faraway land is associated with evil smells. The remote world of the swamps of the Delta is represented by

---

[13] The narrative is very similar to the Story of Sinuhe. The principal theme in both literary works is homesickness in a faraway place. Both Au and Sinuhe return home after years of being abroad and find themselves clothed in fine linen and anointed with scented unguent.

the stench of fish and fowl.[14] The homeland, Thebes, on the other, is described by the notion of being with one's family and cleanliness: being anointed with the myrrh of Punt, having the smell of perfume and being dressed in fresh garments. The homeland is associated with the sweet scents of unguents, the fragrance of civilized life. That the word *ḫnmw* ("smell") indeed refers to the smell of home is unequivocally demonstrated by the house classifier (O1) in the OBrussels E3208 version of the text.[15] Such a classification of smell is not attested in any other text.

The fact that the fish and birds mentioned in the Book of Kemit symbolize the abominable stench of the marshes of the Delta is unequivocally confirmed by a scribal mistake. In the version oIFAO 1115, *ḫnmw* is written with a fish classifier (K5). Since the word clearly has a positive connotation, this must be a scribal mistake. However, it can be easily explained why the scribe made this mistake. The scribe knew that after mentioning the fragrances of the homeland, the odors of the remote land will be described, which were symbolized in the composition by the fish and fowl of the swamps of the Delta. Bad smells were almost always classified with the fish classifier. The scribe added in haste the fish classifier to the word *smell*, since he was already thinking about the next sentences to come. This scribal mistake clearly shows that the scribe understood the opposition between the good scents of the homeland and the malodors of the faraway land.

[FISH]

In the hieroglyphic script, every word related to unpleasant smell was classified with the fish classifier (K5). Malodors were expressed with the words *ḥns*[16] ("to stink"), *sḥnš*[17] ("to make stink"), or *šnt*[18] ("stench"), and they were all followed by the fish classifier (K5).

---

[14] The reason why the Nile Delta represents the idea of a foreign land in this compendium must be the historical memory of the fact that Delta wildlands succumbed to man much later than their Nile Valley counterparts. Despite government incentives for colonization, the region was settled sparsely and slowly. See Steven M. Goodman and Peter L. Meininger, *Birds of Egypt* (Oxford: Oxford University Press, 1989), 33–34.

[15] The member "smell of home" can be added to Goldwasser's [HABITAT] category classified with the house classifier (O1). See Orly Goldwasser, "Where Is Metaphor? Conceptual Metaphor and Alternative Classification in the Hieroglyphic Script," *Metaphor and Symbol* 20 (2005): 96–97. This unique classification of the word *ḫnmw* is an example of alternative classification, which is always a motivated process and reflects a change in the focus of the semantic value of the word. For alternative classification, see Goldwasser, "Where Is Metaphor?," 103–4.

[16] *Wb* 3:301.1.

[17] *Wb* 4:255.5.

ḫnš ("to stink")

sḫnš ("to make stink'")

šni ("stench")

šn ("stench")

The classification of words denoting stench shows us that fish served as a pictorial synonym of evil smells. Fish served as "the prototype of stench" in ancient Egypt.[19] In other words, the fish was chosen as the "best member" or "best example" of the category [STENCH].[20]

There were several types of fish in the arsenal of hieroglyphic signs. Now let us inspect what type of fish the K5 sign represents and why it was chosen to embody the [STENCH] category. From the Middle Kingdom on, the same K5 classifier became the prototype of the [FISH] category in the script. It is used as a generic classifier for fish, for example:

rm ("fish")[21]

Thus, in the ancient Egyptian mind, the prototype of fish was at the same time the prototype of stench.

The hieroglyphic sign K5 most likely represents the *Petrocephalus bane*, a kind of freshwater fish that belongs to the *Mormyridae* family. The *Petrocephalus bane* is known from the Nile proper, the Blue Nile, the White Nile, the Chad Basin, and the Niger. The *Petrocephalus bane* is probably the most common species of Mormyr in the Lower Nile, or rather, perhaps, that which is most easily caught by fishermen.[22] Hence, the *Petrocephalus bane* was consciously chosen to represent fish and stench. Being a freshwater fish from the Nile, it was a characteristically Egyptian fish. More specifically, it inhabited the Lower Nile,

---

[18] *Wb* 4:503.3–4.

[19] Goldwasser was the first to note that the fish served as the prototype of the category [STINKING THINGS] ("Where is Metaphor," 106).

[20] For classifiers representing prototypes, see Orly Goldwasser, *Lovers, Prophets and Giraffes: Wor[l]d Classification in Ancient Egypt*, Göttinger Orientforschungen (Wiesbaden: Harrassowitz, 2002), 19–24.

[21] See under K5 in Gardiner's sign-list: Alan H. Gardiner, *Egyptian Grammar*, 3rd rev. ed. (Cambridge: Cambridge University Press, 1957), 477.

[22] George Albert Boulenger, *Zoology of Egypt: The Fishes of the Nile* (Hugh Rees: London, 1907), 33–35.

which abounded in evil-smelling marshes, where the Egyptians went to fish and fowl. Within this geographic area, the *Petrocephalus bane* was the most common species and the most easily caught by fishermen. This made the *Petrocephalus bane* the most representative member of the [FISH] category, the prototype of fish in ancient Egypt.[23] As such, it became the prototype of [STENCH].

The unmistakable odor of fish is considered detestable in many cultures around the world. It is the breaking down of trimethylamine oxide into trimethylamine, when the fish are killed, that causes the characteristic fishy smell. However, the hotter and more humid the climate is, the faster is the natural process of decay, and the stronger is the smell. Therefore, beside the foul-smelling marshes, where the fish were caught, Egypt's particularly hot climate must have also contributed to the fish becoming the prototype of stench.[24]

[BIRD]

The abovementioned written sources demonstrated that besides fish, the Egyptians considered the smell of waterfowl especially repellent. Let us examine the prototypical member of the [BIRD] category in the Egyptian script in order to learn more about why marsh birds became another emblem of evil smells in ancient Egypt.

---

[23] Ingrid Gamer-Wallert does not believe that the fish classifier in the word *rmw* ("fish") represents the *Petrocephalus bane*. She argues that most of the written documents mentioning the word *rmw* are written in cursive hieroglyphic script, which does not allow the identification of the species. Moreover, no photographs have been published of those few inscriptions, which were written in hieroglyphic script. Gamer-Wallert further asserts: "Keine der im 1. Kapitel genannten Fischarten Altägyptens kann mit Sicherheit als Vorbild des Determinativs von *rmw* angesehen werden ... wird man annehmen dürfen, dass ihr Bild von vornherein keine spezielle Art dargestellt, sondern eine allgemeine Vorstellung von 'Fisch' wiedergegeben hat." Ingrid Gamer-Wallert, *Fische und Fischkulte im Alten Ägypten*, Ägyptologische Abhandlungen 21 (Wiesbaden: Harrassowitz, 1970), 17–18. Gamer-Wallert's view on this matter cannot be accepted. Hieroglyphs are picture-characters, miniature icons representing people, animals, plants, astronomical entities, buildings, furniture, vessels, etc. known to the ancient Egyptians. Each sign in the hieroglyphic script is a deliberate choice representing a visual image of an elected concept. A hieroglyphic sign does not only exist, it also signifies. Thus, we must assume that the fish classifier in the word *rmw* ("fish") portrays a species that lived in ancient Egypt and was well-known to its inhabitants.

[24] While the vast majority of written sources do present fish as the prototype of stench, texts, such as The Pleasures of Fishing and Fowling and Report on the Delta Residence that praise fish, watery regions, and fishing and fowling also need to be taken into consideration. It seems that the negative olfactory value attributed to fish is only a part of a more complex overall picture.

The sign G38/G39 representing a duck was the prototype of birds in ancient Egypt. G38 is a goose, a typical Egyptian bird, a type that bears striking similarity to a duck (*Anser albifrons*). G39 is pintail duck (*Anas acuta*), by far the most frequently represented species of waterfowl in Egyptian art.[25] These two signs were interchangeable.[26] *Anas acuta*, the most common waterfowl in Egypt and the prototype of bird in Egypt per se,[27] seems to be an especially smelly bird, or at least, could be especially smelly, when threatened. An experiment conducted by Swennen in 1968 on brown rats and ferrets concluded that faeces from an eider duck released over the nests after disturbance, even in very small amounts, make food unattractive to ferrets and rats. Both species are known as potential egg-predators.[28] However, faeces from non-breeding ducks and from other species, do not have this effect. Thus, it is only the faeces of the *Anas acuta* that is especially repellent, when this species is disturbed. Therefore, it cannot be a coincidence that the Egyptians considered birds a prototype of stench, beside fish, and the prototype of birds at the same time was the smelliest bird of all, the pintail duck, *Anas acuta*.

2. Fish and Fowl as Symbols of the Evil-Smelling World of Chaos

The conflict of sweet and evil smells was a part of Egypt's everyday reality. The ancient Egyptians believed in two concepts that went hand-in-hand: *ma'at* and *isfet*. *Ma'at* was the world of order and justice, while *isfet* was the world of chaos and evil. The sun-god Re entrusted the king with annihilating malodors and bringing pleasant scents to the world, as part of his duty to implement *ma'at*. The king was assigned to the throne in order to put *ma'at* into effect. Without *ma'at*, *isfet* or chaos dominated the world. *Ma'at* could not exist by

---

[25] Patrick F. Houlihan, *The Animal World of the Pharaohs* (Cairo: The American University in Cairo Press, 1995), 139.

[26] The birds represented by the signs G38 and G39 look very similar. Gardiner identifies G38 as *Anser albifrons*, which is a type of goose. He identifies G39 as a pintail duck and notes that "this type may, if preferred, be employed in place of G38 in the indefinite uses where the actual nature of the bird in question is unknown" (*Egyptian Grammar*, 471).

[27] Goldwasser describes how the duck, the basic-level member of the [BIRD] category, becomes the pictorial representation of the superordinate [BIRD]. As the best example of the [BIRD] category, the duck was chosen to classify words, such as *niw* ("ostrich") and *bik* ("falcon") (*Lovers, Prophets and Giraffes*, 19–20).

[28] Cornelis Swennen notes that faeces of eider ducks seem to be effective also against human "predators." A laborer, who had the habit of collecting eggs, revealed to him in a private conversation that he would refuse to collect the eggs of eider ducks because of the repulsive smell of the faeces covering the eggs. Cornelis Swennen, "Nest Protection of Eiderducks and Shovelers by Means of Faeces," *Ardea* 56 (1968): 255.

itself, it needed a central government in order to come into existence and to be maintained. People could not live without *ma'at*, which means that they could not live without the king. The world's natural state was that of *isfet*, a state of chaos, evil, lies, injustice and stench. The world smelled naturally bad. *Isfet* reeked of fish and birds. People alone were incapable of eliminating the malodors of *isfet*. It was the king's duty to annihilate the stench and to bring forth perfume. As a matter of fact, kingship was not introduced in order to create sweet scents, but first and foremost in order to expel the stench of *isfet* so that people could live.

A hymn to Ramesses VI describes the ascension of the king to the throne. The beginning of the hymn portrays the world of *isfet*, which prevailed at the time Ramesses VI was appointed to the throne. The world of chaos is metaphorically described in the text with fish and birds.

> [...] *t-n[t]-š3 ḥri wdw iw.w r ptri p3 nb (ʿnḫ-wd3)-s(nb) n kmt iw.f m n3y.f ḥb-sd knw* [...] *p3 3pdw rm n3 ʿ3 n3y ḫprw pw tw.nn wn (ḥr) [it]3 [im].n (ḥr) (irt) m3ʿkw n* [...] *[ḫ3]ry ʿw d3ty ḥ3t n srwy m-drt n3 ḥnmty iw.n (ḥr) ḥ3ʿ p3 t3 n it.n mwt*
>
> [...] the area of the marshes abounds in *wadj-fish*; they shall behold the Lord—life, prosperity, health—of the Black Land when he celebrates numerous Sed-festivals [...] who ensnares(?)[29] both *fowl and fish*. Momentous things have befallen us. Those who took from us the food of [... are (now)] widows; those who caused to be consumed the best portion of *geese* are in the hands of harlots. We abandoned the territory of our fathers and mothers. (Hymn III to Ramesses VI, 1–3)

Upon his ascension to the throne, Ramesses VI had to expel the stench of fish and birds of *isfet*. After this was achieved, people could go back to their cities, where the sweet smells filled the air and the courts of law functioned again.

> *tw.n iwi r p3y.n dmi r n3y.k stwt sdmyw r ʿš3ty ndm sti*
>
> We have returned to our city, to your audience-halls, to the many sweet-smelling things. (Hymn III to Ramesses VI, 8)

A characteristic of smell with relevance to *ma'at* is that it was connected to areas. The hymn in question states that people went back to their cities, to the sweet scents. What cities and pleasant smells had in common was that they both required a central government. Cities are an artificially created, human-made environment held together by the laws of justice. Cities were created by the king for the people as their home. Without the Crown, there were no cities, chaos

---

[29] Virginia Condon reconstructed *sḥni* ("to arrest"). Virginia Condon, *Seven Royal Hymns of the Ramesside Period: Papyrus Turin CG 54031*, MÄS 37 (München: Deutscher Kunstverlag, 1978), 30.

ruled the world and people had nowhere to live. Sweet scents were similarly the result of the efforts of the king for the society. The entire concept of *ma'at* was an artificially created reality implemented by the king. The natural order of things was chaos and stench.[30]

3. FISHING AND FOWLING AS A SYMBOLIC ACT OF ELIMINATING STENCH

Fishing and Fowling of the King

In the royal battle against the evil forces of *isfet*, the fish and fowl symbolized the stench and danger the king had to defeat. The Middle Kingdom literary work The Sporting King bears a reference to the evil smell of fish with relevance to *isfet*. The text applies the word 𓆷𓈖 *šn* ("stench") with the fish classifier. The text is in a highly fragmentary state and is not easy to understand; however, it is clear that fishing and fowling as a royal sport is presented as a battle against chaos. The king goes to the marshes to suppress the evil forces of *isfet*, which is characterized by fish and fowl.

[...].f[...].k[...].s m33
[...] wd hnt [...] nswt m ʿwy dpt.f
stp-s3 [...] dšrw psh.f šn.f
nwhw [...].f st3w iry
hsr.n [...] ʿnw n whʿw
[...] him/it [...] you [...] she/it seeing
[...] ordering the sailing [...] the king in the arms of his boat,
the palace [...] red fish, when it emits its stench[31],
ropes [...] of him/it the towing of it (?)
[...] drove away [...] the fishers and fowlers[32] returned. (Sporting King C,1)

In the middle of the dangerous, foul-smelling swamps, surrounded by evil fish and birds, the king emerges as Shesmu, the god of perfume and pleasant smells, who cooked fragrant unguents in his laboratory with his own hands.

---

[30] The same opposition between the sweet scents of the urbanized city (of Thebes) and the stench of the wild, unsettled land (of the marshes of the Delta) could be observed in the Book of Kemit, discussed above.

[31] *psh* means "to bite," "to sting." I translated it here as "emit," as in "to emit a smell."

[32] Quirke translated *whʿw* as "hunters" (*Egyptian Literature 1800 BC*, 209). However, a precise translation would be "fishers and fowlers." While the fish (K5) classifier is a reconstruction, the bird classifier (G41), portraying an alighting pintail duck, is preserved. See Orly Goldwasser, *From Icon to Metaphor: Studies in the Semiotics of the Hieroglyphs*, OBO 142 (Fribourg, Switzerland: University Press; Göttingen: Vandenhoeck & Ruprecht, 1995), 91, for the classification of the word *whʿ* ("fisher and fowler").

di.f ḫꜥ[...] ꜣpdw tꜣ š r ḫddw imyw kb[...] [šsm]w nwdty m mrḥt ḫrt ꜥ.f
That he may cause to appear [...] the birds of the Land of the Lake more than the waterbirds, which are in the catara[ct-region ...]. [Shesm]u the ointment-maker, with the oils, which are under his charge. (Sporting King D,2)

Once again, the stench of fish and fowl in the wild marshland is contrasted with the sweet-smelling ointments of civilized life. It is no coincidence that the king is portrayed as the cruel, bloodthirsty god, Shesmu. Besides being the lord of perfume, Shesmu was known for his violent nature. He was worshipped as the lord of blood, a great slaughterer, who dismembered bodies. Thus, by acting as Shesmu, the king successfully slaughtered the fish and fowl, eliminated stench, and brought forth sweet scents.

Being the lord of sweet-smelling perfume and a bloodthirsty butcher at the same time, Shesmu's character has been often labeled "contradictory" in Egyptological literature.[33] However, when we consider the fact that in the ancient Egyptian worldview, the prerequisite of pleasant smells was slaughtering fish and fowl, which incorporated stench, Shesmu's first seemingly conflicting nature becomes all of a sudden self-explanatory.

Fishing and Fowling of the Upper Classes

One of the most frequent scenes encountered on funerary monuments from the Old Kingdom until the end of the pharaonic period is the tomb owner engaging in an idyllic sporting excursion in the papyrus swamps, hunting waterbirds with his boomerangs, while standing in a light raft, often in the company of friends or family.[34] Nevertheless, by the New Kingdom, these scenes had additionally

---

[33] See, for example, Mark Ciccarello, "Shesmu the Letopolite," in *Studies in Honor of George R. Hughes*, ed. Janet H. Johnson and Edward F. Wente, SAOC 39 (Chicago, IL: The Oriental Institute, 1976), 43–54. Ciccarello discusses Shesmu's "changing personality" stating that "he can be a benevolent god, particularly to the dead, or he can be a very cruel god. Shesmu manifests these two sides of his personality by assuming a different role for each side" (43). Furthermore, Ciccarello declares that Shesmu's transference from bloodthirsty butcher to ointment-maker "remains a mystery" (46).

[34] See, for example, the tomb of Kaemankh in Giza from the Old Kingdom. A well-preserved scene shows the tomb owner Kaemankh standing in a light raft, spearing fish. His son, who accompanied him on the fishing and fowling excursion, is holding a bird in his right hand and a harpoon in his left hand, see Hermann Junker, *Gîza IV: Die Mastaba des K'jm'nh (Kai-em-anch)* (Vienna: Hölder-Pichler-Tempsky, 1944), fig. 8. One of the most well-known representations of a nobleman fishing and fowling from the New Kingdom comes from the Theban tomb of Nebamun, depicting him standing in a small boat, holding a spear in one hand and marsh birds in the other. He is accompanied by his wife, daughter, and cat, see Richard Parkinson, *The Painted Tomb-Chapel of Nebamun: Mas-*

acquired a symbolic significance alluding to the deceased magically overcoming dangerous forces that may threaten their welfare in the netherworld. On the level of the upper classes, the deed of overcoming the evil-smelling fish and fowl of *isfet* represented overcoming danger in their own lives.

Fishing and Fowling of the Lower Classes

As seen above, fishing and fowling as a daytime occupation was regarded the most detestable of all professions due to the abominable smell of fish, birds and swamps.[35] Scholarly works of Egyptology neglect to mention what all Egyptian texts highlight: fishing was a smelly activity. Even though the ancient Egyptian sources provide a detailed description of olfactory sensation, the modern scholar excludes these references from the scientific analysis.

Summary

Fishing and fowling manifested itself on three distinct levels of the ancient Egyptian society and at each level, this activity bore a markedly different meaning. For the king, fishing and fowling was a royal duty that was equated with eliminating stench and danger and overcoming the evil forces of *isfet*, so that the rest of the population could live in peace and be surrounded by sweet scents. For the upper classes, fishing and fowling was a pleasurable pastime activity. A successful fishing and fowling excursion in the life of elite men was a symbol of overcoming evil forces and eliminating stench in their own lives. At the lowest levels of society, fishing and fowling was an occupation. It was considered the most detestable of all professions due to the abominable stench of fish, birds, and the natural habitat of these animals, the swamps of the Delta. The fisher and fowler were drenched in stench every day and were not in the power of getting rid of the smell.

4. FISH AND FOWL AS THE ENEMY OF EGYPT

In sacred contexts, fishing and fowling represented the annihilation of the enemy. From the entire pharaonic history of Egypt, four scenes have been preserved from temples that depict the king fishing and fowling. While this topic was very

---

terpieces of Ancient Egyptian Art in the British Museum (London: The British Museum, 2008).

[35] Nevertheless, there is also written evidence of the occupation of the fisher and fowler being presented in a positive manner. The author of the text The Pleasures of Fishing and Fowling praises the profession and longs to be in the company of fishers and fowlers.

popular on tomb-walls of elite men, it was rare in temples, most likely due to the stench associated with fish and birds. A remarkable scene from the Roman temple of Esna shows Emperor Commodus together with the gods Horus, Thoth, Khnum, and Seshat catching fish and birds with a clap-net.[36] By pulling the rope, the two parts of the clap-net appear to fold together, trapping the fish and birds within. The capturing of fish and fowl symbolizes the destruction of the enemies of Egypt. The king is wearing the Red Crown of Lower Egypt, where the marshes abundant in fish and birds were located. The scene is accompanied by the following text:

grg.n.w [rmw m ḫftyw] 3pdw m sbi[w ...] m š3.sn n s[f]ḫ sp ḥtš ibṯt bwt n ḥ ͨkw-ib ḥḏw
[The fish that are enemy] are trapped; the birds that are the rebels [...] out of their marshes. He (the king) doesn't let loose, he tightens[37] the net. The rebels are slaughtered. (Esna VI, 1, 531,1–2)

The Ptolemaic temple of Edfu yielded two scenes of the king fishing and fowling with the help of several deities.[38] Both accompanying inscriptions describe the captured fish and fowl as the traditional enemies of Egypt, the Asiatics and the Nubians.[39] The king, acting as Horus, destroys the opponents.

sti.n.f iss(t).f inḥ.n.f s(y) dr nw-pn-n-sf ini.n.f bw wr m rmw ͨh ͨw ͨš3w m 3pdw ini.n.f irf m wḥ ͨ r nwt.f ḥr [...] ini.n.f n.s rmw m mrš (ḥr) dmḏ n.s 3pdw 3 m swt grg ini.n.f n.s rmw m sttiw p3iw m iwntiw ... rmw im.s m ͨ nhniw ͨ .s ͨ 3pdw ͨ [im.s m] khb ḥr.s
He casted his net, he tightened it at the crack of dawn and fetched a large amount of fish and a great amount of fowl. He took them to his city as a fisher with [...] He brought them fish from the canal and he caught fowl for them at the fowling grounds by bringing them fish as Asiatics and birds as the nomads (from Nubia)[40].... The fish in it are her[41] ͨopponents, the fowl ͨ [in it] do harm[42] to her (Edfu). (Edfu VI, 56,10–13, 57,2)

---

[36] Esna VI, 1, 5.31.

[37] Should be *ḥtš* ("to tighten") and not *ḥtp*. Maurice Alliot, "Les rites de la chasse au filet, aux temples de Karnak, d'Edfou et d'Esneh," *RdE* 5 (1946): 90.2.

[38] Edfu XIII, CCCCXCII and CCCCXCIII; Edfu XIV, DLXXXV and DLXXXV.

[39] Edfu VI, 55,5–57,5, 236,7–237,5.

[40] Dieter Kurth reckons that the Iuntiu refer to the peoples to the south of Egypt. Dieter Kurth, *Edfou VI: Die Inschriften des Tempels von Edfu; Abteilung I Übersetzungen*, vol. 3 (Gladbeck: PeWe), 95.4.

[41] "Her" most likely refers to the city of Edfu (Kurth, *Edfou VI*, 95.9).

[42] Gamer-Wallert translates: "Die Fische (des Netzes) sind die Rebellen! Die Vögel (des Netzes) sind Keheb (Seth), ihr Führer" (*Fische und Fischkulte*, 74; see also Alliot, "Les rites de la chasse au filet," 88). As opposed to Gamer-Wallert and Alliot, Kurth

*ini.n.f n.s wh'w hn' rsf ' rmw` '33t n tnw.sn* [...] ' *hpnpnw*` ? *hdw imiw nww h3iw ii m kbhw ini.n.f n.s mhy(t) m iwntiw 3pdw irf m sttiw*
He brings for her (the throne) the catch of fish and fowl, fish in great quantities, without a number, [...] khepenpenu(?)-fish and khedju-fish from the great waters, migrating birds that come from the marshlands. He brings for her the fish as the nomads (from Nubia) and the fowl as the Asiatics. (Edfu VI, 237,1–3)

In chapter 134 of the Book of the Dead, fish and fowl embody the enemies of the gods that populate the water and the sky. The gods, led by Horus, destroy them by cutting off their heads.

in msw gbb shr.tn hftyw wsir – NN– m3' hrw hmiyw [hmi]t(y).sn m wi3 n r'w š'd.n hrw tpw.sn r pt m 3pdw hpdw.sn diw r š m rmw
It is the children of Geb, who will overthrow the enemy of Osiris NN, true of voice, the opponents, who will attack the sun-bark. Horus has slaughtered them. Their heads belong to the sky as birds. Their rear parts are thrown into the water as fish. (Book of the Dead 134,3–4)

The Lack of Fish-Offering in Temples

Fish was almost never a part of food-offerings in temples.[43] Accordingly, depictions of fish-offerings in temples are scarce. One rare exception is a statue in the Egyptian Museum of Cairo (CG 392) of two offering-bearers holding plates loaded with fish.[44] The fish are covered in lotus flowers, presumably to suppress their unpleasant odor. Lotus flowers were often placed on food-offerings and in beverages to improve their smell.

On festivals, many temples forbad eating fish entirely.[45] The reason behind the lack of fish-offerings in the temples and the prohibition of eating fish during festivals is very likely to be the strong stench of fish, which led to its cultic impurity. Based on all the evidence referring to the stench of fish, I strongly believe that it was its malodor that led to its exclusion from food-offerings in the temple. Patrick F. Houlihan was one of the very few scholars to suppose that it was the abominable smell of fish that led to its prohibition as food-offering in

---

treats *khb* as a verb: "Die Fische darin sind ihre 'Gegner, die Vögel` [darin sind] die, die sie (die Stadt Edfu) angreifen" (*Edfou VI*, 95,12). I followed Kurth's translation.

[43] Fish was almost never a part of funerary offerings either.

[44] See Ludwig Borchardt, *Text und Tafeln zu Nr. 381–653*, vol. 2 of *Statuen und Statuetten von Königen und Privatleuten im Museum von Kairo: Nos. 1–1294*, Catalogue général des antiquités égyptiennes du Musée du Caire (Berlin: Rechtsdruckerei, 1925), 9–11.

[45] Nevertheless, fish was not completely absent from the temple precinct. It could have served as the aliment of temple staff or holy animals.

sacred contexts.[46] Surprisingly, in the book *Fische und Fischkulte im Alten Ägypten*, which still serves as one of the most essential publications on fish and fish cults in ancient Egypt, Ingrid Gamer-Wallert assumes that the reason behind the prohibition of fish in temples was connected to the holy status of some fish in certain cities.[47] Gamer-Wallert failed to analyze the usage of the fish classifier (K5) in the hieroglyphic script and the role of the odor of fish in the ancient Egyptian culture. As a result, she omitted the offensive smell of fish as a possible cause. The evidence at hand teaches us that the Egyptian temple represented a perfect olfactory world (= *ma'at*), where stench (= *isfet*) could not be present. Fish, the prototype of stench and the olfactory representative of *isfet*, naturally, had to be expelled from the temple.

Roast Meat-Offering of Birds in Temples or the Ritual Burning of the Enemy

As opposed to fish, fowl were an essential part of the food-offerings presented to the gods. While marsh birds were considered malodorous animals alive in their natural environment, the smell of their meat grilled on the altar was considered pleasant and served to trigger the appetite of the gods and attract them to the temple. The flames roasting the meat of fowl on the altar was at the same time magically equated with the burning of the enemy.

> *ts iḥt ḥr ḥ3wt dd mdw ḥ3wt ḥwd m ḥ3w nw ḥ3w 3ḥtyt ḥnm.t ḥnmw.sn ḥ3ḥ.tw r ḥm.t nn wn rkyw.t ḥftyw.t ḥr.tw m ḥbt.sn*
> Placing the offerings on the altar. Words to be spoken: The altar is rich in meat. The meat is from the horizon. You smell their scent going up to your shrine. Your opponents don't exist anymore. Your enemies fall in their slaughterhouse.
> (Dendera III, 185,1–4)

The meat of birds (called "meat of the horizon") metaphorically represents the fallen opponents of Egypt that are burnt in the slaughterhouse. The smell of their roast meat signifies victory over the enemy, serving as an olfactory metaphor of the king's incontestable power and authority.

A similar inscription from the Ptolemaic temple of Edfu reveals that the enemy was symbolically burnt in a kiosk on the roof of the temple called Place of First Holiday.

> *stpt sbi.k stp.wt m ʿ irt ḥr [...] js ʿd ḥ3.w im=sn m irt nfrt tit nbd pw ḥftyw.k iw.sn r ḥ3wt.k n st-ḥ3b-tpi.k snsn.k m ḥty.sn*

---

[46] Houlihan, *Animal World of the Pharaohs*, 130.
[47] Gamer-Wallert, *Fische und Fischkulte*, 81–83.

The meat of your opponents is cut with my own hands. The Eye of Horus [...] roasting the meat-offering as a good deed. It is a symbol of evil.[48] Your enemy is (intended) for the altar of your Place of the First Holiday.[49] You smell their smoke. (Edfu I, 565,67–70)

This ritual act must have been visible for most of the population due to the smoke, and the smell must have travelled in the air through the entire city. The smell of roast waterfowl was an olfactory sign of Egypt's conquest over its enemy and a sign of authority and order. It was ultimately a sign of *ma'at*. As long as meat-offerings of birds were being made, Egypt was at peace.

Seth and the Smell of the Enemy

A royal inscription from Medinet Habu called Second Lybian War: Triumphal Poem of Year 11, dating to the Twentieth Dynasty, the reign of Ramesses III, describes the smell of the enemy being burnt in flames in the slaughterhouse.

iw.w ḥr rd.wy dsw r t3 [ḫb]t nty m h3w n stiw gr rkḥ nḥt
They came on their own feet to the [slaughterhouse], which was in flames and odors, burning strongly. (KRI V, 69,15–70,1)

The word denoting the place the enemy went to is unfortunately fragmentary; however, the house classifier (O1) is preserved indicating that some sort of a building was meant. What is meant based on the context is a place where the enemy was burnt. This reference makes sense in light of the previous Ptolemaic inscriptions from the temple of Dendera and Edfu, which state that the enemy, symbolized by the meat of the bird-offerings, is set in flames and burnt (on the altar). The strong smell and the smoke rising from both the roof of the temple and the slaughterhouse of the enemy must have accounted for an intensive olfactory and visual experience that was intentionally created to emphasize the defeat of the enemy and Egypt's indisputable authority.

The word *stiw* ("odors") is written with the sign of the animal of Seth (E20) and clearly has a negative connotation based on the context. The negative meaning is further emphasized by the Aa2 classifier, which is used to classify the word *sti*[50] when it has a negative connotation, meaning "odor" or "stench."[51] The beginning of the text states that the enemy was "bearing their tribute, making and paying homage to Seth," unequivocally demonstrating that

---

[48] *nbd* was also an epithet of Seth meaning "The Evil One."
[49] TLA lemma-no. 858644. *st-h3b-tpi* ("Place of the First Holiday") was a kiosk on the roof of the Edfu temple.
[50] *Wb* 4:349.5–350.1.
[51] Common in medical papyri, for example.

the god Seth is associated with the enemy and represents the villain of the narrative. Seth was the god of evil, chaos, disease, weather disturbances (storm, thunder), aggressive behavior, and foreigners, and he was often equated with the enemy. The fact that the word meaning "stench" was written with Seth's sign serves as pictorial and lexical-semantic evidence that Seth was affiliated with evil smells. As a matter of fact, in religious writings, Seth is often associated with fish and birds and is overthrown by being snatched in a net.[52] In spell 535 of the Pyramid Texts, Horus captures his archenemy, Seth, together with his followers, with a net in the marshlands. The verb *issỉ*[53] means "to capture with a net." The spell is an early evidence of the king, or Horus, symbolically destroying the enemy and eliminating stench by fishing and fowling in the swamps.

fḫ n.k ḥrw m šṯ.f iss.f imy-ḫt stš
Horus left the *šṯ*-garment for you and captured the followers of Seth with a net. (PT 535, 1285c)

Just before this section, the spell states that the corpse of King Pepi does not rot and does not sweat. He has no body fluids and his corpse did not turn into dust.

n imk.k ppy pw n fdt.k ppy pw n rḏw.k ppy pw n ḥmw.k ppy pw
Your putrefaction does not exist, Pepi. Your sweat does not exist, Pepi. Your body fluids do not exist, Pepi. Your dust does not exist, Pepi. (PT 535, 1283a–1383b)

One of the biggest challenges of life after death has been conquered. The foul smell of the decaying corpse has been avoided. In fact, one of the main reasons behind mummification was to prevent the unbearable stench of putrefaction.[54] The fact that subsequently the spell describes the defeat of Seth by capturing him with a net unequivocally demonstrates that Seth incorporates the abominable smell of decay, the rotting smell of the corpse. Overcoming the stench of decay in the afterlife meant overcoming Seth and his followers, the enemy.[55]

---

[52] Alliot correctly observed that Seth, incorporating the enemy, is captured with a fishnet in various religious writings. However, he failed to mention Seth's connection to evil smells ("Les rites de la chasse au filet," 114–15).

[53] *Wb* 1:130.3.

[54] See spell 412 from the Pyramid of Queen Neith, which contains the following exclamation: "Flesh of Neith, may you not decay, may you not rot! May your smell not be bad!"

[55] Alexandra von Lieven also treated PT 535 with relevance to negative body fluids, and observed that Seth is associated with materials of inferior quality, while positive gods are related to sweet smells: "Dabei werden mit den positiven Gottheiten wohlriechende Produkte assoziiert, wohingegen dem bösen Seth minderwertige und unbrauchbare Stoffe zugeordnet werden." Alexandra von Lieven, "'Where There Is Dirt There Is System': Zur

The Sporting King also seems to bear a visual (red) and olfactory (fish) reference to the defeat of Seth, who represents the enemy. The literary work mentions that the king, presented as a mighty fisher and fowler, destroys the "red fish, when it emits its stench." Red was the color associated with Seth. By describing the color of the fish, the text employs visual sensation to enhance olfactory sensation.[56]

The New Kingdom date of the Medinet Habu inscription discussing the stench of the enemy with relevance to Seth is significant. The New Kingdom was characterized by an expanding policy. Egypt frequently waged war. During this challenging time, the figure of Seth became more prominent. In the hieroglyphic script, the Seth classifier expanded and came to classify more and different categories, as in previous in periods. Niv Allon discussed the semantic shift the Sethian category underwent in the New Kingdom and the reasons behind this change.[57] Table 1a and 1b from Allon's work illustrate the members in the Sethian category in the New Kingdom. Allon rightfully argues that through its syncretism with Ba'al, a Canaanite weather and warrior god, Seth's identification with *extreme weather conditions*, such as heavy rains, snow, clouds, and thunder, and *aggressive behavior* was accentuated. The Sethian category came to include words, such as *snm* ("rainstorm"), *phph* ("storm"), *srk* ("snow"), *h3h3.ty* ("storm"), *kh3* ("shout"), *nhnh* ("to roar"), and *khb(w)* ("to harm"). In this respect, I would like to add another member to the Sethian category outlined by Allon: *sti* ("stench [of the enemy]"). All members of the Sethian category were conspicuous, out of the ordinary, rapid, undeniably strong, and unpleasant. Moreover, they were all related to sensory perception. Seth manifested himself through several senses at the same time: thunder was his voice, precipitation was his touch, and the stench of the enemy was his smell. While Seth's connection to

---

Ambiguität der Bewertung von körperlichen Ausscheidungen in der ägyptischen Kultur," *SAK* 40 (2011): 290–91.

[56] On a few occasions, ancient Egyptian literature makes use of visual sensation to enhance olfactory sensation. I will provide two further examples here. An inscription from the Ptolemaic temple of Edfu states that the inundation of the Nile makes the fields "shine" through its smell: "I give you the Nile at the time of its inundation. He (the Nile) makes the fields shine through his smell. It is not dirty, and it doesn't stink" (Edfu I, 471,12). An inscription accompanying a censing-scene in Room K of the Hibis Temple discusses the smell of the goddess Shentyt. That goddess' scent refers to the scent of incense is evident by the incense classifier (R7) of the word *sti* ("scent"), which functions as a repeater, and by the wall-painting showing the king with a censer in his hand. Gold is used as an adjective to emphasize the high value of the smell of incense: "The scent is within Shentyt, lady of Busiris. The scent is within Shentyt in the divine boat. The scent of Shentyt is the golden scent" (Hibis, Pl. 22, East Wall, Register II, 3–5).

[57] Niv Allon, "Seth Is Baal—Evidence from the Egyptian Script," *AeL* 17 (2007): 15–22. Prior to Allon, Goldwasser shortly treated the Sethian category ("Where Is Metaphor," 108–9).

the stench of the enemy could have been accentuated in the New Kingdom due to Egypt's expanding policy, spell 535 of the Pyramid Texts demonstrates that the association of Seth with evil smells and the enemy has a long tradition, and in fact, it goes back to the Old Kingdom.

Seth, the god of all evil, incorporated every aspect in his figure we have seen before: fish and fowl, the enemy, and foul smells. Nevertheless, his evil and unpleasant nature was a necessary part of existence.

Summary

An examination of the written evidence on the role of fish and fowl as the prototype of stench revealed a wealth of new information about ancient Egyptian culture. The analysis of a small segment of the olfactory world of the ancient Egyptians in this paper has demonstrated that by studying the way the Egyptians perceived the world through smell, supposedly unclear and mysterious matters become apprehensible.

It is to be assumed that what was presented in this article as having a bad smell reflects the collective olfactory values of ancient Egyptian society, which were culturally shaped. It would be unrealistic to think that the olfactory values presented in the texts were the individual olfactory values of the scribes who wrote them. The texts give us the impression that they make use of general olfactory values, which would have been understandable and obvious for everyone. As in every society, there must have been individual olfactory values in ancient Egypt as well; however, based on the available texts, these cannot be detected.

The weather, geographic formations, and species available as food resources unavoidably shape the olfactory prototypes of a culture. Egypt's particularly hot climate and its swamps in the Nile Delta richly inhabited with fish (*Petrocephalus bane*) and birds (*Anas acuta*) providing the main source of nourishment all contributed to the fish and fowl becoming the prototype of stench.

The approach to the detestable odor of fish and fowl revealed the division and hierarchies of the ancient Egyptian society. The king, who was on the top of the olfactory hierarchy, went fishing and fowling as a royal duty in order to slay the enemy and annihilate evil smells, so that the rest of the population could live. For elite men, coming into contact with stench through fishing and fowling represented a challenging pastime activity. By slaughtering fish and fowl in the foul-smelling and dangerous marshes, they expelled odors from their own lives. Fishers and fowlers, who practiced catching fish and birds as a trade, were drenched in stench every day and were not in the position to remove the smell. Due to their smelly occupation, they were at the lowest level of the social and olfactory hierarchy.

The very core of the ancient Egyptian perception of the world, which divided the universe into *ma'at* and *isfet*, paralleled the mechanism of olfaction. Our brain distinguishes between pleasant and unpleasant smells. The distinction of odors into either good or bad, and nothing in between, has survival value. A significant characteristic of odor memory is called *proactive interference*, in which forming one association with a stimulus may make it more difficult to acquire others subsequently. This characteristic of odor memory is dramatically illustrated by "bait shyness" in the animal world, an animal's avoidance of food that has made it sick. Odor perception also plays a key role in the recognition of food for humans. Many people experience a lifelong aversion to a particular food or drink after overindulging or consuming it coincidentally with the onset of illness.[58] Similarly to the sense of smell, the concept of *ma'at* and *isfet* functioned as a type of knowledge organization or guideline that helped the Egyptians distinguish between good and bad in the world.

Since smells move along an axis of good-bad, olfaction served as a perfect sensory perception to express the very essence of the ancient Egyptian worldview, according to which the world was divided into good-bad/ order-chaos/ justice-injustice/ *ma'at-isfet*. The ideology of *ma'at* and *isfet* incorporated divine, human, sensory, and spatial representatives. Seth was the divine representative of the world of *isfet*, opposing Horus, the divine emblem of *ma'at*. The enemy of Egypt, traditionally the Asiatics and the Nubians, were the human representatives of *isfet*, with the king alone as its counterpart fighting for *ma'at*. Evil smells belonged in *isfet*, whereas *ma'at* was characterized by pleasant scents. Each of these opposing worlds had an olfactory representative. Fish and fowl were the prototype of stench in the world of *isfet*. Unguents were the epitome of the fragrant world of *ma'at*. *Isfet* constituted the idea of dangerous wilderness, with the swamps of the Nile Delta as its spatial representative. *Ma'at* embodied the concept of home, with cities as its spatial representative (table 1).

Main concept	isfet	ma'at
	bad, evil	good
	chaos	order
	injustice	justice
Divine representative	Seth	Horus
Human representative	enemy	king
Sensory concept	stench	sweet smells
Olfactory representative	fish and fowl	unguents
Spatial concept	wilderness	home
Spatial representative	swamps of the Delta	cities

Table 1. Concepts belonging to the world *ma'at* and *isfet* and their representatives

---

[58] Trygg Engen, *The Perception of Odors* (Toronto: Academic Press, 1982), 110.

All members listed respectively under *isfet* and *ma'at* in table 1 can be equated with each other. Any member combined with another member will produce a true sentence. Horus is good. Seth is evil. Horus is the king. Seth is the enemy. The king creates sweet scents. The enemy stinks. Cities represent order. Swamps represent chaos. Unguents are found in cities. Fish and fowl are found in the swamps. The king, acting as Shesmu, is responsible for making unguents. The enemy is fish and fowl.

Seth, the divine representative of *isfet*, incorporated all concepts related to *isfet* in his figure. He was associated with all bad smells. He and his followers equaled the enemy, as well as fish and fowl, and were captured with a net in the marshes and slaughtered. The meat of fowl, but not the fish, was burnt in the slaughterhouse, representing another act of victory over the enemy. Seth was the source of the smell of fish and fowl, the smell of burning of the flesh of the enemy, and the smell of the decaying, rotting corpse. Seth's attribution to evil smells goes back to as early as the Old Kingdom. During the wartimes of the New Kingdom, Seth's connection to stench was further strengthened by phonetically writing the word *sṯi* ("stench") with Seth's hieroglyphic sign.

The ancient Egyptian sources demonstrated that smells did not only have prototypes, but also had spatial representatives. The idea of the stench of the faraway land, the foul odor of uncivilized life, was represented by the swamps of the Nile Delta. The concept of the sweet, familiar smell of home was embodied by cities, the fragrance of civilized life. The fact that smells were connected to areas with relevance to *ma'at* and *isfet* can be explained by how odor and context-dependent memory functions in the brain. Olfactory memory proves to be the strongest type of memory. Olfactory information is processed more quickly and with less editing than visual and auditory information and lasts longer. Modern experiments show that odor memory does not decline over time. It is largely the same after five minutes, as one year later.[59] Context-dependent memory is based on the principle that environmental features encoded as part of a memory trace can facilitate memory for stored material when subsequently encountered. When odor memory is combined with context-dependent memory, memory cues are unusually strong and effective.[60]

The ancient Egyptians imagined the world naturally as a chaotic, dangerous, unjust, and evil-smelling environment. The world in its natural state smelled bad. *Isfet* reeked of fish and fowl. It was the Egyptian civilization that brought order, justice, cities, and sweet smells to the world. Nevertheless, the stench of *isfet* was an essential part of existence. There was no *ma'at* without *isfet*. There was no perfume without stench.

---

[59] Engen, *Perception of Odors*, 106–9.
[60] Rachel S. Herz and Trygg Engen, "Odor Memory: Review and Analysis," *Psychonomic Bulletin & Review* 3 (1996): 307–8.

Written Sources

Book of the Dead, Chapter 134
  Lapp, Günther. *The Papyrus of Nu (BM EA 10477)*. Catalogue of Books of the Dead in the British Museum I. London: British Museum, 1997.
Dendera
  Chassinat, Émile. *Le temple de Dendara*. Vol. 3. Cairo: Institut Français d'Archéologie Orientale, 1935.
Dispute
  Barta, Winfried. *Das Gespräch eines Mannes mit seinem BA (Papyrus Berlin 3024)*. MÄS 18. Berlin: Hessling, 1969.
  Goedicke, Hans. *The Report about the Dispute of a Man with His BA: Papyrus Berlin 3024*. Baltimore: Johns Hopkins Press, 1970.
  Allen, James P. *The Debate between a Man and His Soul: A Masterpiece of Ancient Egyptian Literature*. Leiden: Brill, 2011.
Edfu
  Chassinat, Émile. *Le temple d'Edfou I,2*. 2. éd. Cairo: Institut Français d'Archéologie Orientale, 1984.
  ———. *Le temple d'Edfou VI*. Cairo: Institut Français d'Archéologie Orientale, 1931.
  ———. *Le temple d'Edfou XIII*. Cairo: Institut Français d'Archéologie Orientale, 1934.
  ———. *Le temple d'Edfou XIV*. Cairo: Institut Français d'Archéologie Orientale, 1934.
Esna
  Sauneron, Serge. *Le temple d'Esna, Textes nos 473–546, Esna VI,1*. Cairo: Institut Français d'Archéologie Orientale, 1975.
Hibis
  Davies, Norman de Garis. *The Decoration*. Vol. 3 of *The Temple of Hibis in El Khargeh Oasis*. The Metropolitan Museum of Art, Egyptian Expedition Publications 17, 1953.
Hymn III to Ramesses VI
  Rossi, Franceso, and Willem Pleyte. *Papyrus de Turin: Planches*, 1869–1876.
  Condon, Virginia. *Seven Royal Hymns of the Ramesside Period: Papyrus Turin CG 54031*. MÄS 37. München: Deutscher Kunstverlag, 1978.
Kemit
  Posener, Georges, and Annie Gasse. *Catalogue des ostraca hiératiques littéraires de Deir el-Médina, Tome 2: Nos. 1109–1167*. Documents de fouilles 18.2. Cairo: Institut Français d'Archéologie Orientale, 1951.
  Hayes, William C. "A Much-Copied Letter of the Early Middle Kingdom." *JNES* 7 (1948): pl. 1–3.
Kitchen Ramesside Inscriptions (KRI)
  Kitchen, Kenneth Anderson. *Ramesside Inscriptions V: Historical and Biographical*. Oxford: Blackwell, 1983.
Pleasures of Fishing and Fowling
  Caminos, Ricardo Augusto. *Literary Fragments in the Hieratic Script*. Oxford: University Press, 1956.
Pyramid Texts, Spell 535
  Sethe, Kurt. *Text, zweite Hälfte, Spruch 469–714 (Pyr. 906–2217)*. Vol. 2 of *Die altägyptischen Pyramidentexte*. Leipzig, 1910.

Report on the Delta Residence
  Gardiner, Sir Alan H. *Late-Egyptian Miscellanies*. Bibliotheca Aegyptiaca VII. Brussels: Édition de la Fondation Égyptologique, 1937.
Satire of Trades
  Helck, Wolfgang. *Die Lehre des Dw'-Ḥtjj*. Kleine Ägyptische Texte 3. Wiesbaden: Harrassowitz, 1970.
  Jäger, Stephan. *Altägyptische Berufstypologien*. Lingua Aegyptia Studia Monographica 4. Göttingen: Seminar für Koptologie und Ägyptologie, 2004.
Sporting King
  Caminos, Ricardo Augusto. *Literary Fragments in the Hieratic Script*. Oxford: University Press, 1956.

BIBLIOGRAPHY

Alliot, Maurice. "Les rites de la chasse au filet, aux temples de Karnak, d'Edfou et d'Esneh." *RdE* 5 (1946): 57–118.
Allon, Niv. "Seth Is Baal—Evidence from the Egyptian Script." *AeL* 17 (2007): 15–22.
Beaux, Nathalie. "Odeur, souffle et vie." Pages 61–73 in *Mélanges offerts à Ola el-Aguizy*. Edited by Faiza Haykal. Bibliothèque d'étude 164. Cairo: Institut français d'archéologie orientale, 2015.
Borchardt, Ludwig. *Text und Tafeln zu Nr. 381–653*. Vol. 2 of *Statuen und Statuetten von Königen und Privatleuten im Museum von Kairo: Nos. 1–1294*. Catalogue général des antiquités égyptiennes du Musée du Caire. Berlin: Rechtsdruckerei, 1925.
Boulenger, George Albert. *Zoology of Egypt: The Fishes of the Nile*. London: Hugh Rees, 1907.
Ciccarello, Mark. "Shesmu the Letopolite." Pages 43–54 in *Studies in Honor of George R. Hughes*. Edited by Janet H. Johnson and Edward F. Wente. SAOC 39. Chicago: The Oriental Institute, 1976.
Classen, Constance. "Foundations for an Anthropology of the Senses." *International Social Science Journal* 153 (1997): 401–12.
Emerit, Sibylle. "La musique pharaonique, un patrimoine plurimillénaire." Pages 48–61 in *Musiques! Échos de l'Antiquité*. Edited by Sibylle Emerit, Hélène Guichard, Violene Jeammet, Sylvain Perrot, Ariane Thomas, Christophe Vendries, Alexandre Vincent, and Nele Ziegler. Musée du Louvre-Lens, Gand: Snoeck, 2017.
———. "Music and Musicians." In *UCLA Encyclopedia of Egyptology*. Edited by Willeke Wendrich. Los Angeles: University of California, Department of Near Eastern Languages and Cultures, 2013.
Engen, Trygg. *The Perception of Odors*. Toronto: Academic Press, 1982.
Finnestad, Ragnhild Bjerre. "Enjoying the Pleasures of Sensation: Reflections on a Significant Feature of Egyptian Religion." Pages 111–19 in *Gold of Praise: Studies on Ancient Egypt in Honor of Edward F. Wente*. Edited by Emily Teeter and John A. Larson. SAOC 58. Chicago: Oriental Institute, 1999.
Foster, John L. *Ancient Egyptian Literature: An Anthology*. Austin: University of Texas Press, 2007.

Herz, Rachel S., and Trygg Engen. "Odor Memory: Review and Analysis." *Psychonomic Bulletin & Review* 3 (1996): 300–313.

Houlihan, Patrick F. *The Animal World of the Pharaohs*. Cairo: The American University in Cairo Press, 1995.

Gamer-Wallert, Ingrid. *Fische und Fischkulte im Alten Ägypten*. Ägyptologische Abhandlungen 21. Wiesbaden: Harrassowitz, 1970.

Gardiner, Alan H. *Egyptian Grammar*. 3rd rev. ed. Cambridge: Cambridge University Press, 1957.

Goldwasser, Orly. *From Icon to Metaphor: Studies in the Semiotics of the Hieroglyphs*. OBO 142. Fribourg, Switzerland: University Press; Göttingen: Vandenhoeck & Ruprecht, 1995.

———. *Lovers, Prophets and Giraffes: Wor[l]d Classification in Ancient Egypt*. Göttinger Orientforschungen. Wiesbaden: Harrassowitz, 2002.

———. "Where Is Metaphor? Conceptual Metaphor and Alternative Classification in the Hieroglyphic Script." *Metaphor and Symbol* 20 (2005): 95–113.

Goodman, Steven M., and Peter L. Meininger. *Birds of Egypt*. Oxford: Oxford University Press, 1989.

Grässler, Nadine. *Konzepte des Auges im alten Ägypten*. SAK.B 20. Hamburg: Helmut Buske, 2017.

Junker, Hermann. *Gîza IV: Die Mastaba des KAjm'nh (Kai-em-anch)*. Vienna: Hölder-Pichler-Tempsky, 1944.

Kurth, Dieter. *Edfou VI: Die Inschriften des Tempels von Edfu; Abteilung I Übersetzungen*. Vol. 3. Gladbeck: PeWe.

Lichtheim, Miriam. *The Old and Middle Kingdoms*. Vol. 1 of *Ancient Egyptian Literature: A Book of Readings*. Berkeley: University of California Press, 1973.

Manniche, Lise. *Music and Musicians in Ancient Egypt*. London: British Museum, 1991.

———. *Sacred Luxuries: Fragrance, Aromatherapy and Cosmetics in Ancient Egypt*. London: Opus Publishing Limited, 1999.

———. *Sexual Life in Ancient Egypt*. Zürich: Artemis, 1987.

Meyer-Dietrich, Erika, ed. *Laut und Leise: Der Gebrauch von Stimme und Klang in historischen Kulturen*. Mainzer Historische Kulturwissenschaften 7. Bielefeld: transcript, 2011.

Parkinson, Richard. *The Painted Tomb-Chapel of Nebamun: Masterpieces of Ancient Egyptian Art in the British Museum*. London: The British Museum, 2008.

Price, Robyn. "Sniffing out the Gods: Archaeology with the Senses." *JAEI* 17 (2018): 137–55.

Quirke, Stephen. *Egyptian Literature 1800 BC: Questions and Readings*. Egyptology 2. London: Golden House, 2004.

Steinbach-Eicke, Elizabeth. "Experiencing Is Tasting: Perception Metaphors of Taste in Ancient Egyptian." *Lingua Aegyptia* 25 (2017): 373–90.

———. "'Ich habe seinen Anblick geschmeckt …': Verben der Wahrnehmung und die semantischen Beziehungen zwischen Perzeption und Kognition." Pages 209–25 in *Wissen-Wirkung Wahrnehmung: Beiträge des vierten Münchner Arbeitskreises Junge Aegyptologie*. Edited by Gregor Neunert, Henrike Simon, Alexandra Verbovsek, and Kathrin Gabler. MAJA 4. Wiesbaden: Harrassowitz, 2015.

Sutton, David E. *Remembrance of Repasts: An Anthropology of Food and Memory*. Oxford: Berg, 2001.
Swennen, Cornelis. "Nest Protection of Eiderducks and Shovelers by Means of Faeces." *Ardea* 56 (1968): 248–58.
Verhoeven, Ursula. *Grillen, Kochen, Backen im Alltag und im Ritual Altägyptens: Ein lexikographischer Beitrag*. Bruxelles: Fondation Egyptologique Reine Elisabeth, 1984.
von Lieven, Alexandra. "'Thy Fragrance Is in All My Limbs:' On the Olfactory Sense in Ancient Egyptian Religion." Pages 309–25 in *Religion für die Sinne—Religion for the Senses*. Edited by Phillip Reichling and Meret Strothmann. Artificium 58. Oberhausen: Athena, 2016.
———. "'Where There Is Dirt There Is System': Zur Ambiguität der Bewertung von körperlichen Ausscheidungen in der ägyptischen Kultur." *SAK* 40 (2011): 287–300.

SMELLING FAT AND HEARING FLAME: SENSORY EXPERIENCE OF ARTIFICIAL LIGHT IN ANCIENT EGYPT

Meghan E. Strong

BLINDED BY THE LIGHT

Those of us fortunate enough to live in the modern Western world rarely think about artificial lighting. With the flick of a switch or the press of a button, illumination is at our fingertips. Only in rare instances of power outages do we consider how many candles there might be in the house and how many hours of light that might provide. This, however, is a very rare point in civilization. For the majority of human history, the procurement and maintenance of artificial light has been at the forefront of daily life—stoking fires, making candles, even risking life and limb to hunt whales for lamp oil.[1] Artificial light is also typically viewed as a passive source of illumination that is shed on to objects. Rarely, is it seen as an active agent. Recently, however, it has become increasingly apparent that artificial light has very powerful effects and, when applied in large quantities, acts as a pollutant that negatively impacts human health, energy consumption, wildlife, and appreciation of the night sky.[2] To an extent, light pollution has also crept into museums and archaeological sites, as well as the minds of scholars of the ancient

---

[1] William Thomas O'Dea, *The Social History of Lighting* (London: Routledge & Paul, 1958); Jane Brox, *Brilliant: The Evolution of Artificial Light* (London: Souvenir, 2011).

[2] Yongmin Cho et al., "Effects of Artificial Light at Night on Human Health: A Literature Review of Observational and Experimental Studies Applied to Exposure Assessment," *Chronobiology International* 32 (2015): 1294–1310; Fabio Falchi et al., "The New World Atlas of Artificial Night Sky Brightness," *Science Advances* 2 (2016): doi:10.1126/sciadv.1600377; Jonathan Bennie et al., "Ecological Effects of Artificial Light at Night on Wild Plants," *Journal of Ecology* 104 (2016): 611–20; Paul Bogard, *The End of Night: Searching for Natural Darkness in an Age of Artificial Light* (London: Fourth Estate, 2014).

world. The prevalence of a (natural) light-centric view, particularly in archaeology, has obscured the interactions between material culture and day or night, light or dark, and natural versus artificial light.[3]

I would also suggest that the over-abundance of artificial light in modern society has negatively affected the understanding of how artificial light impacts the senses. Electric lighting is sterile, producing textureless, odorless illumination at a consistent intensity and color temperature. Artificial light that relies on a flame, as in ancient Egyptian culture, is far more dynamic and would have impacted the personal sensorium in a variety of ways. This article will examine the sensory profile of artificial light in ancient Egypt by exploring the offering of light during the illumination of the thrones of Upper and Lower Egypt during the royal *sed*-festival. Specifically, this study will focus on the varying sensory experiences of making a lighting device for this ritual occasion, as well as the impact of artificial light on performers, attendants, and the objects to which light is offered within this sacred context. Contrary to modern preconceptions, textual, archaeological, and iconographic evidence from Egypt suggests that artificial light was not only employed to affect visual perception. Instead, lighting implements created a contrasting lightscape to that of natural light, which required different sensory engagement of ritual participants and witnesses with sacred objects.[4] As a result, artificial light is viewed here as a participant in these ritual performances.

As much as possible the experience of light in ancient Egypt is approached from an emic perspective in this article. This breaks away from the Western, ocular-centric view of light and moves toward a multisensory perspective of ancient Egyptian lighting. To investigate the function of lighting in the *sed*-festival, this article will incorporate extant archaeological, textual, and iconographic data with information gathered from reproducing and utilizing ancient lighting devices. Experimental archaeology is particularly beneficial in investigating ancient technologies and has been employed by Egyptologists to provide insights into the mummification process, pottery production, and furniture craftsmanship, among other subjects.[5] Experimental work is well-suited to a sensory examination of artificial lighting devices as it allows for personal experience of the construction

---

[3] Nancy Gonlin and April Nowell, eds., *Archaeology of the Night: Life after Dark in the Ancient World* (Boulder: University Press of Colorado, 2018); Marion Dowd and Robert Hensey, eds., *The Archaeology of Darkness* (Oxford: Oxbow Books, 2016).

[4] I adopt the definition of *lightscape* as the "changing landscapes of light and darkness." This term is introduced in Mikkel Bille and Tim Flohr Sørensen, "An Anthropology of Luminosity: The Agency of Light," *Journal of Material Culture* 12 (2007): 267.

[5] John Coles, *Experimental Archaeology* (London: Academic Press, 1979); Carolyn Graves-Brown, ed., *Egyptology in the Present: Experiential and Experimental Methods in Archaeology* (Swansea: Classical Press of Wales, 2015).

and utilization of the implements to be included in the analysis. A reflexive approach in this type of investigation is vital, as I cannot say how the ancient Egyptians structured a sensory hierarchy, if they even had one. Nevertheless, visual, haptic, olfactory, and aural senses all would have played a part in not only the experience of artificial lighting devices themselves, but in the perception of objects illuminated by them.

The primary function of an artificial light source is to illuminate a space lacking in or devoid of natural light. In ancient Egypt, the reason for this illumination varied from a practical application of allowing workers to see during construction of the underground tombs in the Valley of the Kings to serving as an offering for a sacred occasion in a temple or tomb chapel.[6] In all of these instances, artificial lighting not only facilitated the visual navigation of these built environments, but also impacted the viewer's perception of the space and objects within it. Scholars have previously discussed the role of light, both natural and artificial, as the means by which humans experience the world.[7] It is only recently, however, that anthropologists, archaeologists, and art historians have begun to examine how lighting, particularly artificial lighting, is used and manipulated within individual cultures to impact material culture.[8] Specifically, as Mikkel Bille and Tim Flohr discuss in their introduction of an "anthropology of luminosity," scholars are now beginning to examine "how light is *used* socially to illuminate places, people and things, and hence affect the experiences and materiality of these, in culturally specific ways."[9] This type of examination allows for a consideration of how light impacts and/or creates shadow, sheen, color, and movement when interacting with different spaces and surfaces.

---

[6] Jaroslav Černý, *The Valley of the Kings: Fragments d'un Manuscrit Inachevé*, Bibliothèque d'étude 61 (Cairo: Institut français d'archéologie orientale du Caire, 1973); Harold H. Nelson, "Certain Reliefs at Karnak and Medinet Habu and the Ritual of Amenophis I (Concluded)," *JNES* 8 (1949): 321–23.

[7] Maurice Merleau-Ponty, *Phenomenology of Perception*, trans. Donald A. Landes (London: Routledge, Taylor & Francis, 1964); Tim Ingold, "Stop, Look and Listen! Vision, Hearing and Human Movement," in *The Perception of the Environment: Essays on Livelihood, Dwelling and Skill* (London: Routledge, 2000), 243–87.

[8] Liz James, *Light and Colour in Byzantine Art*, Clarendon Studies in the History of Art 15 (Oxford: Clarendon, 1996); Bissera V. Pentcheva, *The Sensual Icon: Space, Ritual and the Senses in Byzantium* (University Park: The Pennsylvania State University Press, 2010); Claire Nesbitt, "Shaping the Sacred: Light and the Experience of Worship in Middle Byzantine Churches," *Byzantine and Modern Greek Studies* 36 (2012): 139–60; Bissera V. Pentcheva, "Phenomenology of Light: The Glitter of Salvation in Bessarion's Cross," *The Oxford Handbook of Light in Archaeology*, ed. Costas Papadopoulos and Holly Moyes (Oxford: Oxford University Press, 2017).

[9] Bille and Sørensen, "Anthropology of Luminosity," 265.

While not previously applied in Egyptology, this line of inquiry could provide new insights into ancient Egyptian material culture as Egyptologists rarely have the opportunity to appreciate these objects in their originally intended lighting environment. Tomb chapels and burial chambers in Egypt, for example, are lit with crude, fluorescent floor lamps that drown out color and illuminate a space in its entirety. This is far from the lighting conditions that the ancient Egyptians would have experienced. The light from lamps or hand-held lighting devices would have flickered, moved, and interacted with the carved and/or painted surfaces of the wall. They would have created shadows and varying levels of darkness, only illuminating small portions of a tomb at a time. Similarly, viewing a cult statue, a faience shabti, or a burnished ceramic bowl in a glass case under static LED lighting, as opposed to a soft flickering flame, creates a very different visual impression on the viewer. While ancient Egyptians would not have seen their world under the glow of an LED or a fluorescent lightbulb, they would have experienced different perceptions of an object under the glare of the bright Egyptian sun versus the dim, erratic glow of an artificial lighting device. It is this interplay of different lighting conditions that will be explored below.

MAKING LIGHT

Procuring the Raw Materials

The primary components of an Egyptian lighting implement are a wick and an illuminant. This is made clear from extant lighting devices, such as open-vessel lamps from an Eighteenth Dynasty cemetery at Qurnet Murai on the west bank of Luxor, which consisted of a twisted linen wick and a piece of animal fat placed inside a wheel-made, Nile-silt-ware ceramic bowl.[10] A different type of lighting device, which I have designated as the wick-on-stick type, is an alternative to a lamp and commonly appears in New Kingdom tomb and temple scenes.[11] Relevant to the purposes of this article, this type of lighting device is frequently shown being offered for ritual occasions both to deceased individuals in tomb chapels and to gods on temple walls. To my knowledge, only one physical example of this

---

[10] Bernard Bruyère, *Rapport Sur Les Fouilles de Deir El Medineh, 1934–1935; La Necropole de l'Est. (2e Pt)*, Fouilles de l'Institut Français d'archéologie Orientale 15 (Cairo: Institut français d'archéologie orientale, 1937), 99, figs. 50, 136; Guillemette Andreu and Christophe Barbotin, *Les Artistes de Pharaon: Deir El-Médineh et La Vallée Des Rois* (Paris: Réunion des musées nationaux, Brepols, 2002), 107–8.

[11] Meghan E. Strong, "Illuminating the Path of Darkness: Social and Sacred Power of Artificial Light in Pharaonic Period Egypt" (PhD diss., University of Cambridge, 2018), 60–66.

type of lighting implement survives in the archaeological record, uncovered during excavations in the tomb of Tutankhamun (JE62356, Egyptian Museum Cairo).[12] I will focus on the production and utilization of this type of lighting device for the remainder of the article as it is the one featured in offerings for the *sed*-festival.

To understand the sensory experience of making a wick-on-stick type implement, I chose to recreate my own, modeled after the piece from Tutankhamun's tomb. For my experiments, I utilized organic, untreated, roughly-woven linen for wicks in keeping with G. M. Eastwood's discussion of wicks excavated at the site of Amarna.[13] Her examination indicated that most wicks were made from reused linen, suggesting that strips could easily be torn off of old clothing or bed linen. This corroborates with ostracon Toronto A 11 from the New Kingdom village site of Deir el-Medina, which states that *ḥbs jss* ("old clothes") were used to make wicks for use in construction of the tombs in the Valley of the Kings.[14]

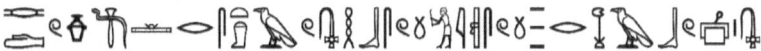

ᶜnḏ wꜣ ḏ r stꜣ ḥbs jss r ḥbs
fresh fat for lighting and old clothes for *ḥbs*
(Letter from Inheretkhau to Userkai, oToronto A 11, line 11[15])

The method of twisting a wick is straightforward and requires holding the length of linen at one end and then twisting the entire strand between the fingers and thumb. While holding the two ends, in order to prevent the piece from unraveling, the length of linen is folded in half, allowing the two halves to twist around each other. The twisting action is sufficient to hold the wick together with only the very ends slightly separating from each other. The end result is a wick that very closely resembles the hieroglyph

𓂂.

---

[12] Howard Carter's original notes for this object, as well as photos of the object *in situ* and after removal from the tomb can be accessed online in the Howard Carter Archives through The Griffith Institute: http://www.griffith.ox.ac.uk/discoveringTut/.

[13] Gillian M. Eastwood, "Preliminary Report on the Textiles," in *Amarna Reports 2*, ed. Barry J. Kemp et al., Occasional Publications; Egypt Exploration Society 2 (London: Egypt Exploration Society, 1985), 226–30.

[14] Černý, *Valley of the Kings*.

[15] Kenneth A. Kitchen, ed., *Ramesside Inscriptions, Series A, Translations III: Ramesses II, His Contemporaries* (Oxford: Blackwell, 2000), 30, 43,1–44,4.

Textual and archaeological evidence suggests that a variety of vegetable oils and animal fats could be used as illuminants by the ancient Egyptians.[16] Vegetable oils included castor, linseed, sesame, and olive, along with rendered animal fats from cattle, geese, and pigs. I will focus here on the production and use of beef tallow, which I rendered myself from organic, free-range cattle suet. I chose to render my own tallow as raw suet from cattle was easy to obtain and, according to a festival calendar at the site of Gebel Silsila, tallow or *sgnn* from cows was of the highest quality (*ḥȝtj*).[17]

There are two extant scenes that possibly represent the process of fat rendering: one from a subsidiary chamber (Room C) in the tomb of Ramesses III (KV11), which shows the processing of an ox, and the other from Room 17, located off the butcher's yard in Seti I's temple at Abydos.[18] To my knowledge, only the Abydos scene has been published.[19] In the scene, a scribe oversees a group of workmen or priests who chop up pieces of fat (*ʿḏ*), place them over a flame in a large pot, and then strain the fat through twisted fabric into a vat for collection. Because there is negligible accompanying text to provide any more detail to the scene, I corroborated this ancient evidence with discussion of fat rendering techniques from Salima Ikram, Margaret Serpico, and blog posts for home rendering.[20] The modern process of rendering closely parallels the Abydos temple

---

[16] Basma Koura, *Die "7-heiligen Öle" und andere Öl- und Fettnamen: Eine lexikographische Untersuchung zu den Bezeichnungen von Ölen, Fetten und Salben bei den alten Ägyptern von der Frühzeit bis zum Anfang der Ptolemäerzeit (von 3000 v. Chr.–ca. 305 v. Chr.)*, Aegyptiaca Monasteriensia 2 (Aachen: Shaker Verlag, 1999); Margaret Serpico and Raymond White, "Oil, Fat and Wax," in *Ancient Egyptian Materials and Technology*, ed. Paul T. Nicholson and Ian Shaw (Cambridge: Cambridge University Press, 2000), 390–429; M. S. Copley et al., "Gas Chromatographic, Mass Spectrometric and Stable Carbon Isotopic Investigations of Organic Residues of Plant Oils and Animal Fats Employed as Illuminants in Archaeological Lamps from Egypt," *The Analyst* 130 (2005): 860–71; Daniel Zohary, Maria Hopf, and Ehud Weiss, *Domestication of Plants in the Old World: The Origin and Spread of Domesticated Plants in Southwest Asia, Europe, and the Mediterranean Basin*, 4th ed. (Oxford: Oxford University Press, 2012).

[17] Carl Richard Lepsius, *Denkmäler aus Aegypten und Aethiopien* (Berlin: Nicolaische Buchhandlung, 1849), Abth. III, Bl. 200d.

[18] Salima Ikram, *Choice Cuts: Meat Production in Ancient Egypt*, OLA 69 (Leuven: Peeters, 1995), 177–79. Ikram also suggests that Middle Kingdom tomb models, such as the butchering scene of Meketre, may depict fat rendering by the inclusion of a pot filled with mixed red and white contents in the context of animal butchery (179).

[19] Édouard Naville, *Détails relevés dans les ruines de quelques temples égyptiens: 1re partie: Abydos, 2e partie: Behbeit-el-Hagher, Appendix: Samanoud* (Paris: Geuthner, 1930), 9.

[20] Ikram, *Choice Cuts*, 176. Serpico and White, "Oil, Fat and Wax," 408–9. The most thorough description of beef tallow production that I found was: http://www.theprairiehomestead.com/2012/02/how-to-render-beef-tallow.html.

scene and indicates that the first crucial step in the process is chopping the suet into very small cubes. This is suggested by piles of fat in front of the two Abydene priests, who appear to be vigorously hacking at it with knives. The online blog post I consulted states that keeping the fat cold aides in this process as it prevents the fat from melting and sliding all over the chopping board. As the ancient Egyptians would have had no means of refrigeration to chill the fat, I allowed my suet to come to room temperature before cutting it into cubes.

The suet became increasingly hard to chop as the radiant heat from my hands began to melt the fat. After a couple close calls of cutting off my thumb, I did resort to keeping the suet in the refrigerator and only removing small portions at a time that could be cubed quickly. After cubing all the suet and placing it in a cast-iron pot, I rendered it slowly over a low flame. After approximately fifteen minutes, a greasy odor began to permeate the kitchen. Within half an hour the smell was so intense that I had to close the kitchen door and open a window in an attempt to keep the meaty aroma from permeating the entire house. In total 2 kg of fat took approximately an hour and fifteen minutes to render, at which point the small burnt remaining pieces of tissue could be strained away. After allowing the rendered fat to cool for a few minutes, I poured it into glass jars for storage. It quite quickly set into a slightly viscous, pale yellow tallow.

Perceiving Fabric and Fat

The production of a wick from a strip of linen was quite a straight-forward process and could be easily understood from observing extant examples. After a few practice attempts, it was quite a mindless task and something committed to kinaesthetic or muscle memory. The process was dominated by haptic perception of the woven linen between the fingertips and the tautness in the twist of the fabric. As Deir el-Medina ostracon Toronto A 11 indicates, the use of old clothes for wicks would suggest that the feel of the linen was a familiar texture. However, textual evidence from the Middle Kingdom tomb contracts of Hepdjefa suggests that wicks made for offerings or for festival occasions were made from finer, high-quality fabrics.[21] Specifically, in Contract 5 it is stipulated that individuals should go to the temple and obtain wicks for lighting from the *šnḏty* (the "keeper of the

---

[21] Francis Llewellyn Griffith, *The Inscriptions of Siût and Dêr Rîfeh* (London: Trübner, 1889); George A. Reisner, "The Tomb of Hepzefa, Nomarch of Siût," *Journal of Egyptian Archaeology* 5 (1918): 79–98; Jochem Kahl, *Ancient Asyut: The First Synthesis after Three Hundred Years of Research*, The Asyut Project 1 (Wiesbaden: Harrassowitz Verlag, 2007); Kahl, *Ornamente in Bewegung: Die Deckendekoration Der Grossen Querhalle Im Grab von Djefai-Hapi I. in Assiut*, The Asyut Project 6 (Wiesbaden: Harrassowitz Verlag, 2016).

wardrobe").²² This individual was likely in charge of all the fabrics used in the temple, which were presumably of high-quality since they would be used to clothe the statue of the god, among other ritual functions. The maker(s) of wicks for ritual offerings, such as for the *sed*-festival, may have then perceived them to be special by the fine texture of the linen, which would have contrasted in feel to more utilitarian textiles. Additionally, the term used for "wick," $ḥ$ / $ḥ^ct$, seems to relate to twisting or braiding. This is explicitly stated in a line of accompanying text to a scene of light offering from the temple of Karnak, which describes the act of

$sḫt\ ḥ^ct$ ("twisting the wick")²³

The term may also relate to the visual appearance of these objects, which is further complemented by the haptic sensation of twisting the fabric between one's fingers, as well as twisting the fabric around itself in order to produce a wick.

The production of an animal fat illuminant, such as beef tallow, is much more of a multisensory experience, in addition to being labor intensive. The basic act of chopping animal fat from a logistical sense must have been rather complicated in the Egyptian heat. As the fat warmed from the atmospheric temperature and the body heat of the person chopping it, the suet would have become increasingly slippery. This would not only have made the fat itself more difficult to cut, but would have coated the hands of the worker making it difficult and dangerous to grasp the knife needed for the task. A pungent, meaty aroma also would have emanated from the raw fat as it warmed and melted. From the depiction in Seti's temple at Abydos, as well as Middle Kingdom tomb models, such as the model of a slaughterhouse from the tomb of Meketre (20.3.10, Metropolitan Museum of Art), it appears that the rendering process was done outside or in an unroofed building.²⁴ This certainly would have allowed the oily smell to dissipate, although the odor would likely have set into the kilts of the workers charged with overseeing the rendering. The scent produced from rendering fat in my own home lingered for about a week. As the fat heated, it sizzled and spit, which meant that the cooking surface surrounding the pot was coated in a thin layer of grease by the end of the rendering process. The rendering suet also needed to be stirred intermittently. This process required that I come in more direct contact with the bubbling fat, hearing the constant sizzle, breathing in the thick steam, and feeling the sting of the hot fat splattering my hands. Those who participated in fat rendering on a regular basis may very well have carried the scent, and perhaps the scars from burning, home with them. As previously stated, beef tallow was considered

---

[22] Griffith, *Inscriptions of Siût and Dêr Rîfeh*, plate 7, line 296.

[23] Nelson, "Certain Reliefs at Karnak and Medinet Habu," 325.

[24] Adela Oppenheim et al., *Ancient Egypt Transformed: The Middle Kingdom* (New York: Metropolitan Museum of Art, 2015), cat. 143.

to be a high-quality product and so the presence of a greasy, meaty cologne may have served as an olfactory reminder of an individual's association with high commodity items and perhaps afforded them a higher status in the community. The Egyptians might have also found the scent of rendered animal fat quite pleasing, correlating it to the aroma of grilled meats, which were offered and consumed on festival occasions and for funerary banquets.

Assembling a Lighting Device

The production of a wick-on-stick type lighting device was fairly time consuming, primarily because it involved several steps for proper assembly. I used two different types of reeds for my experiments based on availability. Initial tests utilized lengths of bamboo acquired from a local garden supply store, which are in the same family as common reeds and are the same thickness as the reed visible on the Tutankahmun lighting implement. Additional experiments utilized reeds procured from a Nile Delta farm in Egypt.[25] Based on dimensions of the Tutankhamun lighting device, I made most wicks approximately 38 cm in length. A 38 cm wick required approximately 76 cm of linen to produce, since the length of textile needed to be folded in half. The longer the completed wick, the longer the original strip of linen. Due to the length of material that needed to be twisted, producing a wick for a wick-on-stick device was more complicated and unwieldy than a lamp wick. Quite frequently I, or other experiment participants, lost hold of one end of the fabric while twisting, which resulted in the linen unraveling and necessitating a fresh start. As with the twisting of lamp wicks, however, I am sure this would be committed to kinaesthetic memory with practice.

Once the wick was assembled, it needed to be attached to a reed with an additional strip of linen. Again, using the Tutankahmun lighting device as an example, I placed the open end of the wick at the top of the stick and secured it to the reed by wrapping the extra strip of linen tightly around them both. It was not necessary to tie a knot to hold the wick in place as long as the additional strip of linen was wound tight enough. The remainder of the linen strip was then wound around the reed, leaving a few centimeters gap between each turn. The final wick-on-stick devices were not as elegant in appearance as Tutankhamun's piece, but they were a close approximation (fig. 1).

After the wick was attached to the reed a selected illuminant needed to be applied. For vegetable oils, it was easiest to submerge the entire lighting implement into a glass or jar of the illuminant. This allowed the wick to absorb the maximum amount of oil. Pouring the oil over the device also worked but took much longer for the wick to become saturated. This method also necessitated a

---

[25] My thanks to Dr. Mennat Allah el-Dorry for procuring the reeds from her family farm in Egypt and to Dr. Giulio Lucarini for transporting them from Cairo to Cambridge.

receptacle to be placed underneath the device in order to avoid wasting oil. Animal fats were fairly time-consuming to apply. However, because the fat had to be applied by hand it allowed the maker of the device to ensure that every inch of the fabric and reed were coated in illuminant. For some wick-on-stick lighting experiments, I applied the illuminant and then immediately lit the devices, while for other experiments I stored the implements for twenty-four to forty-eight hours and then lit them.[26] Storage did not make any difference in their ability to burn, nor did the device dry out over this period of time.

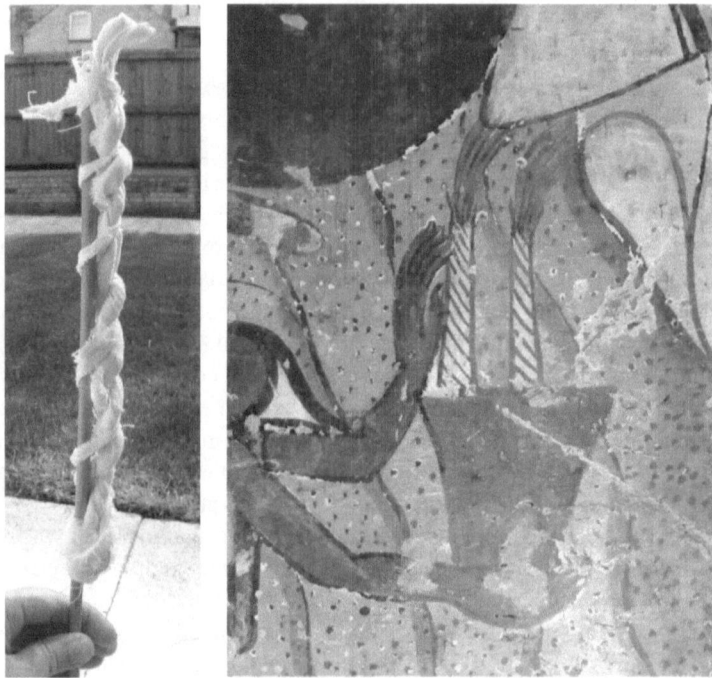

Fig. 1 (left). Example of recreated wick-on-stick device used in experiments. Photograph by author.

Fig. 2 (right). Detail of twists painted onto depiction of wicks in an offering scene from the tomb of Amunnakht (TT218); Luxor, west bank, Deir el-Medina. Photograph by Author.

---

[26] Since conducting my experiments in the spring and summer of 2016, I have learned that fabric soaked in linseed oil and left to sit has the capability to spontaneously combust. I would therefore strongly discourage other scholars from soaking wicks in linseed oil and storing them for future use.

Feeling Light

The making of wick-on-stick implements impacts quite heavily on haptic sensation. This includes the feel of the textile used for the wick, as well as the contrasting smooth almost silky texture of the reed to which it is attached. It is also important to note the time spent procuring materials, as well as manipulating wick and illuminant with one's hands in order to create a lighting device. The reeds must be procured, the wick must be made to an appropriate length, and then the two are tightly lashed together with additional linen. This may not take more than a few minutes with a fair amount of practice, but it requires both manual dexterity and a tactile experience with two differing textures. The application of illuminant, particularly animal fat, also adds to the haptic perception of the object. The easiest mode of application is to scoop the fat out of the jar with one's fingers and then rub the tallow into the wick and onto the reed. To ensure the illuminant is thoroughly worked into the wick, several applications of tallow are required. As the tallow warms, the applicant's hands also become thoroughly coated in fat, which impart a lingering mild greasy smell and act as an excellent moisturizer. The silky, greasy texture of the fat, as well as the subsequent suppleness of the light maker's hands, was likely quite different from the majority of tactile sensations experienced by ancient Egyptians. The heat and sun would sap moisture from the skin, while building materials such as sand, mudbrick, and stone were rough and jagged. Textures in the natural landscape, such as palm trees, animal hair, and other plants and grasses, would also all share a coarse, fibrous quality. Making a wick-on-stick lighting device would therefore create a completely different sensory experience, separating it from textures in the everyday vernacular and perhaps lending to the perceived importance of the item.

The investment of time and craftsmanship in wick-on-stick lighting implements also seems appropriate for an item used in ritual offerings. Perhaps this is one reason, in addition to their portability, why they are commonly depicted in sacred celebrations. The action of twisting fabric, as with the manufacture of lamp wicks, also plays a significant role in constructing wick-on-stick devices. An added layer of twisting or wrapping is also needed to attach the wick to the reed in order to complete the piece. The manual twisting of the fabric seems to have been a significant detail as it is not only referenced in terminology, it is consistently carved and/or painted onto representations of wick-on-stick devices (fig. 2).

Hearing Fat and Smelling Oil

Burning the wick-on-stick implements to test the illuminants described above made it apparent that not all potential Pharaonic period fats and oils produced the same amount or quality of light, nor were they all equally pleasant to burn. They also produced very different sensory experiences. Castor oil, for example, would have been extremely disagreeable in a confined space. The smell, which was akin to burning tires, accompanied by thick, black smoke would have likely produced coughing, a stinging throat and burning eyes to individuals in the same room. Linseed oil, which produced the same amount of smoke as castor, had an unexpected scent of grilled or charred meat, which may have been an appealing quality to an ancient Egyptian. Grilled meat and fowl in particular are commonly depicted and recorded as desirable offerings to the gods and the deceased. Perhaps burning a lamp or wick-on-stick device coated in linseed oil would mimic this delectable aroma. If using a lighting device in an enclosed space, it seems likely that animal fats would be preferred as they produced minimal to no smoke or scent.[27] This in fact corroborates textual evidence from Deir el-Medina that *sgnn*, rendered animal tallow, or *ᶜḏ wḏȝ*, fresh fat, were requested illuminants for artificial lighting devices used in the construction of the tombs in the Valley of the Kings.[28]

In addition to smoke or scent, burning wick-on-stick devices would also emit a hissing sound at irregular intervals. The spitting or hissing sound produced by these implements is particularly interesting. Putting this sound in context, however, requires an understanding that wick-on-stick devices are most commonly labeled as *tkȝ* in ritual offering scenes. Based on extant textual evidence, *tkȝ* seems to be a potent sacred artificial light source that can be wielded by snake goddesses as a protective flame. Several mentions of goddesses using *tkȝ* or *tkȝw* (plural) are made in the Book of Overthrowing Apep, including:

𓅓𓏤𓏏𓇋𓇋𓊃𓃀𓇋𓇋𓏏𓁐 𓁷𓏤 𓏏𓎡𓏛

ȝsbyt ḥry tk
the goddess, Asbet, who presides over the *tkȝw* (line 22, 22)[29]

The flame of the *tkȝ* itself is also associated with fire spit from the mouth of the *uraeus*, the reared cobra frequently depicted on the brow of the king.

---

[27] Lighting experiments in Altamira cave achieved similar results when burning fat obtained from a cow tibia in a stone, open-vessel oil lamp Matilde Múzquiz Pérez-Seoane et al., *The Cave of Altamira* (New York: Abrams, 1999).

[28] Černý, *Valley of the Kings*, 45.

[29] Raymond O. Faulkner, *The Papyrus Bremner-Rhind (British Museum No. 10188)*, Bibliotheca Aegyptiaca 3 (Bruxelles: Édition de la Fondation égyptologique Reine Élisabeth, 1933), 45.

bš ḥr-tp=f tk₃ r wptw si₃ ᶜwt wnm=s ḥᶜw
His uraeus spits tk₃ on foreheads, she consumes bodies and devours limbs.[30]

It is possible that the hissing, spitting sound from *tk₃* in wick-on-stick form reinforced this association with snakes and/or snake goddesses. This aural connection between light offerings and the protective power of snakes may have also strengthened the perception that light was an appropriate gift to provide on the occasion of the *sed*-festival, which commemorated the renewal of kingship.

ILLUMINATING THE THRONES FOR THE *SED*-FESTIVAL

After a wick-on-stick device was made, it could have been used in a variety of rituals, including funerals, New Year's eve and New Year's day celebrations, and for daily offerings to the deceased or the gods.[31] A relatively rare ritual occasion on which artificial light was offered was during the *sed*-festival or *heb sed*. This ritual, attested as early as the First Dynasty (ca. 3000 BCE), was a celebration of kingship intended to renew the physical and spiritual energy of the king after thirty years of rule.[32] Various accounts of *sed*-festivals survive, but some of the most detailed date to the reign of Amenhotep III.[33] There is, however, only one register of scenes in the temple of Soleb that speaks directly to the role of artificial light in the *sed*-festival.[34] The scenes are greatly damaged resulting in significant loss to the text and imagery, in addition to a reduction in the information that can be

---

[30] Samuel Birch, *Inscriptions in the Hieratic and Demotic Character, from the Collections of the British Museum* (London: Woodfall & Kinder, 1868), XXIX.

[31] Nelson, "Certain Reliefs at Karnak and Medinet Habu"; Adolphe Gutbub, "Un Emprunt Aux Textes Des Pyramides Dans l'hymne à Hathor, Dame de l'ivresse," in *Mélanges Maspero I—Orient Ancien*, vol. 4, MIFAO 66 (Cairo: Institut français d'archéologie orientale, 1961), 31–72; Fayza Haikal, "Preliminary Studies on the Tomb of Thay in Thebes: The Hymn to the Light," in *Melanges Gamal Eddin Mokhtar*, ed. Paule Posener-Kriéger, vol. 1, Bibliothèque d'étude 97 (Cairo: Institut français d'archéologie orientale du Caire, 1985), 361–74; Daniela C. Luft, *Das Anzünden der Fackel: Untersuchungen zu Spruch 137 des Totenbuches* (Wiesbaden: Otto Harrassowitz, 2009); Meghan E. Strong, "A Great Secret of the West: Transformative Aspects of Artificial Light in Dynastic Egypt," in *Archaeology of the Night*, ed. Nancy Gonlin and April Nowell (Boulder: University Press of Colorado, 2018), 249–64; Strong, "Illuminating the Path of Darkness," 135–93.

[32] Eric Uphill, "The Egyptian Sed-Festival Rites," *JNES* 24 (1965): 365–83.

[33] David B. O'Connor and Eric H. Cline, eds., *Amenhotep III: Perspectives on His Reign* (Ann Arbor: University of Michigan Press, 1998); Arielle P. Kozloff, *Amenhotep III: Egypt's Radiant Pharaoh* (Cambridge: Cambridge University Press, 2012).

[34] John A. Wilson, "Illuminating the Thrones at the Egyptian Jubilee," *JAOS* 56 (1936): 293–96; Michela Schiff Giorgini, *Soleb III: Le Temple Description* (Cairo: Institut français d'archéologie orientale du Caire, 2002), 218–22; Schiff Giorgini, *Soleb V: Le Temple Bas-Reliefs et Inscriptions* (Cairo: Institut français d'archéologie orientale, 1998), pl. 33–38.

gleaned from such an isolated context. Nevertheless, valuable data on the offering of light can still be surmised. What is clear is that the visual focal point of the register is the shrine that contains the two thrones, symbol of the *heb sed* and representative of the king's rule over Upper and Lower Egypt.[35] Specifically, the left side of the kiosk, which is on the northern part of the wall, contains the throne of Lower Egypt indicated by four papyriform columns that support a cavetto cornice topped with a row of *uraei*. The right side of the kiosk, on the southern portion of the wall, contains the throne of Upper Egypt and is decorated with four lotiform columns. From the traces of decoration still visible on the wall, it appears that the entire container was decorated with emblems of kingship including figures wearing the crowns of Upper and Lower Egypt, Horus and Seth, the "mighty bull," another figure carrying the crook and flail, and two rows of solar-crowned *uraei*. The carving of the right side of the shrine, which is better preserved, indicates that the thrones are placed on a raised dais and carry an enthroned figure who holds a scepter of some kind in his hand. This may indicate that the thrones each bore a figure of the king wrapped tightly in the *heb sed*-cloak wearing the crowns of Upper and Lower Egypt in their respective sides of the shrine. This harkens back to some of the earliest depictions of the *sed*-festival such as the ebony label of Den (EA32650, British Museum) and the Narmer macehead (E. 3631, Ashmolean Museum).[36]

Appropriately, the depictions on either side of the central shrine are mirror images of each other, in order that the same rite may be performed before both thrones. The primary ritual performer is Amenhotep III who, accompanied by Queen Tiye, presents a very tall wick-on-stick type lighting implement, referred to as a *tkꜣ* in the surrounding text, before the open doors of the kiosk containing the thrones.[37] Between the king and the kiosk is a mound-shaped container labeled as a *sḥ n mrḥt štt* (a "booth of secret oils"), which was likely provided in order to *ḥft tnṯꜣt* ("fill the kiosk with light").[38] Presumably then, these oils are meant to serve as illuminants for the *tkꜣ*.

While the focal point of the scene is the shrine and thrones, the emphasis of the accompanying text is on the light source, the *tkꜣ*. The text follows a formulaic

---

[35] Schiff Giorgini, *Soleb V*, pl. 36.

[36] Nigel Strudwick, *Masterpieces of Ancient Egypt* (London: British Museum Press, 2006), 38–39; John Baines, "Origins of Egyptian Kingship," in *Ancient Egyptian Kingship*, ed. David O'Connor and David P. Silverman (Leiden: Brill, 1995), 118–19, 3.8.

[37] Schiff Giorgini, *Soleb V*, pl. 35, 37.

[38] Schiff Giorgini, *Soleb III*, 220–21; Schiff Giorgini, *Soleb V*, pl. 35. This phrase was translated by Wilson as "illuminate the thrones"; however, I believe "fill the shrine with light" is a more accurate translation as *tnṯꜣt* refers to the container that holds the thrones, not the thrones themselves. For a discussion of this see Strong, "Illuminating the Path of Darkness," 186–89.

pattern by requesting that one individual brings a flame (*bs*) in order to give the fire (*st*) of the *tkꜣ* to another individual so that they might fill the kiosk with light. The first person to do this is, of course, the king and so the rite begins as the lector priest, Nebermeretef, says:

sm jn bs dw n nswt nswt šsp st m tkꜣ ḥft [*tnt ꜥt*]
O sem-priest (Mery), bring a flame and give (it) to the king. O King, take the fire of the *tkꜣ* (for) filling the shrine with light. (column 2)[39]

This pattern continues so that a lector priest, the "guardian of the place" and the "guardian of the *wsḫt*," along with others whose titles are lost, are asked to bring a flame and give it to a *sem*-priest, the "Great One of Upper Egypt," the chief of magicians, and the "god's mother" so that they may illuminate the throne.[40] The inscription is only preserved on the southern portion of the wall, but presumably the inscription on the northern side would have listed individuals from Lower Egypt. This inscription, though fragmentary, appears to establish that only certain individuals may offer the light before the thrones. Significantly, the first part of the invocation refers to the light source as *bs*, a flame. Only in the second half of the phrase, when it is received by an individual is it called a *tkꜣ*. As mentioned previously, *tkꜣ* is a term used to refer to a light source offered in a ritual context, or in relation to a powerful flame issued from a *uraeus* or snake goddess. The term *bs*, on the other hand, I have not found used in texts referencing light offerings, nor is it recorded in any light offering scenes that I have identified. It is then possible that *bs*, in this context, is used to create a distinction between a less potent light source that is brought to the ritual performers, and a *tkꜣ* that is presented before the thrones. This hierarchy of power is also suggested by the individuals who bring the light source and those who ultimately present it. Lower ranking priests, as well as guardians of the place and the *wsḫt*, bring the *bs*, while the "Great One of Upper Egypt," the chief of magicians and the "god's mother," perhaps referring to the mother of Amenhotep III or her representative, take the "fire of the *tkꜣ*" and present it as an offering.

I would suggest that those who present the *tkꜣ* before the thrones are considered to be more powerful and/or important because of the effect that the light had on the thrones. The illumination of a throne in an enclosed shrine by a flickering light source would have created a luminous, glimmering effect. The thrones representing Upper and Lower Egypt likely would have been covered in sheets of

---

[39] Schiff Giorgini, *Soleb V*, pl. 37.
[40] Wilson, "Illuminating the Thrones at the Egyptian Jubilee," 295; Schiff Giorgini, *Soleb III*, 220.

metal, semi-precious stones, and glass-like inlays, similar to the golden throne of Tutankhamun (JE62028, Egyptian Museum, Cairo).[41] These would have glistened under the warm glow of artificial light, with carved detail and/or raised relief creating variations in shadow and texture. The light also would have moved and played off the walls of the shrine, perhaps creating even more of a coruscating effect if the shrine itself was covered in metal and glassy inlaid decoration. Additionally, the presentation of the light required the ritual performer to be within close proximity to the object to which light is presented. In this case, it appears that an individual would step up just in front of the opened doors of the shrine, as the depiction of Amenhotep III indicates. This may have involved a priest or other high-ranking official stepping out of the rows of ritual attendants and individually walking forward to "fill the shrine with light." This would have separated them out as individuals worthy of offering *tk3*, in addition to allowing other attendants to witness the effect that their light had on the throne and setting. Additionally, those offering *tk3* may have applied one or a selection of the illuminants from the "booth of secret oils" to their light, exposing them to the silky, greasy texture of the oil and any perfume that may have been added to them. As the offering bearers stepped back into the crowd, they would have carried this scent with them—a lingering reminder to those near them that they were selected to offer light. Viewed within the larger context of the *sed*-festival, those individuals who presented light before the thrones of Upper and Lower Egypt may have been regarded as taking part in the rejuvenation of the king and the legitimacy of his rule. This was particularly relevant for the *heb sed* depicted at Soleb as it marked Amenhotep III's first jubilee celebration, which commemorated a new thirty-year cycle of kingship, in addition to his transition to a deified form of the sun god, Ra.[42]

It seems likely that one purpose of offering light during the *sed*-festival was that it caused a transition, or alteration, in perception of the objects illuminated by an artificial lighting device. This ritual was a multisensory experience that made the most of contrasts. This included contrasting light conditions between the enclosed darkness of a shrine versus the glitter of thrones illuminated by a flickering flame. Additionally, the differing lighting environments would not only have impacted the visual perception of an object, but also caused ritual performers and attendants to interact with objects in a different way, thus impacting other senses. The light offering would likely have given off some amount of heat, but it would have been an isolated fleeting warmth different from the heat of the sun or the

---

[41] Details available online under "throne (ceremonial chair)" Carter No. 91: http://www.griffith.ox.ac.uk/discoveringTut/

[42] W. Raymond Johnson, "Amenhotep III and Amarna: Some New Considerations," *The Journal of Egyptian Archaeology* 82 (1996): 66; O'Connor and Cline, *Amenhotep III*; Kozloff, *Amenhotep III*, 120–22, 182–96.

coolness of an enclosed temple courtyard. The application of illuminants, as indicated in the relief at Soleb, would have put the offering bearer in contact with the smooth, greasy texture of various fats and oils, as well as any added perfumes. In the scene, light is presented directly in front of the shrine containing the thrones, requiring the offering bearer to be in close proximity to the offering recipient. This would ensure that the full effect of the flickering light would be visible across the surface of the object and that the ritual performer would be able to witness this effect. This may also have put the offering bearer much closer to a royal throne than they had ever been before, allowing them to pick out details in texture, carving, or color that may not be visible from a distance. The effect of a lighting device on thrones must have been particularly arresting, highlighting the glint of metal or the shimmer of a semi-precious stone. The enclosure of these objects within a gilded shrine would only have enhanced the interplay of light, dark, glitter and shadow. This interpretation supports my theory that lighting was an active agent in light offering rituals, not a passive source of illumination. Significantly, the transformative effect of light offerings impacted many senses in the ritual performer and attendants. This multisensory effect enhanced the perceived power of lighting implements, as well as the social status of the individual(s) worthy of using and presenting light offerings.

Conclusions

The material presented in this article suggests that artificial lighting in ancient Egypt produced a multisensory experience that extended from the procurement of the raw materials to the construction of the device through the burning of the light itself. I cannot comment on what ancient Egyptian senses would have been impacted the most by artificial lighting. What is crucial to consider is that there are visual, haptic, olfactory, and aural sensations created by artificial lighting that are distinct, particularly when viewed in comparison to natural lighting or complete darkness. While sunlight in Egypt is glaring, hot, flattening, and static, artificial lighting produces a warm glow, which is erratic and soft. Artificial light also draws one closer to an object or surface due to its minimal amount of light. The flame of an artificial light source picks out carved details, creates a sense of movement, and illuminates only small portions of a surface at a time, casting portions of a room or object into deep shadow while highlighting others. The required proximity between the viewer and the flame also exposes the viewer to the heat of the flame, the smell of the illuminant, and the texture of the illuminated surface. Significantly, conclusions drawn about the sensory experience of artificial lighting are supported by textual evidence and religious ideology, providing a richer understanding of ancient Egyptian culture. As discussed, the act of twisting linen for wicks, for example, may be related to the term h / $h^{c}t$ (a "twisted/braided thing"), which is also consistently depicted in images of wick-on-stick lighting devices. Similarly, it is also possible that the greasy, beefy smell of rendered tallow added to the prestige of an individual in charge of producing illuminant or that the hissing sound from a burning wick-on-stick implement would support the correlation between the flame of a *tk₃* and divine snake goddesses. All of this evidence suggests that sensory archaeology, and experimental archaeology, can add to and enhance Egyptological scholarship. Additionally, viewing artificial light as an active agent can provide exciting avenues for future research in material culture, ritual studies, and consideration of the role of luminosity in ancient Egypt.

BIBLIOGRAPHY

Andreu, Guillemette, and Christophe Barbotin. *Les Artistes de Pharaon: Deir El-Médineh et La Vallée Des Rois.* Paris: Réunion des musées nationaux, Brepols, 2002.

Baines, John. "Origins of Egyptian Kingship." Pages 95–156 in *Ancient Egyptian Kingship*. Edited by David O'Connor and David P. Silverman. Leiden: Brill, 1995.

Bennie, Jonathan, Thomas W. Davies, David Cruse, and Kevin J. Gaston. "Ecological Effects of Artificial Light at Night on Wild Plants." *Journal of Ecology* 104 (2016): 611–20.

Bille, Mikkel, and Tim Flohr Sørensen. "An Anthropology of Luminosity: The Agency of Light." *Journal of Material Culture* 12 (2007): 263–84.

Birch, Samuel. *Inscriptions in the Hieratic and Demotic Character, from the Collections of the British Museum*. London: Woodfall & Kinder, 1868.

Bogard, Paul. *The End of Night: Searching for Natural Darkness in an Age of Artificial Light*. London: Fourth Estate, 2014.

Brox, Jane. *Brilliant: The Evolution of Artificial Light*. London: Souvenir, 2011.

Bruyère, Bernard. *Rapport Sur Les Fouilles de Deir El Medineh, 1934–1935; La Necropole de l'Est. (2e Pt)*. Fouilles de l'Institut Français d'archéologie Orientale 15. Cairo: Institut français d'archéologie orientale, 1937.

Černý, Jaroslav. *The Valley of the Kings: Fragments d'un Manuscrit Inachevé*. Bibliothèque d'étude 61. Cairo: Institut français d'archéologie orientale du Caire, 1973.

Cho, Yongmin, Seung-Hun Ryu, Byeo Ri Lee, Kyung Hee Kim, Eunil Lee, and Jaewook Choi. "Effects of Artificial Light at Night on Human Health: A Literature Review of Observational and Experimental Studies Applied to Exposure Assessment." *Chronobiology International* 32 (2015): 1294–1310.

Coles, John. *Experimental Archaeology*. London: Academic Press, 1979.

Copley, M. S., H. A. Bland, P. Rose, M. Horton, R. P. Evershed. "Gas Chromatographic, Mass Spectrometric and Stable Carbon Isotopic Investigations of Organic Residues of Plant Oils and Animal Fats Employed as Illuminants in Archaeological Lamps from Egypt." *The Analyst* 130 (2005): 860–71.

Dowd, Marion, and Robert Hensey, eds. *The Archaeology of Darkness*. Oxford: Oxbow Books, 2016.

Eastwood, Gillian M. "Preliminary Report on the Textiles." Pages 226–30 in *Amarna Reports 2*. Edited by Barry J. Kemp et al. Occasional Publications; Egypt Exploration Society 2. London: Egypt Exploration Society, 1985.

Falchi, Fabio, Pierantonio Cinzano, Dan Duriscoe, Christopher C. M. Kyba, Christopher D. Elvidge, Kimberly Baugh, Boris A. Portnov, Nataliya A. Rybnikova, and Riccardo Furgoni. "The New World Atlas of Artificial Night Sky Brightness." *Science Advances* 2 (2016): doi:10.1126/sciadv.1600377.

Faulkner, Raymond O. *The Papyrus Bremner-Rhind (British Museum No. 10188)*. Bibliotheca Aegyptiaca 3. Bruxelles: Édition de la Fondation égyptologique Reine Élisabeth, 1933.

Gonlin, Nancy, and April Nowell, eds. *Archaeology of the Night: Life after Dark in the Ancient World*. Boulder: University Press of Colorado, 2018.

Graves-Brown, Carolyn, ed. *Egyptology in the Present: Experiential and Experimental Methods in Archaeology*. Swansea: Classical Press of Wales, 2015.

Griffith, Francis Llewellyn. *The Inscriptions of Siût and Dêr Rîfeh*. London: Trübner, 1889.

Gutbub, Adolphe. "Un Emprunt Aux Textes Des Pyramides Dans l'hymne à Hathor, Dame de l'ivresse." Pages 31–72 in *Mélanges Maspero I—Orient Ancien*. Vol. 4. MIFAO 66. Cairo: Institut français d'archéologie orientale, 1961.

Haikal, Fayza. "Preliminary Studies on the Tomb of Thay in Thebes: The Hymn to the Light." Pages 361–74 in *Melanges Gamal Eddin Mokhtar*. Edited by Paule Posener-Kriéger. Vol. 1. Bibliothèque d'étude 97. Cairo: Institut français d'archéologie orientale du Caire, 1985.

Ikram, Salima, *Choice Cuts: Meat Production in Ancient Egypt*. OLA 69. Leuven: Peeters, 1995.

Ingold, Tim. "Stop, Look and Listen! Vision, Hearing and Human Movement." Pages 243–87 in *The Perception of the Environment: Essays on Livelihood, Dwelling and Skill*. London: Routledge, 2000.

James, Liz. *Light and Colour in Byzantine Art*. Clarendon Studies in the History of Art 15. Oxford: Clarendon, 1996.

Johnson, W. Raymond. "Amenhotep III and Amarna: Some New Considerations." *The Journal of Egyptian Archaeology* 82 (1996): 65–82.

Kahl, Jochem. *Ancient Asyut: The First Synthesis after Three Hundred Years of Research*. The Asyut Project 1. Wiesbaden: Harrassowitz Verlag, 2007.

———. *Ornamente in Bewegung: Die Deckendekoration Der Grossen Querhalle Im Grab von Djefai-Hapi I. in Assiut*. The Asyut Project 6. Wiesbaden: Harrassowitz Verlag, 2016.

Kitchen, Kenneth A., ed. *Ramesside Inscriptions, Series A, Translations III: Ramesses II, His Contemporaries*. Oxford: Blackwell, 2000.

Koura, Basma. *Die "7-heiligen Öle" und andere Öl- und Fettnamen: Eine lexikographische Untersuchung zu den Bezeichnungen von Ölen, Fetten und Salben bei den alten Ägyptern von der Frühzeit bis zum Anfang der Ptolemäerzeit (von 3000 v. Chr.–ca. 305 v. Chr.)*. Aegyptiaca Monasteriensia 2. Aachen: Shaker Verlag, 1999.

Kozloff, Arielle P. *Amenhotep III: Egypt's Radiant Pharaoh*. Cambridge: Cambridge University Press, 2012.

Lepsius, Carl Richard. *Denkmäler aus Aegypten und Aethiopien*. Berlin: Nicolaische Buchhandlung, 1849.

O'Dea, William Thomas. *The Social History of Lighting*. London: Routledge & Paul, 1958.

Luft, Daniela C. *Das Anzünden der Fackel: Untersuchungen zu Spruch 137 des Totenbuches*. Wiesbaden: Otto Harrassowitz, 2009.

Merleau-Ponty, Maurice. *Phenomenology of Perception*. Translated by Donald A. Landes. London: Routledge, Taylor & Francis, 1964.

Múzquiz Pérez-Seoane, Matilde, et al. *The Cave of Altamira*. New York: Abrams, 1999.

Naville, Édouard. *Détails relevés dans les ruines de quelques temples égyptiens: 1re partie: Abydos, 2e partie: Behbeit-el-Hagher, Appendix: Samanoud*. Paris: Geuthner, 1930.

Nelson, Harold H. "Certain Reliefs at Karnak and Medinet Habu and the Ritual of Amenophis I (Concluded)." *JNES* 8 (1949): 321–23.

Nesbitt, Claire. "Shaping the Sacred: Light and the Experience of Worship in Middle Byzantine Churches." *Byzantine and Modern Greek Studies* 36 (2012): 139–60.

O'Connor, David B., and Eric H. Cline, eds. *Amenhotep III: Perspectives on His Reign*. Ann Arbor: University of Michigan Press, 1998.

Oppenheim, Adela, Dorothea Arnold, Dieter Arnold, and Kei Yamamoto. *Ancient Egypt Transformed: The Middle Kingdom*. New York: Metropolitan Museum of Art, 2015.

Pentcheva, Bissera V. "Phenomenology of Light: The Glitter of Salvation in Bessarion's Cross." In *The Oxford Handbook of Light in Archaeology*. Edited by Costas Papadopoulos and Holly Moyes. Oxford: Oxford University Press, 2017.

———. *The Sensual Icon: Space, Ritual and the Senses in Byzantium*. University Park: The Pennsylvania State University Press, 2010.

Reisner, George A. "The Tomb of Hepzefa, Nomarch of Siût." *Journal of Egyptian Archaeology* 5 (1918): 79–98.

Schiff Giorgini, Michela. *Soleb III: Le Temple Description*. Cairo: Institut français d'archéologie orientale du Caire, 2002.

———. *Soleb V: Le Temple Bas-Reliefs et Inscriptions*. Cairo: Institut français d'archéologie orientale, 1998.

Serpico, Margaret, and Raymond White. "Oil, Fat and Wax." Pages 390–429 in *Ancient Egyptian Materials and Technology*. Edited by Paul T. Nicholson and Ian Shaw. Cambridge: Cambridge University Press, 2000.

Strong, Meghan E. "A Great Secret of the West: Transformative Aspects of Artificial Light in Dynastic Egypt." Pages 249–64 in *Archaeology of the Night*. Edited by Nancy Gonlin and April Nowell. Boulder: University Press of Colorado, 2018.

———. "Illuminating the Path of Darkness: Social and Sacred Power of Artificial Light in Pharaonic Period Egypt." PhD diss., University of Cambridge, 2018.

Strudwick, Nigel. *Masterpieces of Ancient Egypt*. London: British Museum Press, 2006.

Uphill, Eric. "The Egyptian Sed-Festival Rites." *JNES* 24 (1965): 365–83.

Wilson, John A. "Illuminating the Thrones at the Egyptian Jubilee." *JAOS* 56 (1936): 293–96.

Zohary, Daniel, Maria Hopf, and Ehud Weiss. *Domestication of Plants in the Old World: The Origin and Spread of Domesticated Plants in Southwest Asia, Europe, and the Mediterranean Basin*. 4th ed. Oxford: Oxford University Press, 2012.

Contributors

Constance Classen: Centre for Sensory Studies, Concordia University, Montreal (Canada).

Nicla De Zorzi: Department of Near Eastern Studies, University of Vienna (Austria).

Jan Dietrich: Department of Theology, School of Culture and Society, Aarhus University (Denmark).

Dorothée Elwart: Laboratoire d'Excellence Histoire et anthropologie des savoirs, des techniques et des croyances, École pratique des hautes études, Paris (France).

Sibylle Emerit: Laboratoire Histoire et Sources des Mondes Antiques, Centre national de la recherche scientifique, UMR 5189, Lyon (France).

Dorothea Erbele-Küster: Faculty of Protestant Theological, Johannes Gutenberg-University, Mainz (Germany).

Greg Schmidt Goering: Department of Religious Studies, University of Virginia, Charlottesville (United States).

Dora Goldsmith: Egyptological Seminar, Freie Universität, Berlin (Germany).

Marianne Grohmann: Faculty of Protestant Theology, University of Vienna (Austria).

David Howes: Department of Sociology and Anthropology, Concordia University, Montréal (Canada).

Kirsty L. Jones: Department of Theology and Religious Studies, Georgetown University, Washington DC (United States).

Thomas Krüger: Faculty of Theology, University of Zurich (Switzerland).

Kiersten Neumann: Oriental Institute, University of Chicago (United States).

Anne-Caroline Rendu Loisel: Institut d'Histoire et d'Archéologie de l'Orient ancien, Université de Strasbourg (France).

Annette Schellenberg: Faculty of Protestant Theology, University of Vienna (Austria).

Thomas Staubli: Faculty of Theology, University of Fribourg (Switzerland).

Meghan E. Strong: Division of Archaeology, University of Cambridge (United Kingdom).

Allison Thomason: Department of Historical Studies, Southern Illinois University Edwardsville (United States).

Pierre Van Hecke: Faculty of Theology and Religious Studies and Faculty of Arts, Catholic University of Leuven (Belgium).

Index of Ancient Sources

Hebrew Bible/Old Testament
Genesis
1	151
2–3	145–46, 148, 150, 153, 156–57
2:7	149, 194
2:9	149–50
2:12	150
2:16–17	149–50
2:18	150
2:19	99
3	146, 149, 157–58
3:3	150
3:5	150, 171
3:6	149, 151
3:7	151, 171
3:22	150
6:14ff	50
8:21	115
21:14	77
21:19	171
24:16	151
26:7	151
27:34	109
34:30	119
37:15	77
43:32	113, 124
46:34	124
49:20	190

Exodus
4:11	176
5:21	119
8:22	113, 124
16:31	107
56:10	176

Leviticus
5:1	59
13:45	195
18:28	139
18:30	138
21:1	195
25:35	90, 96
26:29	192
26:30	137

Numbers
4:20	206
6:26	187
11:8	107
19:10–22	195

Deuteronomy
1:12	183
1:39	148
4	71
4:9–10	66
4:24	193
7	138
7:26	137
11:2	66
11:7	66
14:3	113
21:15–17	63
23:13–15	122
23:24	123
26:17	174
28:29	79
28:53–57	192
29:16	137
32:13	191
32:35	90

Judges		18:27	63
3:24	121	19:12	125
9:11	191	21:26	137
18:25	109		
		2 Kings	
Ruth		6:17	171
1:20	109	6:25	123
		6:26–30	192
1 Samuel		17:12	137
2:8	193	18:27	123, 135
13:4	119	21:21	137
14:24	105	23:24	137
14:29	105		
14:34	105	2 Chronicles	
15:32	109	6:40	172
16:2	151	7:15	172
21:14	107, 110	28:15	90
22:2	109		
24:5	122	Nehemiah	
25	155	1:6	172
25:22	122		
25:33	107	Esther	
25:34	122	1:2–3	151
28	133		
		Job	
2 Samuel		1:22	111
1:26	133	3:20	109
3:35	105	4:4	90, 96
7:2	60	6:4	110
7:10	192	6:5	110
10:6	119	6:6	100, 110–11
11:2	151	6:7	110
12:17	192	6:30	116
13:7	192	12:5	96
17:8	109	12:11	103, 105–6
19:36	105	12:15	90
22:8	95	12:20	107
22:30	174	12:24–25	90
22:43	123	18:7–10	91
		19:17	119
1 Kings		20:2	88
1:41	76	20:7	134
3:9	99	20:12–15	109
10	204	22:2	151
14:5	94	26:11	95
14:10	122, 135	29:10	190
14:15	90–91	29:15	70

30:29	189	68:12	175
33:20	151	69:22	192
34:3	105–6	73:2	91
34:27	151	73:2–3	93
34:35	151	75	94
39:13–17	190	75:4	94
42:5–6	60	77:4	206–7
		82:5	96
Psalms		93:1	94
10:17	151	99:1	94–95
16:8	92	104	94
17:5	76, 81	104:5	94
18:8	95	104:32	94
18:30	174	104:34	200
19:11	151	105:37	90
22:16	190	107	89
26:1	93	107:4	77
27:2	92	107:23–27	89
30:7	92	113:7	193
31:19	176	115	71
34	101, 107	115:4–7	71
34:1	107	119:66	107
34:9	99–100, 103, 105–6	119:82	188
36:10	186	119:103	109
37:23–24	96	119:105	186
38:14	176	119:123	188
38:18	92	125:1	94
39:3	176	135	71
39:10	176	137:6	190
42:6	206–7	145:15	99
42:12	206		
43:5	206	Proverbs	
46	95	1:3	151
46:1–7	96	1:11	82
46:6	94	1:15	82
46:7	94, 207	1:16	76–78, 82
48:8–9	60	1:17	77
51:16	176	1:18–19	82
55:18	206	1:21	76
59:7	206–7	2:2	78, 83
59:15	206–7	2:10	78, 83
60:3–5	90	2:12–15	80
60:4	95	2:13	79
60:5	94	3:18	153
62:3	92	3:23	80
62:7	92	3:24	112, 200
64:4	110	4	93

4:1–2	212	14:35	151
4:4	212	15:24	151
4:6	212	15:32	157
4:10–19	78–79	16:1	64
4:11–12	78, 93	16:20	151
4:14–17	78, 80	16:23	151
4:18–19	79	17:2	151
4:19	93	17:8	151
4:20–27	79–81	17:27	125
5:1–23	81	18:10	78
5:4	110	18:21	157
5:5	81	19:2	70, 82
5:6	80–81	19:14	151
5:7	174	19:17	63
5:10–16	211	19:22	151
5:18–23	90	20:12	51
6:12–20	77	20:17	112, 200
6:18	76–78, 82	20:19	125
6:23	79	20:20	62
7	75–79	21:5	70
7:1	77	21:10	153
7:2	83, 212	21:11–12	151
7:7	75	21:15	153
7:10	76	21:16	151
7:11	76, 207	21:20	151
7:12	76	21:25–26	151
7:13–20	77	23	89
7:15	81	23:9	125
7:21	77	23:33–34	88
7:25	77, 83	24	154
8:32	174	24:13–14	108, 153, 156
10:5	151	24:16	96
10:19	151	25:8	76
10:24	151	25:9–10	125
10:30	93, 96	25:26	94
11:12–13	125	26:7	174
11:22	83, 107, 155	26:16	83, 107, 155
11:23	151	27:17	190
11:30	153	28:20	70
12:3	80	28:22	70
12:16	125	29:20	70
12:23	125	30:12	123
13	153	30:32–33	125
13:5	153	31:6	109
13:12	151, 153	31:8	176
13:19	11, 151	31:18	83, 88, 101, 105–6, 155
13:25	153		

Ecclesiastes		5:4	206–7
2:13–14	79	5:5	202–3
9:11	81	5:6	200
11:3–6	65	5:9–16	211
		5:10–16	185, 201, 211
Song of Songs		5:13	201–2
1:2	203	5:14–15	203
1:2–3	200, 202	5:15	201
1:3	202, 204	5:16	203
1:4	203–4	6:2–3	202
1:5	201	6:4–5	201
1:6	205	6:5	206
1:7	183, 200	6:5–7	211
1:8	201	6:7	203
1:10	201	6:11	201–2, 204
1:12	202–4	7:2	203
1:13–14	202–3	7:2–6	211
1:15–16	201	7:2–7	201
1:17	202	7:3	202–3
2:1–3	203	7:6	204
2:5–7	203	7:8–9	203
2:8	174, 200	7:9	202–3
2:8–9	175, 211	7:9–10	199, 204
2:10	200–201	7:10	202–3
2:12–13	201	7:11–13	203
2:13	203	7:12–13	202
2:14	112, 200–201	7:13	201–2
2:15–16	202	7:13–14	204
2:16	203	7:14	202–3
3:6	202	8:1	203–4
4:1–7	201, 211	8:2	202–3
4:2	201	8:3	200–203
4:3	203	8:13	200–201
4:6	202–3	8:14	202–3
4:7	175		
4:9	206	Isaiah	
4:10	201–3	1:3	81
4:10–11	202	2:1	166
4:10–5:1	204	3:8	94
4:11	199, 203–4	4:4	123, 135
4:12–5:1	203	5:2	119
4:13	202–3	5:4	119
4:13–16	202	5:20	110
4:15	206	5:22	168
4:16	203	5:26–28	92
5:1	202–4	5:27	90
5:2	200	6	171

6:4–7	171	40:16	171
6:9–10	167	40:20	90
8:14	94	41:7	90
8:14–15	90	42:7	171
9:1	171	42:18	171–72
9:15	171	42:19	172, 178
9:18	171	42:20	171
11	48	43:8	167, 172
13:1	166	44:18	167
13:17	171	45:2	164
13:21	189	45:13	164
14:11	206	48:8	168
14:17	171	49:18	171
16:11	119, 207	50:5	168
17:12	207	51:1–2	171
19:13	94	51:6	171
19:13–14	90	51:17	94
22:2	76	51:17–23	90
24:19–20	90	51:22	94
24:20	94	53:7	176
26:6	76	53:10	162, 176
26:7	164	54:1	175
27:6	191	54:10	96
28:7–8	89, 135	56:10	81, 167, 176, 186
28:8	123	57:20	123
29:9–10	90	59:3	171
29:18	172	59:7	82
30:5	119	59:10	176
30:30	193	59:11	206
31:8	170	59:14	96
31:16	171	60:4	171
32:7	171	63:15	171
33:15	174	64:7	194
33:23	175	65:11	64
34:3	119	66:3	137
35	165–66, 172, 174, 176		
35:1–2	176	Jeremiah	
35:3	96	1:1–13	166
35:4–10	165	1:6	174
35:5	167, 171–73, 177	2:19	109
35:5–8	161–63, 172–73, 175, 177	2:20	174
35:6	173–74, 176	2:23	168
35:8–9	174	3:21	162
36:12	123	4:19	207
37:17	171	5:21	170–71
38:9	171	5:22	206
40:3	164	6:20	112, 200

7:23–24	174	51:32	162
7:24	173	51:55	207
7:26	173	52:11	171
9:4	169		
9:13	174	Lamentations	
10:1	169	1:7–12	188
11:8	173–74	1:10	194
13:10	174	1:11	189
15:16	109	1:14	194
15:17	169	1:17	194
15:19	169	1:18	188
16:7	162	1:20	188
16:12	174	2	184
17:23	173	2:4	194
18:6	194	2:5	184
18:15	94	2:7	184, 194
19:5	138	2:10	184
19:9	192	2:11	188
20:11	90, 92	2:12	189
23:12	90–91, 169	2:15	184
23:13	111	2:16	184, 188
24:6	174	2:18	184
25:4	173	2:20	188, 192
25:15–28	90	3:1	188
25:16	94	3:36	188
31	165–66, 172–75	3:45	123
31:7–9	161–65, 171, 175, 177	3:50	188
31:8	162	3:59–60	188
31:9	91	3:63	188
31:20	64	4	181–98
31:26	112	4:1	184–185
32:23	174	4:1–16	183
34:14	173	4:2	183–85, 194
35:15	173–74	4:3–4	189, 191
38:6	123	4:3–5	189
38:9	162	4:4	189, 192
39–40	190	4:5	185–86, 190–91, 193, 196
39:7	171	4:5–9	191
44:5	173	4:7	184–86
44:23	174	4:8	184–85
46:6	90	4:9	188, 191
46:12	91	4:9–11	189
48:11	108	4:10	189, 191–92, 194
48:36	207	4:11	188, 190, 193–94
50:32	90	4:12	188
50:39	189	4:13	186, 195
50:42	206–7	4:14	186, 188, 195–96

4:14–15	183, 195	Jonah	
4:15	195	3:7	105, 107–8
4:16	186–88		
4:17	187–88	Micah	
4:17–20	183	1:8	189
4:20	188, 193–94	7:10	123
4:21–22	183		
4:21	196	Nahum	
5:1	188	3:3	91
5:13	90, 92		
		Habakkuk	
Ezekiel		1:6	109
3:1	116	2:15–16	89–90
3:1–3	109	2:18	176
3:26	176, 190		
4:9–15	134	Zephaniah	
4:12	123	1:9	174
5:10	192	1:12	108
7:16	206–7	1:17	186
11:21	138		
14:6	137	Zechariah	
14:12–23	63	9:3	123, 135
15:7	193	10:5	123
16:36	137	12:2	94
16:37	112, 200	12:2–3	90
20:7–8	137		
24:27	176	Malachi	
33:22	176	3:4	112
36:18	137		
36:25	137	**New Testament**	
36:30	191	Matthew	
		5:13	110
Daniel			
3:10	107	Mark	
10:15	176	9:50	110
Hosea		Luke	
4:5	90	14:34	110
9:4	112, 200		
		Ephesians	
Amos		5:2	119
2:13	90, 94		
4:8	94	Philippians	
8:12	94	4:18	119
9:5	90		
		Colossians	
		4:6	110

INDEX OF ANCIENT SOURCES 391

Revelation
2:7 153
5:8 119
8:3–4 119
22:1–2, 14, 19 153

Deuterocanon and Septuagint
Sirach
10:9 134
17:6–7 151
36:31 174
42:8 90
51:21 207

1 Maccabees
1:54 137
6:7 137

4 Maccabees
16:18 153

Old Testament Pseudepigrapha
4 Ezra
8:52 153

Testament of Levi
18:10–11 153

Dead Sea Scrolls
1QSa
2:7 90

11QT 123
46:13–16 122

Ancient Jewish Writers
Josephus Flavius, *Jewish War*
148–149 122–123

Jewish Texts from Egypt
TAD
A4.7–9 113

Rabbinic Works
b. Yoma
30a 134

Mesopotamian Sources
4R 17.r.11 285

81-2-4 294.o.11–17 225

AbB
2.115 obv. 9–14 217, 222–23
14.29 38–39 219

ABL
3.301 obv. 20–22 220

AfK
2 100.i.16–17 263

Agušaya
A v.23′–vii.9′ 241
B i.18 242

Alamdimmû
2:63–64 221
6:64 221
8:92 221

ARM
26.1:375 n. 13 233
26.198 234

Ashurbanipal Prism A
ix.37 230

BM
98743 ii.5–10 224

CT
15:45–47 237, 244–45
15:104–107 237
15:222–223 241
41:30–31 231

Curse of Agade
249 191

Ebla
Letter G 47 130

Enuma Elish		Lamaštu	
3:129–138	284	1:62	243
		1:63–66	244
Erm		1:104–109	243
15639	286	2:31–33	239
		2:38	244
Erra		3:64–68	239
4:56	130		
		Lamentation over Sumer and Ur	
ETCSL		389	191
c.5.3.5	222, 231		
c.5.4.11	232	*LKA*	
c.5.4.12	222	23.r.14–15	285
		63.o.13'	240
Father and His Disobedient Son		92.o.11–17	225
147–158	223		
		Ludlul	
Gilgamesh		2:106–107	233
5:99–106	281		
7:109–117	132	MAD	
7:117, 119	236	5.7–12	288–89
7:182–192	245		
9:172–190	282–83	Maqlû	
10:304–307	282	4:73	219
12:134–135	245	5:57–72	238
		5:73–75	238
Iqqur īpuš	261		
		MSL	
K		13:245	221
48+	265	15:126, 132–143	221
2000+	262		
3397+	264	Nergal and Ereškigal	
3664+	261	149–157	245
3810	263	O.174//W.20030/15, BE.13987	260
4592+	264		
5668 ii.5–10	224	Pazuzu	
6082 B.10–11	225	57, 16	245
6082 B.14–16	225	58, 37–41	243
KAR		Proverbs of Ancient Sumer	
1.r.20	236	9 n.1.12	224
174.r.iii.5–16	233		
		RIM	
KBo		3.1:19 (Ur-Bau E3/1.1.6.5.ii.8–iii.2)	261
1:67, 38 r.12'–16'	221	3.1:39 (Gudea E3/1.1.7.StC.iii.6–7)	261

INDEX OF ANCIENT SOURCES

RIMA
1:167 (Adad-nerari I A.0.76.35) 260
1:189 (Shalmaneser I. A.0.77.2.5–13, 21–24) 261
2:153 (Ashurnasirpal A.0.101.30) 294
2:296 (Ashurnaṣirpal II A.0.101.32.9) 261
3:56 (Shalmaneser III A.0.102.10.iv.51–55) 263
3:133–134 (Shalmaneser III A.0.102.53) 260

RIMB
2:148 (Sargon II B.6.22.3.i.39–40) 265
2:207 (Ashurbanipal B.6.32.6.26–30) 261

RINAP
3.1:34 (Sennacherib 1.35) 306
3.1:82–83 (Sennacherib 10.23–25) 259
3.1:98 (Sennacherib 15.iv.33'–34') 301
3.1:111 (Sennacherib 16.i.25–6) 301
3.1:133 (Sennacherib 17.iii.52) 301
3.1:139 (Sennacherib 17.vi.30–36) 270
3.1:184 (Sennacherib 22.vi.24–31) 229
3.1:224 (Sennacherib 34, 53b–55a) 229
3.2:315–316 (Sennacherib 223, 34b–40a) 229
3.2:334 (Sennacherib 230, 95b–98a) 229
4:21 (Esarhaddon 1.iv.85–v.1) 230
4:33–34 (Esarhaddon 2.v.27–32) 270
4:125 (Esarhaddon 57.iii.16–41) 261
4:125 (Esarhaddon 57.iii.42–iv.6) 259
4:125–126 (Esarhaddon 57.iv.16–26) 263
4:126 (Esarhaddon 57.v.3–14) 262
4:126 (Esarhaddon 57.v.23–28) 263
4:126 (Esarhaddon 57.v.25) 260
4:126–127 (Esarhaddon 57.v.31–38.vi.20–27) 265
4:136 (Esarhaddon 60.22'–23') 272
4:155 (Esarhaddon 77.10–11) 270
4:201 (Esarhaddon 104.vii.19–29) 261
4:206 (Esarhaddon 105.v.23–28) 265
4:230 (Esarhaddon 113.24–26) 263

SAA
2:6, 547–550 192
2:11, 2.iv.14–16 235–236
2:49, 6.490–492 235
2:55, 6.603–605 220
3:14 267
3:29 228
3:30 226
3:32 282
3:37, 23' 267
3:39 267
3:39, r.24–25 267
3:64, 29.o.l. 226
3:64, 29.o.4 227
3:65, 29.o.10, 13–14 227
3:66 227
3:72, 32 r.13 245
13:78 308
17:49, 53r.4'–5' 223

SBTU
3 n. 69 §30 244

ST II 232 263

STT
252.r.23–25 231

Šumma ālu 260–61, 301
46:10 230–31
49:4 230–31
49:71–90 232
49: 77' 231

Šumma izbu
22:159 231
22:153 232

Udug-hul
6:175' 222

YOS
3 19 r.20–21 224
11 11:5a.o.1–3 232

Egyptian Sources
Book of the Dead 123, 125
17 S5 128
28a S1 127
28b S2 127
29A 126
30B 338

33 S		129	Dendera
40 P1		128	III, 185,1–4	350
40 S1		128		
47 S var.		128	Dispute of a Man with his BA
51		127	88–90	338
51 S		127	91–93	338
52a S		127	93–95	339
52b S2		128		
53b S1		127	EA	138
53b S2		128	8	372–73
82b S		127		
85a S1–2		128	Edfu	
85b		126	I, 471,12	353
90 S2		129	I, 565,67–70	350–51
102b S		127	VI, 56,10–13, 57,2	348
109b S2		126	VI, 237,1–3	349
116 T		127		
124b S		127	Esna	
126		128	VI, 1, 531,1–2	348
130b S2		129		
130b S6		129	Hibis	
134		349	Pl. 22, East Wall, Register II, 3–5	353
137 A T11		126		
144e S		126	Hymn III to Ramesses VI
153c S2		128	1–3	344
160 S1		126	8	344
162 T5		126		
168b S9		129	Kemit	
168e S54		127	6–8	339
176 S		127		
178f S2		127	KRI	
178g S		128	III, 43,1–44,4	365
178n S		128	V, 69,15–70,1	351
182a S1		128		
183b S1		128	pBremner-Rhind	
184b S2		128	22,22	372
186Ba S1		129		
189		127	Pleasures of Fishing and Fowling	337, 342
189a.d.f.i S		127		
			Pyramid Texts	
Coffin Texts			210	127
173		127	409	127
216		127	412	352
581		127	535	352
1011		127		
			Report on the Delta Residence	337, 342

Satire of Trades
20   338–39
21   338

Sporting King
C,1   345
D,2   346

Greek Sources
Aphthonius, *Progymnasmata*
36–37   211

Archilochus
fragment 201   57

Aristotle, *Poetics*
21.1457b6–7   100
22.1458a21–23   100

Aristotle, *Rhetoric*
3.2   100

Herodas, *Mimes*
6.37   224

Quintillian, *Institutio oratoria*
8.3.67–69   209–210

Index of Modern Authors

Abusch, Tzvi 219, 238, 246
Adams, Charles 28, 36
Aitken, Kenneth T. 171, 178
Al-Fouadi, Abdul-Hadi A. 281, 290
Albenda, Pauline 295–96, 299–300, 309
Albertz, Rainer 149, 158
Allan, Frank 30, 36
Allen, James P. 357
Allen, Thomas George 125–26, 139
Alliot, Maurice 348, 352, 358
Allon, Niv 353, 358
Alster, Bendt 223–24, 246
Altman, Charles B. 272, 276
Alvarez-Mon, Javier 307–9
Ambos, Claus 258, 260–65, 267, 275
Ames, Michael M. 15, 37
Andermann, Lisa 8, 30, 37
Anderson, Robert D. 320, 322–23, 332
Andrae, Walter 266, 269, 275
Andreu, Guillemette 364, 278
Angyal, András 120, 140
Ankersmit, Frank 44, 52
Annus, Amar 233, 246
Appadurai, Arjun 23, 37
Archi, Alfonso 130, 140
Arnold, Dieter 380
Arnold, Dorothea 380
Aro, Jussi 259, 277
Assmann, Jan 319, 332
Aster, Shawn Z. 218, 240, 246
Ataç, Mehmet-Ali 264–65, 275, 293, 307–9
Augustin, Matthias 151, 158

Avrahami, Yael vii, 51–53, 58–59, 61, 66–67, 71–72, 78, 84, 87, 97, 105, 116, 152, 154–56, 158, 166, 172, 175–76, 178, 181–82, 186, 193, 196–97
Bahrani, Zainab 295, 309
Baines, John 374, 378
Barack, Sarah 274, 278
Barbotin, Christophe 364, 378
Barnett, Richard David 299, 310
Barr, James 51, 53, 114, 117
Barrelet, Marie-Thérèse 131–32, 140
Barrett, Caitlín E. 307, 310
Barstad, Hans M. 164, 178
Barta, Winfried 357
Barth, Christoph 90–91, 93, 97
Barth, Fredrik 28, 37
Barton, John 147, 158
Basso, Ellen Becker 15, 37
Baugh, Kimberly 379
Bauks, Michaela 149, 159
Baudrillard, Jean 15, 37
Baumann, Arnulf 90, 97, 206, 212
Baumann, Gerlinde 193, 197
Baumgarten, Albert I. 123, 140
Beaux, Nathalie 336, 358
Bell, Catherine M. 256, 275
Bellisle, France 117
Ben Zvi, Ehud 161, 178
Bénazeth, Dominique 320, 332
Bennie, Jonathan 361, 378
Benzel, Kim 267, 275
Berges, Ulrich 183, 197
Berlejung, Angelika 245–46

Berlin, Adele	183, 185–92, 195, 197	Butler, Shane	218
Berlin, Isaiah	57, 67	Cagni, Luigi	264, 275
Berndt, Ronald M.	7, 24, 37	Calame-Griaule, Geneviève	16, 37
Berry, John W.	18, 25–26, 37	Caminos, Ricardo Augusto	357–58
Biggs, Robert D.	237, 246	Campbell, Donald T.	26
Bille, Mikkel	362–63, 378	Carasik, Michael	58–60, 64–67
Biocca, Ettore	19–20, 37	Carpenter, Edmund	5, 12–14, 19, 27, 37
Biran, Adam	119, 140	Carr, David M.	162, 178
Birch, Samuel	373, 378	Carroll, Robert P.	166, 171, 178
Black, Jeremy	281, 290	Carter, Howard	365
Bland, H. A.	378	Cassin, Elena	218, 240, 242, 246
Blenkinsopp, Joseph	173, 178	Castaing-Taylor, Lucien	44
Blesser, Barry	326, 330, 332	Cauville, Sylvie	328–329, 332
Bligh, John	205, 212	Cavigneaux, Antoine	265, 275
Blocher, Felix	131, 140	Černý, Jaroslav	363, 365, 372, 378
Bloom, Lois	75	Cesara, Manda	6, 37
Boas, Franz	12–13, 37	Chamberlain, Alexander	23, 37
Böck, Barbara	220–21, 227, 246	Chapman, Cynthia R.	228, 246
Bogard, Paul	361, 378	Chassinat, Émile	327, 329, 332, 357
Boman, Thorleif	45, 49–51, 53, 58, 67, 181, 197	Cho, Yongmin	361, 378
		Choi, Jaewok	378
Borchardt, Ludwig	349, 358	Ciccarello, Mark	346, 358
Borger, Rykle	230, 246	Cinzano, Pierantonio	379
Bosman, Hendrik Ludolph	192, 197	Cirillo, Thomas	138, 140
Bottéro, Jean	283, 290	Civil, Miguel	130, 143
Boulenger, George Albert	341, 358	Clair, Colin	26, 37
Bourdieu, Pierre	69–70, 84	Clark, Elizabeth A.	146, 159
Bozak, Barbara A.	162, 178	Classen, Constance	vii 9, 14, 21, 25, 30, 33, 37, 39, 43–45, 48–49, 52–53, 146, 152, 156–57, 159, 181–82, 197, 336, 358
Bradley, Mark	218		
Brain, Robert	17, 37		
Breniquet, Catherine	295, 310		
Brenner, Athalya	202, 209, 212	Clay, Albert T.	224, 247
Briggs, Jean	19, 22, 37	Clemens, Ashley	224, 247
Brockmole, James R.	304, 310	Clements, Ronald Ernest	164–66, 171, 173, 178
Brose, Patrick	322, 333		
Brown, Michael	35, 37	Clements, Ruth E.	112, 117
Brox, Jane	361, 378	Clifford, James	45, 52
Bruyère, Bernard	364, 378	Clifford, Richard John	112, 117
Budde, Karl	148, 159	Cline, Eric H.	373, 376, 380
Buddle, Kathleen	32, 37	Cohen, Yoram	217
Bull, Cynthia J.	73, 84	Cole, Michael	23, 41
Butler, Sally A. L.	280, 290	Cole, Steven W.	308, 310

Coles, John	362, 378	Dowd, Marion	362, 378
Collins, Paul	299, 310	Drewnowski, Adam	108, 117
Condon, Virginia	344, 357	Driver, Samuel R.	148, 159
Cook, Michael	120, 142	Dubuisson, Daniel	318, 332
Cooper, Jerrold S.	191, 197, 224, 247	Duhm, Bernard	164, 178
Copley, M. S.	366, 378	Dundes, Alan	3, 38
Corballis, Michael C.	254, 278	Durand, Jean-Marie	219–20, 234, 247
Corbin, Alain	24, 27, 38, 49	Duriscoe, Dan	379
Cornill, Carl Heinrich	162, 178	Eastwood, Gillian M.	365, 378
Cox, Rupert	45, 53	Ebeid, Nabil I.	129, 140
Crawford, Cory D.	303, 310	Eck, Diana	9
Crouch, Carly L.	112–13, 117, 136, 140	Edzard, Dietz Otto	131, 140, 225, 247
Cruse, David	378	Elliott, Denielle	44, 53
Crüsemann, Frank	152, 159	Ellis, Richard S.	258, 260–63, 268, 275
Culhane, Dara	44, 53	Elwart, Dorothée	323–25, 332
Curtis, Valerie	119, 140	Elvidge, Christopher D.	379
Dahood, Mitchell	106, 117	Elwood, Lisa S.	119, 140
Dalley, Stephanie	236, 247	Emerit, Sibylle	316–17, 328, 331, 333, 335–36, 358
Damerji, Muayad Said Basim	263, 275		
Daniel, E. Valentine	7–8, 29, 38	Endicott, Kirk M.	34–35, 38
Darwin, Charles	119–20, 140	Engen, Trygg	355–56, 358–59
Daube, David	59	Epping, Joseph	267, 275
Daumas, François	322, 329, 332	Erbele-Küster, Dorothea	152, 154, 159
Davies, Norman de Garis	357	Evans, Jean	295, 310
Davies, Thomas W.	378	Evershed, R. P.	378
de Joode, Johan	104, 107, 109, 117	Falchi, Fabio	361, 379
De Zorzi, Nicla	193, 226, 228–33, 245, 247, 306, 310	Fales, Mario	229, 247
		Fallon, April E.	120, 140, 142
DeClaissé-Walford, Nancy	106, 117	Farber, Walter	239, 242–44, 247
Delattre, Alain	320, 332	Faulkner, Raymond O.	372, 379
Delitzsch, Franz	106, 117	Febvre, Lucien	32, 38, 50, 53
Deller, Karlheinz	300, 310	Feder, Yitzhaq	136, 140, 218–219, 232, 242, 248
Deregowski, Jan B.	26, 38		
Diaconu, Mădălina	87, 97	Feld, Steven	8, 15, 38
Dietrich, Jan	65–67, 181, 302	Feldman, Marian	293, 309–310
Dijk, Jan van	232, 247	Ferguson, Priscilla Parkhurst	103, 117
Dobbs-Allsopp, Frederick William	183–84, 191, 197, 211, 213	Fernando, Nathalie	316, 333
		Fessler, Daniel M. T.	120, 140
Donald, Merlin	66–67	Fincke, Jeanette C.	227, 248
Dorsey, David A.	163, 178	Fink, Sebastian	61, 68
Douglas, Mary	23, 38, 136	Finkel, Irving L.	272, 274–75
Dow, James	14, 38	Finnestad, Ragnhild Bjerre	336, 358

Fischer, Georg	108, 117	Gericke, Jaco	63–64, 68
Fishbane, Michael	162, 178	Gerlemann, Gillis	206, 213
Flückiger-Hawker, Esther	244, 248	Geurts, Kathryn Linn	44, 53, 71, 84, 87, 97
Forrest, Barbara	302, 310		
Forti, Tova	105, 109, 117	Gill, Sam D.	12, 38
Foster, Benjamin R.	218, 225–27, 232, 248, 288, 290	Glenn, H. Patrick	52–53
		Goedicke, Hans	357
Foster, John L.	338, 358	Goetze, Albrecht	232, 247
Foster, Susan Leigh	73, 240–43	Goldie, Peter	208, 214
Foucault, Michel	27, 38	Goldingay, John	165, 178
Fox, Michael V.	62–63, 65, 68, 75–77, 80–84	Goldstein, E. Bruce	304, 310
		Goldwasser, Orly	340–41, 343, 345, 353, 359
Frahm, Eckart	130, 140, 229–30, 248		
Frake, Charles	23, 38	Gonlin, Nancy	362, 379
Frame, Grant	226, 248	González Holquín, Diego	9, 38
Frandsen, Paul John	124–25, 127, 140–41	Goodman, Steven M.	340, 359
		Gordis, Robert	149, 159
Frankfort, Henri	147, 159	Graff, Sarah B.	301, 310
Frazer, James G.	120	Grässler, Nadine	335, 359
Freedman, Sally	148, 231–32, 260–61, 275	Gravelle, Karen	4, 41
		Graves-Brown, Carolyn	362, 379
Frevel, Christian	181–85, 190, 193, 197	Green, Anthony	264, 275
Furgoni, Riccardo	379	Greenstein, Edward	64, 68
Gabbay, Uri	187, 197	Gregor, Thomas	18–19, 35, 38
Gadotti, Alhena	237, 248	Griffin, Kit	28, 35, 38
Gamer-Wallert, Ingrid	342, 348, 350, 359	Griffith, Francis Llewellyn	367–68, 379
		Groneberg, Brigitte	130, 141, 240–42, 248, 288, 290
Gardiner, Alan H.	341, 343, 358–59		
Gardner, Howard	18, 38	Grünbaum, Thor	208, 213
Gasse, Annie	357	Guichard, Michaël	218, 238, 248
Gaston, Kevin J.	378	Guillebaud, Christine	331
Gaut, Berys N.	147, 159	Guinan, Ann	301, 310
Gauthier, Baptiste	254, 275	Guralnick, Eleanor	272, 275
Gebhart-Sayer, Angelika	11–14, 16, 38	Gutbub, Adolphe	373, 379
Gelb, Ignace	288	Haag, E.	164, 178–79
Geller, Mark	222, 248–49	Haas, Volkert	131
Geller, Markham	222–23	Hahn, Tomie	73, 77, 84
Geller, Stephen	61, 68	Haidt, Jonathan	120–21, 141, 143
Genders, Roy	17, 38	Haikal, Fayza	373, 379
Gendler, Tamar	208, 213	Hall, Edward T.	6, 17, 38
George, Andrew R.	132, 141, 222, 231, 233–34, 236, 242, 245, 248, 281, 290	Hamilakis, Yannis	218, 249, 294, 310
		Hannig, Rainer	126, 141

Harmanşah, Ömür	294, 310	Huxley, Aldous	279
Hartenstein, Friedhelm	187, 197	Ihde, Don	13, 39
Harvey, Susan Ashbrook	48, 53	Ikram, Salima	366, 379
Hasenfratz, Hans-Peter	126, 141	Imada, Sumio	141
Hatton, Peter	83, 85	Inbar, Yoel	121, 142
Haul, Michael	130, 141, 230, 249	Ingold, Tim	363, 379
Hayes, William C.	357	Irvine, Sidney H.	25, 37
Heeßel, Nils P.	243, 245, 249, 260, 275	Irving, Andrew	45, 53
Heimpel, Wolfgang	234, 237, 249	Izre'el, Shlomo	281, 290
Helck, Wolfgang	358	Jackson, Bernard S.	62, 68
Helfmeyer, Franz Josef	188, 197	Jackson, Michael	31, 39
Helion, Chelsea	121, 142	Jacobson, Rolf	106, 117
Heller, Robert	254, 275	Jäger, Stephan	358
Hensey, Robert	362, 378	Jahnow, Hedwig	186, 197
Herrmann, Christian	137, 141	James, Elaine T.	211, 213
Herskovits, Melville J.	26	James, Liz	363, 379
Herz, Rachel S.	111, 117, 356, 359	James, Wendy	35, 39
Herzfeld, Michael	45, 53	James, William	6, 39
Hickmann, Hans	316, 320–21, 323, 333	Janowski, Bernd	58, 60, 68, 154, 159
Hinds, Alden	111, 117	Jaques, Margaret	218, 242, 249, 284, 290
Hinson, Benjamin	321–22, 333		
Hopf, Maria	366, 380	Jastrow, Marcus	110
Hornung, Erik	127, 141	Jiménez, Enrique	232, 249
Horowitz, Wayne	287, 290	Joachim, Heinrich	125, 141
Horton, M.	378	Johnson, Dru	66–68
Houlihan, Patrick F.	343, 349–50, 359	Johnson, Justin Cale	222–23, 249
Höver-Johag, Ingeborg	151, 155, 159	Johnson, Mark	60, 68, 83, 85, 100–102, 115, 117
Howell, Signe	34, 38		
Howes, David	vii, 3, 5, 7, 12, 16, 29, 31, 35, 38–39, 43, 45, 47–49, 52–53, 146, 152, 156–57, 159, 181–82, 197	Johnson, Susan L.	117
		Johnson, W. Raymond	376, 379
		Jones, Douglas Rawlinson	162, 179
Hrůša, Ivan	245, 249	Joyce, James	6, 39
Hugh-Jones, Christine	36, 39	Junker, Hermann	325, 333, 346, 359
Hugh-Jones, Stephen	20, 36, 39	Jursa, Michael	217, 224, 237, 249
Huizinga, Johan	44	Jütte, Robert	205, 213
Humbert, Paul	112, 114–15, 117, 151, 159	Kadish, Gerald E.	127, 141
		Kahl, Jochem	335, 367, 379
Hunt, Earl B.	25, 37	Kahn, Miriam	33, 39
Hunt, John	303, 310	Kaiser, Otto	163, 165, 179
Hunt, Patrick	200, 209, 213	Kammerer, Thomas R.	284, 290
Hurowitz, Victor	240, 249	Karasik, Carol	35, 39
Hussey, Mary I.	232, 247	Karlsson, Matthias	228–29, 249

Katz, Dina	244, 249	Lambert, Wilfred G.	130, 142,
Kaufman, Stephen A.	108, 117	224–25, 233, 249, 284, 290	
Kazen, Thomas	136, 141–42	Lane, Edward William	115
Keck, Frédéric	331	LaNeel Tanner, Beth	106, 117
Keel, Othmar	139, 142, 201, 205, 213	Lanfranchi, Giovanni B.	257, 276
Kelly, Daniel	111, 117	Langdon, Stephen	268, 276
Kennedy, John G.	36, 39	Lapinkivi, Pirjo	236–37, 243–45, 249
Keown, Gerald L.	174, 179	Laplantine, François	43, 53
Kessler, Dieter	322, 333	Lapp, Günther	357
Kessler, Rainer	191, 197	Larsen, Mogens Trolle	262, 276
Kieran, Matthew	208, 213	Larson, Greger	133, 142
Kilmer, Anne D.	236, 249	Lateiner, Donald	138, 142, 217, 249
Kim, Eunjung	161, 179	Lavandier, Catherine	331
Kim, Kyung Hee	378	Lawson, Rebecca	208, 213
King, Leonard William	255, 275	Layard, Austen H.	271, 276
Kirkby, John T.	100, 117	Le Poidevin, Robin	255, 276
Kitchen, Kenneth A.	357, 365, 379	Leach, Edmund	28, 39
Knauft, Bruce M.	28, 39	Lee, B. R.	378
Knohl, Israel	125, 142, 184, 197	Lee, Eunil	378
Koch, Klaus	82–83, 85, 151, 159	Leenhardt, Maurice	5, 39
Koch, Ulla Susanne	255, 259, 275	Legrain, Leon	131, 142
Koenen, Klaus	183–85, 187–88,	Leick, Gwendolyn	225, 250
190, 192–95, 197		Lenzi, Alan	viii, 233, 259, 276
Kogan, Leonid	230	Leppert, Richard	49, 54
Kolbe, Dieter	264, 276	Lepsius, Carl Richard	366, 379
Kondo, Dorinne	29, 39	Lévi-Bruhl, Lucien	64
Koura, Basma	366, 379	Lévi-Strauss, Claude	31, 34, 39–40
Kozloff, Arielle P.	373, 379	Lewis, Gilbert	25, 40
Kramer, Samuel Noah	306, 310	Lichtheim, Miriam	338, 359
Kraus, Hans-Joachim	172, 179, 186, 197	Lim, Bo H.	164, 173, 179
Krebernik, Manfred	265, 275	Lindberg, David C.	205, 213
Krüger, Thomas	43, 181	Lindow, Wolfgang	136, 142
Kugel, James L.	70, 85	Lipschits, Oded	191, 197
Kuipers, Joel C.	8, 39	Little, Kenneth	7, 40
Kurth, Dieter	348–49, 359	Livingstone, Alasdair	227, 255, 267, 276
Kyba, Christopher C. M.	379	Llinás, Rodolfo R.	73–74, 77–78, 85
Labat, René	260, 276	Lopes, Dominic McIver	208, 213
Lacey, Simon	208, 213	López Austin, Alfredo	20–21, 40
Lackenbacher, Sylvie	258, 276	Loret, Victor	316
Lakoff, George	60, 68, 83, 85,	Loud, Gordon	272, 276
100–102, 115, 117		Luckenbill, Daniel D.	262, 276
Lam, Joseph	114, 117	Luft, Daniela C.	373, 379

Lukko, Mikko 245, 250
Lund, Øystein 164, 179
Lyon, David G. 262, 276
MacDonald, Nathan 162, 179
MacGinn, Colin 121, 142
Machinist, Peter 245, 250, 308, 310
Mackenzie Brown, Cheever 5, 40
Mallgrave, Harry Francis 303, 310
Mallowan, Max Edgar Lucien 268, 276
Malul, Meir 147, 149, 151, 155, 157, 159, 235, 237, 250
Manniche, Lise 335–36, 359
Marböck, Johannes 110, 117
Marcus, George E. 45, 53
Marcus, Michelle I. 293, 310
Marks, Lawrence 10, 40
Marti, Lionel 218, 238
Masetti-Rouault, Maria Grazia 228, 250, 284, 290
Masson, Aurélia 321, 333
Matthews, Claire R. 173, 179
Maul, Stefan M. 131, 142, 236, 250
Mayer, Walter 227, 250
Mayer-Opificius, Ruth 132, 142
McCauley, Clark R. 120, 140, 143
McCown, Donald Eugene 132, 142
McGinn, Colin 208, 213
McKane, William 111, 117
McLuhan, Eric 45, 54
McLuhan, Marshall 22, 45–47, 54
Meigs, Anna Stokes 20, 40
Meininger, Peter L. 340, 359
Meissner, Bruno 131, 142, 221, 250
Mennella, Julie A. 117
Menzel, Brigitte 258, 276
Merleau-Ponty, Maurice 7, 40, 363, 380
Métraux, Rhoda 6, 40
Metzler, Kai A. 284, 290
Meyer-Dietrich, Erika 317, 333, 335, 359
Michalowski, Piotr 284–85, 290
Milano, Lucio 229, 250

Militarev, Alexander 230, 250
Miller, William Ian 111, 118, 120, 142
Millman, Linda 120, 143
Milton, John 145, 148, 157, 159
Mineka, Susan 120, 142
Miscall, Peter D. 163, 179
Montagu, Ashley 18, 40
Morenz, Ludwig D. 319, 333
Morgan, John 23, 40
Mortier, Roland 104, 118
Munn, Nancy D. 25, 40
Munro, Jill M. 202, 213
Muraoka, Joüon 114
Muros, Vanessa 272, 276, 278
Múzquiz Pérez-Seoane, Matilde 372, 380
Nadali, Davide 257, 276, 299, 303–4, 311
Nakamura, Carolyn 268, 276
Nanay, Bence 208, 213
Nassouhi, Essad 263, 277
Nattiez, Jean-Jacques 316, 333
Naville, Édouard 366, 380
Nelson, Harold H. 363, 368, 373, 380
Nemeroff, Carol 120, 143
Nesbitt, Claire 363, 380
Neumann, Kiersten 270, 272, 277, 293
Nissinen, Martti 234, 236, 250
Novotny, Jamie R. 258, 262, 277
Nowell, April 362, 379
Nussbaum, Martha C. 120, 142
O'Connor, David B. 373, 376, 380
O'Connor, Kathleen 164, 179
O'Dea, William Thomas 361, 379
O'Dowd, Ryan 61, 68
Ohnuki-Tierney, Emiko 7, 25, 34, 40
Olatunji, Bunmi O. 119, 140
Olkes, Cheryl 23, 41
Olyan, Saul M. 113, 118, 170, 174–75, 179
Ong, Walter J. 18, 22, 31, 40

Oppenheim, A. Leo   280, 286–87, 291, 294–95, 302, 309, 311
Oppenheim, Adela   368, 380
Oshima, Takayoshi   233, 245, 250
Oswalt, John N.   163, 165, 179
Otto, Eckart   62, 68, 147, 153, 159–60
Otto, Nina   210, 213
Papineau, David   302, 311
Parayre, Dominique   131, 142
Parkinson, Richard   346, 359
Parpola, Simo   192, 197, 220, 226, 250, 257, 259, 270, 277
Parry, Vicki   272, 276
Patnaik, Naveen   29, 40
Paul, Shalom M.   203, 213
Paulson, William   21, 40
Peck, Jason Michael   147, 160
Peetz, Melanie   208, 213
Peled, Ilan   217, 225, 236, 241–42, 250
Penfield, Wilder   46, 54
Pentcheva, Bissera V.   363, 380
Pérez Arroyo, Rafael   335
Perrot, Sylvain   316–17, 333
Petrie, William Matthew Flinders   320, 333
Pinard, Sylvain   5, 9, 40
Pink, Sarah   44, 54
Pizaro, David   121, 142
Place, Victor   268, 273, 277
Pleyte, Willem   357
Pliner, Patricia   120, 140
Ponchia, Simonetta   245, 250
Pongratz-Leisten, Beate   228, 236, 250, 259, 277, 295, 308, 311
Porten, Bezalel   113, 118
Porteous, J. Douglas   7, 19, 40
Portnov, Boris A.   379
Posener, Georges   357
Powell, Marvin A.   284, 291
Price, Robyn   336, 359
Quack, Joachim Friedrich   325, 333
Quirke, Stephen   338, 345, 359

Rabb, Lauren   303, 311
Rad, Gerhard von   145, 160, 170, 179
Radner, Karen   235, 250, 308, 311
Rahiem, Mohamed Abdel   320, 333
Rajadell, Àngel   256, 277
Ramharter, Esther   211, 213
Raphael, Rachel   170, 179
Rasmussen, Theodore   46, 54
Raux, Sophie   318, 332
Raven, Marteen   321, 333
Rawlinson, Andrew   7, 40
Reade, Julian E.   272, 274–75, 277, 296, 299, 311
Reichel-Dolmatoff, Gerardo   4, 14, 24, 30, 33, 40–41
Reicke, Bo   149, 160
Reiner, Erica   231, 236, 242, 251, 295
Reisner, George A.   367, 380
Rendu Loisel, Anne-Caroline   218, 240, 251, 286, 289, 291, 300–301, 308, 311
Renkema, Johan   186–87, 192, 194, 197
Reynders, Marleen   322, 333
Richter, Barbara   327, 334
Rippl, Gabriele   209–10, 213
Ritchie, Ian   3, 33, 41, 48, 54
Rivlin, Robert   4, 41
Robben, Antonius C. G. M.   44, 54
Robson, Eleanor   255, 260–62, 277
Roby, Courtney   210, 214
Rochberg, Francesca   267, 277
Romano, James F.   321, 334
Romanyshyn, Robert D.   32, 41
Römer, Willem H. Ph.   223
Rose, P.   378
Rossi, Franceso   357
Roy, Arundhaty   133, 142
Royzman, Edward B.   136, 142
Rozin, Paul   120, 140–43
Rubio, Gonzalo   256, 277
Russell, John Malcolm   270, 277, 299, 311

Rybnikova, Nataliya A. 379
Ryholt, Kim 325, 333
Ryu, S. H. 378
Sabini, John 136, 142
Sachs, Curt 316
Sacks, Oliver W. 21, 41
Salgues, Emmanuelle 232, 248
Sallaberger, Walther 130, 143
Salter, Linda-Ruth 326, 330, 332
Samet, Nili 183, 185, 198
Sander, Friedrich 26
Sauneron, Serge 357
Savran, George 59–60, 68
Scalise, Pamela J. 174, 179
Schafer, R. Murray 7, 41
Schart, Aaron 155, 160
Schellekens, Elisabeth 208, 214
Schellenberg, Annette 43, 58, 65, 68, 158, 160, 184, 195, 198–201, 206–207, 214
Schieffelin, Edward L. 34, 41
Schiff Giorgini, Michela 373–75, 380
Schifferstein, Hendrik N. J. 208, 214
Schiffmann, Harvey Richard 72, 85
Schipper, Jeremy 162, 168, 179
Schmidt Goering, Greg 77, 84, 88, 105, 109, 118, 145–46, 154–55, 160, 181
Schmitt, Aaron W. 268, 277
Schroer, Silvia 139, 142, 187, 198
Schweitzer, Stephan James 161, 179
Scribner, Sylvia 23, 41
Scurlock, Jo Ann 235, 251
Seeger, Anthony 5, 16, 21, 27–28, 34, 41
Segal, Marshall H. 26, 41
Serpico, Margaret 366, 380
Sethe, Kurt 357
Seyfried, Friederike 335
Shafer, Ann 293, 309, 312
Sharon, Douglas 4, 41
Sheets-Johnstone, Maxine 74–75, 80, 85
Shupak, Nili 124, 143, 156, 160
Siskind, Janet 21, 41
Sjøberg, Åke W. 222–23, 227, 232, 251, 306, 312
Sladek, William R. 241, 251
Sloterdijk, Peter 135–36, 143
Sluka, Jeffrey A. 44, 54
Smith, Gary V. 164, 173, 180
Smith, Mark M. 181, 198
Smothers, Thomas G. 174, 179
Sneed, Mark R. 146, 160
Snell, Bruno 50
Sommer, Benjamin D. 165–66, 180
Sonik, Karen 264, 277
Sørensen, Tim Flohr 362–63, 378
Soulen, Richard N. 202, 211, 214
Spatharas, Dimos 138, 142, 217, 249
Sperling, David 64, 68
Spieckermann, Hermann 158, 160
Spiegelberg, Wilhelm 325, 334
Stacey, David 173, 180
Stackert, Jeffrey viii
Stallybrass, Peter 27, 41
Starr, Ivan 259, 277
Staubli, Thomas 121, 133, 136, 139, 143, 187, 198
Stein, Diana 279, 291
Steinbach-Eicke 336, 359
Steinert, Ulrike 182, 194, 198, 219, 233, 251
Steinkeller, Piotr 287, 291
Stern, Herold 148, 160
Sterne, Jonathan 318, 334
Stewart, Anne 153–54, 160
Steymans, Hans U. 234, 251
Stöckl, Jonathan 234, 237, 251
Stol, Marten 225–26, 251
Stoller, Paul 23, 41, 45, 54, 73, 85
Stone, Ruth 28, 41
Strassmaier, Johann N. 267, 275
Strawn, Brent A. 296, 312
Streck, Michael 232, 240–42, 251
Strong, Meghan E. 364, 373–74, 380
Strudwick, Nigel 374, 380

Suddendorf, Thomas	254, 278	Verhoeven-van Elsbergen, Ursula	336, 360
Sulzmann, Sven	255, 278		
Sumi, Akiko Motoyoshi	211, 214	Vermès, Géza	122, 143
Sutton, David E.	337, 360	Vignemont, Frédérique de	87, 97
Swennen, Cornelis	343, 360	Villard, Pierre	226, 252
Synnott, Anthony	6, 11, 31, 42	Vincent, Alexandre	316–17, 333–34
Tadmor, Hayim	228, 251	Vogt, Evon	8
Takács, Gábor	126, 143	Voigt, Karlheinz	205, 212
Talon, Philippe	284, 291	Volk, Konrad	222, 252
Tambiah, Stanley J.	239–40, 251–52	von Lieven, Alexandra	127–28, 143, 317, 334, 336, 352, 359–60
Tedlock, Barbara	7, 41		
Tennant, Frederick R.	146, 160	Von Soden, Wolfram	287, 291
Thomas, Nigel J. T.	208, 214	Walker, Christopher B. F.	226, 252
Thomason, Allison	293–94, 299–300, 312	Warner, William Lloyd	24, 42
		Wasserman, Nathan	225, 232, 234, 252, 287–88, 291
Tiemeyer, Lena-Sofia	186, 198		
Tigay, Jeffrey H.	122, 143, 236–37, 252	Watanabe, Chiko	295–96, 306, 312
Tilford, Nicole L.	vii–viii, 72, 85, 87, 97, 150, 154, 160	Watanabe, Kazuko	192, 197
		Watts, John D. W.	165, 173, 180
Toner, Jerry	218, 252	Webb, Ruth	209–11, 214
Tooman, William A.	162, 180	Weeks, Stuart	65, 68
Topman, Doris	127–28, 143	Weiss, Ehud	366, 380
Tov, Emanuel	162, 180	Weissert, Elnathan	306, 312
Trible, Phyllis	145, 160	Wellhausen, Julius	148, 150, 160
Tsevat, Matitiahu	63, 68	Welton, Peter	23, 40
Tudeau, Johanna	234, 252	West, Martin L.	57, 68
Tzamalikos, Panayiotis	254, 278	Westbrook, Deanne	146, 160
Uphill, Eric	373, 380	Westenholz, Age	288, 291
Van De Mieroop, Marc	61–62, 68, 228, 250, 302, 312	Westenholz, Joan Goodnick	225–26, 230, 240, 249, 252, 288, 291
Van der Toorn, Karel	218, 238, 252	Whiston, William	141
Van Hecke, Pierre	103, 118, 189, 193, 205–6, 213	Whitaker, Robyn J.	209–10, 214
		White, Allon	27, 41
van Loon, Hanneke	110, 118	White, Raymond	366, 380
van Wassenhove, Virginie	254, 275	Whitrow, Gerald James	254, 278
Vatsyayan, Sachchidanand Hiranand	254, 278	Whorf, Benjamin Lee	32, 42
		Whyte, Alison	272, 276, 278
Veenhof, Klaas R.	233, 252	Widmaier, Kai	318–19, 334
Veenker, Ronald A.	204, 214	Wiggermann, Frans Anton Maria	242, 252, 264, 268, 278
Veldhuis, Niek	231–32, 252		
Verderame, Lorenzo	257, 276, 278	Wilbert, Werner	31, 42

Williamson, Hugh Godfrey Maturin 171, 180
Wilson, John A. 373–75, 380
Winter, Irene J. 267–67, 278, 293, 295, 299, 308, 312
Wischnowsky, Marc 183, 198
Witherspoon, Gary 12, 42
Wober, J. Mallory 18, 23, 42, 46–47, 54
Wolff, Hans Walter 58, 68, 156–57, 160
Woods, Christopher 256, 278
Wright, Chris 45, 53
Yamamoto, Kei 380
Young, Michael W. 33, 42
Zandee, Jan 127, 143
Zawadzki, Stefan 228–29, 252
Zgoll, Annette 280, 291
Ziegler, Christiane 322–23, 334
Ziegler, Nele 220, 252
Zignani, Pierre 327, 334
Zimmer, Carl 46, 54
Zohary, Daniel 366, 380
Zsolnay, Ilona 234, 252
Zubek, John 30, 42
Zwickel, Wolfgang 185, 198, 237, 252